Child Health
A Textbook for the DCH

Child Health
A Textbook for the
DCH

Edited by

David Harvey MB FRCP DCH
Senior Lecturer in Paediatrics, Institute of Obstetrics
and Gynaecology; Consultant Paediatrician, Queen
Charlotte's Maternity Hospital, London and St Charles'
Hospital, London

and

Ilya Kovar MB MRCP FRCP(C) FAAP
Senior Lecturer in Child Health, Charing Cross and
Westminster Medical School; Consultant Paediatrician,
Charing Cross Hospital, London

CHURCHILL LIVINGSTONE
EDINBURGH LONDON MELBOURNE AND NEW YORK 1985

CHURCHILL LIVINGSTONE
Medical Division of Longman Group Limited

Distributed in the United States of America by Churchill
Livingstone Inc., 1560 Broadway, New York, N.Y. 10036, and
by associated companies, branches and representatives
throughout the world.

First published 1985

ISBN 0 443 02358 1

British Library Cataloguing in Publication Data
Child health: a textbook for the DCH.
  1. Pediatrics
  I. Harvey, David   II. Kovar, Ilya
  618.92   RJ45

Library of Congress Cataloging in Publication Data
Main entry under title:
Child health.
  Includes index.
  1. Pediatrics.   I. Harvey, David (David Robert)
II. Kovar, Ilya. [DNLM: 1. Pediatrics. WS 100 C5363]
RJ45.C533   1984   618.92   84–19954

Produced by Longman Singapore Publishers (Pte) Limited
Printed in Singapore

Preface

This book is intended primarily for doctors interested in preparing for the Diploma in Child Health examinations. We hope that family doctors, even if not taking the examination, will also find it useful in their everyday practice. We have asked contributors to include sufficient information on hospital practice so that general practitioners will know the sort of management their patients may receive if referred to a paediatric department.

Since this book began its gestation there have been several changes in the regulations, and aims, of the various diplomas of child health; the London examination is now supervised by the Royal College of Physicians, while there is a totally new examination of community child health in Edinburgh. The new regulations stress the importance of community child health and the role of both preventative and therapeutic aspects of primary care. The DCH has assumed a useful and important place in the training and accreditation of general practitioners and community paediatricians and is no longer to be regarded as a mini MRCP.

We thank our contributors and the staff at Churchill Livingstone for their patience; we hope that the reader will find the information from the various contributions on general practice, development and the subspecialities useful.

London   D.H.
1985   I.K.

Contributors

A. J. Barrett MD, MRCPath (*Haematology*)
Professor of Haematology, Charing Cross and
Westminster Medical School, London, UK

Jane Baxter MB, MRCP (*Endocrine and metabolic
disease*)
Formerly Fellow in Endocrinology, Hospital for
Sick Children, Toronto, Canada

M. J. Brueton MSc, MD, MRCP, DCH (*Infant
feeding, Gastrointestinal disorders*)
Senior Lecturer in Child Health, Charing Cross
and Westminster Medical School, London, UK

Sarah Bundey MB, FRCP, DCH (*Genetic
disorders*)
Lecturer in Clinical Genetics, Queen Elizabeth
Medical Centre, Birmingham, UK

A. Butterfill MB, MRCP, DCH (*The handicapped
child*)
Consultant Paediatrician, Hereford, UK

M. C. K. Chan MD, FRACP (*Tropical child
health*)
Senior Lecturer, School of Tropical Medicine,
Liverpool, UK

Christine E. Cooper OBE, MB, FRCP, DCH
(*Accidents non-accidental injury and child abuse*)
Formerly Consultant Paediatrician, Department of
Child Health, University of Newcastle-upon-Tyne,
UK

Mary Cummins MB, MRCP, DCH (*History
taking, Emergency procedures*)
Senior Paediatric Registrar, Queen Charlotte's
Maternity Hospital, London, UK

Professor Sir John Dewhurst MD, FRCS,
FRCOG (*Gynaecological disorders*)
Professor of Obstetrics and Gynaecology, Institute
of Obstetrics and Gynaecology, Queen Charlotte's
Maternity Hospital, London, UK

J.A.S. Dickson FRCS (*Surgical disorders*)
Consultant Paediatric Surgeon, Children's
Hospital, Sheffield, UK

R. Dinwiddie MB, FRCP, DCH (*Respiratory
disease*)
Consultant Paediatrician, Hospital for Sick
Children, Great Ormond Street, London, UK

Elspeth Earle MB, MRCPsych, DPM (*Behaviour
disorders*)
Formerly Consultant Psychiatrist, Queen
Charlotte's Maternity Hospital, London, UK

Janet Goodall MB, FRCP, DCH (*The dying
child*)
Consultant Paediatrician, City Hospital,
Stoke-on-Trent, UK

A. W. Goodwin MB, MRCP, DCH (*Heart
disease*)
Senior Registrar, Newcastle General Hospital,
Newcastle-upon-Tyne, UK

D. Harvey MB, FRCP, DCH
Senior Lecturer in Paediatrics, Institute of
Obstetrics and Gynaecology, Queen Charlotte's
Maternity Hospital; Consultant Paediatrician, St
Charles' Hospital, London, UK

A. S. Hunter MB, MRCP, DCH (*Heart disease*)
Paediatric Cardiologist, Freeman Hospital,
Newcastle-upon-Tyne, UK

I. Kovar MB, MRCP, FRCP (C), FAAP
Senior Lecturer in Child Health, Charing Cross
and Westminster Medical School; Consultant
Paediatrician, Charing Cross Hospital, London, UK

S. Lingam MD, MRCP (*Neurology*)
Locum Consultant Paediatrician, Barking
Hospital, London, UK

T. Lissauer MB, MRCP (*Infectious diseases*)
Consultant Paediatrician, St Mary's Hospital,
London, UK

J. MacKinnon BSc, MB, MRCP (*Miscellaneous
problems*)
Consultant Paediatrician, Sydenham Children's
Hospital, London, UK

The late **W. Marshall** PhD, MD, FRACP, DCH
(*Infectious diseases*)
Formerly Consultant Paediatrician, Hospital for
Sick Children, Great Ormond Street, London,
UK

Patricia Morris-Jones MB, FRCP, DCH
(*Oncology*)
Senior Lecturer in Paediatric Oncology,
University of Manchester, UK

G. Rylance MB, MRCP (*Pharmacology*)
Consultant Paediatrician, Children's Hospital,
Birmingham, UK

W. McN. Styles MB, MRCGP (*Demography,
Prevention of illness, Caring for children in general
practice*)
General Practitioner, The Grove Health Centre,
London, UK

R. S. Trompeter MB, MRCP (*Disorders of the
kidney*)
Senior Lecturer in Paediatrics, Royal Free
Hospital Medical School, London, UK

Shelagh Tyrell MD, MFCM, DPH, DCH
(*Demography*)
Principal Child Health Physician, Paddington and
North Kensington Health District, London, UK

Sheila Wallis MB, MRCP, DCH (*Growth and
development*)
Senior Paediatric Registrar, Royal Berkshire
Hospital, Reading, and Wolfson Centre, Institute
of Child Health, London, UK

J. Warner MD, MRCP, DCH (*Allergic and other
immunological disorders*)
Consultant Paediatrician, Brompton Hospital,
London, UK

A. Whitelaw MD, MRCP (*The newborn baby*)
Consultant Neonatologist, Hammersmith
Hospital, London, UK

Contents

Demography

STATISTICS AND MORTALITY RATE

Vital statistics is the detailed study of life and death in the community, and this became a practical possibility in this country with the first census of 1801. A few far-sighted doctors recognised that information collected on a national scale could be used for the benefit of all citizens.

Demographic considerations

The population of the UK in 1978, with the percentage of children in that population, is given in Table 1.1. The *birth rate* has been falling steadily since the beginning of this century; in recent years, both birth rate and *fertility rate* (that is the number of births per 1000 women between

Table 1.1 The population with the percentage of children (0–14 years) in the UK

	Approximate number of persons in 1978 (millions)	0–14 years (percentage)
UK	55.8	22
England & Wales	49.1	22
Scotland	5.2	23
Northern Ireland	1.5	28

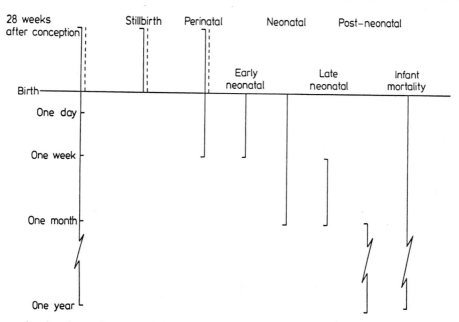

Fig. 1.1 Infant and perinatal mortality rates and their subgroups

the ages of 15 and 44) have fallen since a high peak in 1964. In 1978, however, there was an upturn in both, with a 4 per cent increase in the number of babies born. In 1981 it seemed to have started to drop again.

Place of confinement

When families choose to have fewer children, it is especially important to ensure a successful outcome for every confinement, and the small but finite risk of having a baby at home is no longer considered acceptable by most obstetricians and paediatricians. In 1976, 97.5 per cent of mothers in England and Wales had their babies in hospital. Not all mothers welcome this trend, and if their cooperation is to be achieved, they must be reassured that their skills in labour and their opportunities for bonding with their babies are fully respected.

Infant mortality

Once the value of the statistical method was appre-

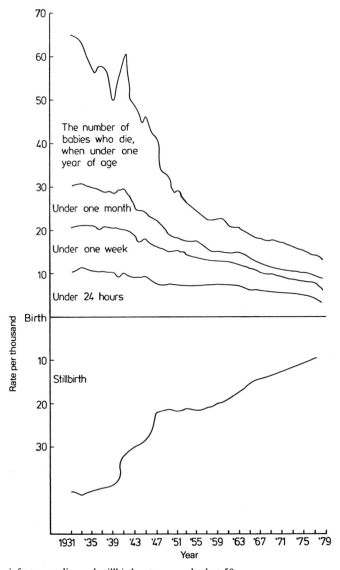

Fig. 1.2 The change in the infant mortality and stillbirth rates over the last 50 years

ciated, doctors began to look at situations over which they previously had no control. Death and disease came under scrutiny, and developments in public health made the country a safer place to live in. But it remained dangerous for infants who, in some big cities, had little more than an even chance of survival until their first birthday. However, with improvements in the social environment in which children were brought up, as well as advances in medical science and accessibility of medical care, the infant mortality rate has declined, at times dramatically, during the twentieth century.

The infant mortality rate is defined as the number of infants who die under one year of age per 100 live births. Included in these figures will be the preterm baby who dies within minutes of birth, and the 11-month-old child who succumbs to pneumonia. The causes of death for each of these babies is very different, so the components of infant mortality are separated to allow for sensible comparison. The two rates most commonly used today are the *perinatal mortality rate* (the number of stillbirths plus the number of babies who die in the first week of life out of every 1000

total births), and the *post-neonatal mortality rate* (the number of babies who die between the ages of 4 weeks and one year out of every 1000 live births) (Figs. 1.1 and 1.2).

Three major conditions account for most of perinatal mortality: prematurity, congenital abnormalities, and hypoxia during labour and birth. While the main causes of death in the perinatal period concern obstetric conditions, this is not so for the post-neonatal deaths.

A study was made of post-neonatal deaths in 1971, in England and Wales and in 8 other countries. Figure 1.3 shows the number of babies that died in those 8 countries for every 100 dying in England and Wales, as well as the proportion of deaths which were due to congenital malformation. The actual number of deaths from this last cause remains relatively constant, but the proportion is higher in the countries with low post-neonatal mortality rates.

It is the deaths not due to congenital abnormalities that cause most concern. The commonest of these is variously described in different countries as either respiratory disease, ill-defined symptoms or accidental death. Many of these deaths are

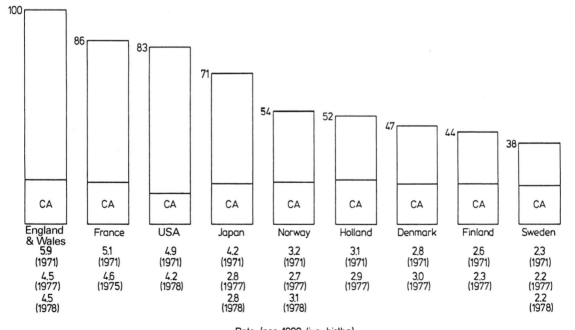

Rate (per 1000 live births)

Fig. 1.3 International comparison of post-neonatal deaths as a percentage of England and Wales in 1971. The post-neonatal rates per thousand live births is shown in figures. (CA shows the number of deaths from congenital abnormalities)

never satisfactorily explained, and most present as cot death, or sudden death in infancy.

International Comparisons

Comparisons of mortality rates between countries provide interest and a spur to the competitive spirit, but their value is necessarily limited. Populations are not always comparable in terms of health or height of the womenfolk. In some countries, such as Sweden, there appears to be an overwhelming willingness to conform, and this includes attendance at antenatal and child health clinics. There are, again, fundamental differences in registration practice. In France, deaths of infants between birth and the third day of life, by which time registration is required, are classified as false stillbirths. In England and Wales any baby born alive, of whatever gestation, must be registered, but this only applies to stillbirths if the gestation period is 28 weeks or longer. Registration has financial advantages for the mother, who can then collect her maternity grant, and a tax rebate. These considerations could influence the doctor faced with an equivocal live birth.

Sharing information of this sort does mean that each country learns from the experiences of the others, and can adopt good practices. There are currently several international ventures which should improve data and recording and allow for real comparisons to be made.

History-taking; clinical examination and basic investigations

HISTORY-TAKING, CLINICAL EXAMINATION AND BASIC INVESTIGATIONS

INTRODUCTION
The aim of history-taking and clinical examination in paediatrics is the total assessment of the child and his physical complaint in the context of his family and social circumstances. Any medical problem is greatly affected by previous illness, family relationships, housing conditions and schooling difficulties.

HISTORY-TAKING

The correct diagnosis and comprehensive management of illness is impossible without an accurate history. In children, this is usually obtained from the mother or father. As soon as they are old enough, children should be encouraged to give their own account of the problem; even a young child can, for example, identify the site of pain. During the interview the child should gain confidence from watching friendly communication between the doctor and his parents. Appropriate toys and a small table should be available in the consulting room. All but the illest child will enjoy some distraction. The doctor may gain valuable information about the child's abilities and general state by simple observation during this period.

It is important to learn and listen carefully. One should remember that the parents are usually right, they have had much more time to watch the child than the doctor.

Outline of history

1. Name and personal details of child including school and local child health centre where appropriate
2. Name and relationship of informant
3. Referring doctor or agency
4. Presenting complaint
5. Details of present complaint
6. Direct systematic questioning
7. Recent contact with infectious disease
8. Past history
   a. Birth history
   b. Feeding history
   c. Medical history
   d. Hospital admissions
   e. Development
   f. Immunisations
9. Family history: names, ages, occupations of immediate family.
Illness in family. Is there any consanguinity?
10. Social history: details of housing and particularly bathroom and cooking facilities. Facilities for play. Number of bedrooms. Financial situation. Behaviour and relationships.
11. Schooling: performance, attendance, difficulties, special teaching required.

Model history

Rosemary X (known as
Rosie)   Date of birth 6.2.80
58 Hamilton Road,
London W6   Aged 10 months
Referred by Dr Y
Informant — mother. Rosie's sister also present.

Presenting complaint

Cough for 5 days

History of present complaint

Well until 5 days ago when she developed a cough. Appetite decreased for 3 days when wheezing began. Listless and febrile for 24 hours. Rubbing right ear. Sister aged 3 also has a cold. No diarrhoea or vomiting. Drinking fairly well but not eating. Micturition normal.

Past history

Birth Born at Fishpool Hospital after a normal pregnancy, normal delivery at 41 weeks gestation, induced because of poor weight gain. Birth weight 2.8 kg. No neonatal problems. Forty-eight hour discharge

Illnesses Recurrent chestiness since the age of 3 months. Occurs about every month with colds. Treated with antibiotics and cough linctus on several occasions. Well in between attacks. Mild eczema since 2 months old. No other illnesses. No operations. No hospital admissions.

Immunisations BCG given at birth because of family history of tuberculosis. Triple and polio aged 3 months and 5 months. Third injection recently delayed by a cold.

Development Smiled at 5 weeks. Sat at 7 months. Pulls to standing. Cruises around furniture. Babbles. Waves bye-bye. Plays pat-a-cake. Has passed 8 month developmental test at local clinic and hearing test from Health Visitor.

Feeding Breast fed for 3 months. Mixed feeding at 4 months. Now eats family food, and drinks 'red top' cow's milk not boiled.

Family & social history

Family Mother aged 22, single, English. Healthy. Father aged 24, single. Works on a building site. Healthy. Sister: Jane, aged 3 years (same father).

Family illnesses Maternal grandfather had tuberculosis 2 years ago treated at the local chest clinic. Her mother had bronchitis and eczema as a child. There is no diabetes, epilepsy, or other disease in the family.

Social Rosie and her sister live with their mother in a 2-bedroomed council flat on fifth floor of a block which has its own kitchen and bathroom. Rosie sleeps in bed with her mother; she wakes frequently at night. Their father visits erratically and provides no financial support. Both children go to day nursery. The health visitor sees children regularly. The family had social work help in the past but not at present. Grandparents live locally but both work and do not have much time for the children.

At the end of a well-taken history the doctor should be able to form a list of problems and differential diagnostic possibilities. The clinical examination should then confirm or support one of the possibilities and leave the doctor with a working diagnosis which is then confirmed by further investigation or by response to a clinical trial of therapy.

PHYSICAL EXAMINATION

The methods of examination vary considerably with the age of the child and the clinical situation. Knowledge of what is normal for children of different ages is essential in order to distinguish that which is abnormal see Table 2.1. It is not appropriate to assess the development of an acutely ill child other than by means of the history, whereas a well 4-year-old can cooperate with a detailed neurological examination. Unpleasant procedures are sensibly left to the end of the examination, e.g. examination of ears, throat, rectum. Weighing and measuring of toddlers and infants may be classified as 'unpleasant', but are usually carried out before seeing the doctor. The undressing and dressing involved is not appreciated by children.

Most toddlers are happiest sitting on their mother's knees but may lie on the examination cough once they have gained confidence. Infants should be examined naked, an irreducible inguinal hernia may be missed as the cause of persistent crying, or an undescended testicle may remain undiagnosed if the napkin is not removed. Older children may be embarrassed if completely naked.

General condition

The general condition of the child should first be considered in the light of the particular clinical situation. The alertness, responsiveness, hydration, state of nutrition, colour and temperature must be noted. It is useful to make the general comment whether or not the child 'looks ill'. The skin should be examined closely for rashes and other lesions, for example, it is vital not to miss the petechial rash of meningococcal infection.

Weighing and measuring

These can be distressing for young or ill children. The measurements are, however, essential. Infants must be weighed naked, while older children may keep on underclothing. Length is measured using an infant measuring table up to 2 years of age and height with a standiometer in older children. The measurements should be plotted on a percentile chart.

The head

The size of the head is measured around its maximum circumference using a paper or metal tape measure, plastic tape measures stretch and should not be used. The size of the head must be related to the child's height and weight and plotted on the appropriate percentile chart (Figs. 2.1 & 2.2).

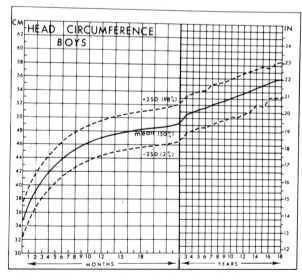

Fig. 2.1 Head circumference for boys from birth to 18 years (Nellhaus 1968)

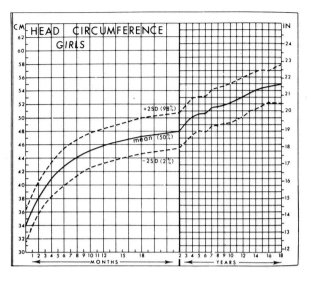

Fig. 2.2 Head circumference for girls from birth to 18 years (Nellhaus 1968)

Size and shape

A big head may be found in a big child, as a familial trait, in hydrocephalus, megalencephaly, subdural effusion or space-occupying lesion. A small head is found in a small child, mental retardation, as a familial tendency and in craniostenosis. Unusual head shape may be related to preterm birth, baby's posture or Down's syndrome. Preterm infants have increased antero-postero diameter (dolichocephaly); cranial asymmetry is commonly seen in normal infants (plagiocephaly); reduced antero-postero diameter (brachycephaly) is associated with Down's syndrome.

The fontanelles

The fontanelles should be palpated. The anterior fontanelle is normally flat and pulsation can be felt. Bulging and loss of pulsation in the resting state suggest raised intracranial pressure. Other signs of raised intracranial pressure are separation of the skull suture lines and the sun-setting sign. The anterior fontanelle usually closes between 10 and 18 months of age, but there is a very wide normal variation. Premature closure, however, occurs in craniostenosis and microcephaly; delayed closure is associated with hydrocephalus, hypothyroidism, rickets and cleidocranial dysostosis. The posterior fontanelle is usually palpable for the first one or 2 months of life. The third fontanelle is a normal variant which lies between the anterior and posterior fontanelles; it occurs more commonly in Down's syndrome than among the general population. Craniotabes or softening of areas of the skull is also common in normal infants but is found frequently in rickets.

The eyes

Convergent squint is abnormal after 6 months of age (see Chapter 24), and ophthalmological referral is indicated. Severe squint may require expert opinion in infants less than one month old. Wide epicanthic folds may cause an apparent convergent squint, but asymmetrical reflection of a light shone into the pupils is seen in true squint. Sticky eyes are common in the first year of life. Gentle bathing with moist cotton wool is usually sufficient treatment. Examination with the ophthalmoscope will exclude lens and vitreous opacities and refractive errors. Examination of the fundi may be difficult and dilatation of the pupils needed. In young infants, it is best to do the examination during sleep. Older children can have their gaze attracted by a toy. Where there is suspicion of a non-accidental injury, retinal haemorrhages may be seen without skull fractures. Congenital ptosis is seen frequently but acquired ptosis suggests third nerve palsy and possibly raised intracranial pressure. Nystagmus is frequently associated with severe visual defect, but may also have a neurological cause. Screening for refractive errors should be a routine part of the developmental examination using Stycar equipment in infants and young children.

The face

The features may be very helpful in diagnosing generalised conditions such as Down's syndrome, hypothyroidism or Hurler's syndrome. Abnormal shapes and relationships of the facial features are described in many congenital syndromes.

The ears

The ears must be inspected for external abnormalities. They are low set if the upper border of the lobe is below a line drawn from the lateral angle of the eye to the external occipital protruberance. Low set ears are found in Down's and other congenital syndromes. It is essential to examine the ears of all sick children with an auriscope. The mother should hold the child firmly (Fig. 2.3), otherwise pain may be caused. The largest speculum possible is used to avoid both discomfort and pushing wax inwards. The ear lobe should be pulled gently outwards. Otitis media causes an inflamed, thickened, immobile, bulging or perforated drum. The symptoms are varied, inconsolable crying, fever, headbanging, feeding difficulties or rubbing ears. Hearing tests appropriate for age should be carried out after recovery.

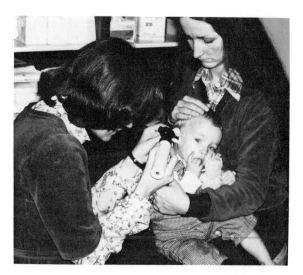

Fig. 2.3 The auriscope examination of a young child

The mouth and throat

This is best left to the end of the examination if tongue depression is needed (Fig. 2.4). Many children will provide a good view of their throats by tilting their heads back, protruding the tongue and saying 'aah'. When the tongue depressor is correctly used gagging is not inevitable. The palate, mucosae and teeth should also be inspected. Tonsillitis may cause abdominal pain, difficulty in swallowing and even respiratory obstruction if there is gross tonsillar enlargement. It is impossible to differentiate bacterial from viral tonsillitis on clinical grounds — viruses are the cause in around 90 per cent of cases. The throat

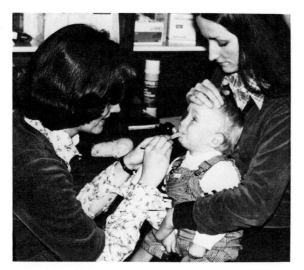

Fig. 2.4 The examination of the mouth and throat of a young child

should not be examined in the presence of stridor as respiratory obstruction may be precipitated. Dental infections may cause facial pain or swelling, ear ache and submandibular swelling.

The neck

In Turner's syndrome the neck is short and webbed. Swellings may be due to lymph node enlargement, salivary gland enlargement, goitre, branchial cyst or cystic hygroma. The latter transilluminates. Torticollis in an infant may be due to sternomastoid tumour which is usually palpable around the midpoint of the muscle. Neck retraction may be present in severe respiratory distress in an infant or at any age due to meningism.

The lymph nodes

Lymph nodes are frequently enlarged in response to local or generalised infection. Occasionally,

more sinister conditions are responsible. Resolution to normal size may take several months. The groin glands may be palpable without evidence of recent infection.

The chest

The shape and symmetry of the chest should be noted. Pigeon chest or barrel-shaped chest are associated with chronic undertreated asthma. Sternal depression (pectus) may be familial. Gynaecomastia is not uncommon in boys at puberty, and the two breasts may be asymmetrical in girls. Wide spaced nipples are seen in Turner's syndrome.

Respiratory distress

Signs of this are tachypnoea (see Table 2.1), cyanosis, flaring of the alae nasi, use of accessory muscles, intercoastal and subcostal recession and pulsus paradoxus. Impaired percussion note may be due to a collection of fluid or gross pulmonary consolidation. Auscultation is often unhelpful, and a cold stethoscope can cause crying. The most ill asthmatics have silent chests but all other signs of severe respiratory distress. Classical signs of consolidation are unusual in childhood, and a chest X-ray must be carried out if pneumonia is suspected. Added sounds heard on auscultation are frequently transmitted from the throat, musical added sounds and coarse crepitations are common in toddlers with upper respiratory tract infection, and do not usually indicate pneumonia or the need for antibiotic treatment.

The heart

Palpation of the pulse for rate and rhythm should be routine. Sinus arrhythmia may be marked and

Table 2.1 Normal values for physiological measurements at different ages

	Birth	6 weeks	1 year	5 years	10 years
Respiratory rate (per minute — mean)	30	30	25	22	20
Heart rate (per minute — mean)	140	135	115	100	90
Systolic blood pressure (mmHg)		95	95	100	105

Table 2.2 Practical aspects of blood pressure measurement

1. Child at rest
2. Cuff: depth at 2/3 length of the upper arm, and bladder length should be the circumference of the arm
3. Technique

ultrasonic	— correlates best with intra-aterial pressures
auscultation	— for older children
palpation	— inaccurate
flush method	— inaccurate

extra-systoles are not unusual. Oedema, clubbing and cyanosis should be sought and the femoral pulses palpated. Blood pressure is measured at rest with the appropriately sized cuff (Table 2.2). The precordium may bulge with cardiac enlargement and palpation may reveal abnormal ventricular impulses and thrills. Heart sounds and murmurs should be listened for carefully. Murmurs are graded from one to six and are timed. Innocent murmurs are common and are accentuated by fever.

The abdomen

Inspection may reveal distension, visible peristalsis, outline of organs, umbilical or inguinal herniae, distended veins and scars. Abdominal breathing is normal in infants, loss of this may indicate peritonitis. The child should be examined lying on a bed or in the mother's arms; flexion of the hips and knees is helpful. The ability of the child to blow out and suck in the abdominal wall freely helps to exclude peritoneal irritation. The child's face should always be watched so that tenderness may be detected. Abdominal organs should be palpated, warm hands are essential. In infants, the normal liver is palpable up to 2 cm below the costal margin and the spleen tip may be felt when the abdominal wall is lax. Rectal examination should be carried out in cases of rectal bleeding, constipation, suspected intussusception and in children with acute abdominal pain.

The genitalia

Male

Both testes are usually descended a birth and are of equal size. Scrotal swelling may be due to hernia, hydrocele, cyst of the cord, etc. Hydro-celes are common, non-tender, transilluminate and often resolve spontaneously. Inguinal herniae will be tender if irreducible or strangulated. Torsion of the testis or epididymities produces a swollen tender scrotum. The foreskin cannot normally be retracted in babies, it can usually be retracted after the age of 6 years. Testes are frequently retractile in older children. If examination is carried out with the boy's hips and knees flexed as in a squatting position, the testes will lie in the scrotum.

Female

The vagina may be imperforate but labial adhesions are a more common cause of a covered vagina.

The skeleton

Knock knees, bow legs, intoeing gait and flat feet are common in infancy, and rarely require treatment. Pain in the knee may be referred from the hip. Limp may originate from the hips, the knees, the spine and intra-abdominal conditions. The spine should be examined. Scoliosis developing during adolescence may require urgent treatment. Minor anomalies of the hands and feet, e.g. extra digits, Simian crease, curvature of fifth finger and syndactyly, particularly of the second and third toes, are common.

The nervous system

The techniques of examination vary enormously with the age of the child, his developmental progress and his state of general health. In addition to standard equipment for neurological examination, it may be useful to have some coloured one inch (2.5 cm) cubes, a bell and a Manchester rattle (for hearing tests). In very young children, seedless raisins may be used to test fine motor skills and very small cake decorations (hundreds and thousands) to test near vision. Small toys and picture books may also be helpful. Observation alone will give a great deal of information, particularly in young or mentally retarded children. Behaviour, apparent intelligence, gait, coordination, power and speech may be assessed by observation.

Full neurological examination includes the state of consciousness and orientation, emotional state and intelligence. Speech, comprehension, reading and writing should also be assessed when appropriate. The cranial nerves, gait, posture, power, tone, coordination, sensation and reflexes are also examined. It may require more than one consultation to complete the examination in detail. Examination methods have been standardised for different age groups and for detecting minor neurological abnormalities (Paine & Oppe 1975).

BASIC INVESTIGATIONS

It is important to remember that even minor procedures may be alarming for young children and their parents. No investigation should be carried out without good reason. When taking blood, all the necessary tests should be made with one venepuncture wherever possible. It is best if a parent holds the child during painful procedures when this is technically possible. Doctors must become accustomed to the presence of parents at such times.

Urine samples for culture are collected as midstream or clean catch specimens. Urine collected into bags stuck on to the perineum is suitable for biochemical testing but not for culture because of contamination with skin organisms. Suprapubic aspiration of the bladder may be necessary in the young infant with suspected urinary tract infection.

It is very important to know or to have access to normal values for investigations which may vary with age (see Appendix 1).

Laboratory investigation for some common conditions

1. Enuresis
     urine culture
     urine glucose
2. Recurrent abdominal pain
     urine culture
     sickle test (in children from areas where sickle cell disease is common)
3. Diarrhoea
     stool culture for bacteria, microscopy for parasites and electron microscopy for rotavirus. Blood urea and electrolytes (if evidence of dehydration) and reducing substances (if symptoms persistent)
4. Failure to thrive
     urine sugar and protein, urine culture and microscopy, haemoglobin, blood urea and electrolytes, stool microscopy and culture
5. Before general anaesthesia
     haemoglobin and sickle test (when ethnic origin indicates)
6. Febrile convulsion
     lumbar puncture essential if child less than 18 months old, or if any clinical suspicion of meningitis
7. Convulsion without fever
     blood glucose and haemoglobin, plasma calcium, urea, amino acids, skull X-ray and EEG
8. Recurrent wheezing
     plasma IgE, blood eosinophil count, chest X-ray, Mantoux test, skin tests.

FURTHER READING

Apley J & MacKeith R 1978 The child and his symptoms, 3rd edn. Blackwell Scientific Publications, Oxford

Illingworth R S 1979 The normal child, 7th edn. Blackwell Scientific Publications, Oxford

Illingworth R S 1979 Common symptoms of disease in children, 6th edn. Churchill Livingstone, Edinburgh.

Nellhaus G 1968 Head circumference from birth to eighteen years; practical composite international and interracial graphs. Pediatrics 41: 106–114.

Paine R S & Oppe T E 1975 Neurological examination of children, 5th edn. Clinics in Developmental Medicine No 20/21, Spastics International Medical Publications with Heinemann Medical Books Ltd, London.

3

Growth and development

Growth and development

Growing up is one of the essential features of childhood. Growth and development usually occur in harmony, each influencing the other. The effects of a loss of this harmony can be clearly seen with the premature onset of puberty in a 6-year-old girl, or the mentally retarded 15-year-old boy, taller than his mother, but with the abilities and understanding of a naughty 3-year-old.

GROWTH

Cell and tissue growth

Why cells divide, and how they know when to start and stop remains a mystery. Three phases of tissue growth have been postulated. In the first phase all cells multiply; during the second phase some cells multiply, but they also increase in size due to the addition of cytoplasm, while in the final phase cell multiplication halts and only cell enlargement occurs. Some cells, such as those of skin and blood, continue to multiply and replace themselves throughout life. Other tissues such as brain, muscle, and lung have only limited phase when cell multiplication can occur and, therefore, are more vulnerable to insults at this time. Animal research has shown that if the supply of nutrients is limited during the whole of this sensitive growth phase then the relevant organ (e.g. the brain) remains small and does not catch up in growth later; if it is only affected for part of the time, catch-up can occur.

Attempts have been made to apply these principles to human growth. It is known that some babies who grow slowly before birth catch up, while others remain small. The evidence suggests these babies are more likely to remain small if slow growth has been severe (affecting head as well as body growth) and prolonged (starting before 34 weeks gestation). Similarly, there has been concern that overfeeding in infancy might lead to excessive multiplication of fat cells, so that the fat child becomes a fat adult; this theory is not proven.

Patterns of human growth

Prenatal growth

Data about prenatal growth have been obtained by carefully examining fetuses aborted because either the fetus or the uterus was defective. Recently, ultrasound has enabled us to measure the fetus in utero. During the first trimester of pregnancy crown-rump measurements are very accurate, from about 13 weeks gestation biparietal diameter measurements of the head can be made, and from midterm head and abdominal circumference measurements. Growth curves have been compiled using this data, and it is clear that growth in utero is extremely rapid with little variation between infants until the last trimester of pregnancy. The first indication of slow growth is a reduction in abdominal circumference, and if very severe, head growth slows. It is suggested that an early ultrasound measurement before 20 weeks to confirm dates, and measurement of head diameter and abdominal circumference at 32 weeks, would detect 90 per cent of all small-for-dates infants.

Variations in fetal growth depend not only on the fetus, but also the mother and the environmental and nutritional circumstances in which she lives. Probably, maternal size has the greatest constraining influence on fetal growth, for the obvious reason that a small mother would have difficulty delivering a large baby. Studies where Shire horses were crossed with Shetland ponies clearly demonstrated this; the foals whose mothers were Shire horses were much larger than those whose mothers were Shetland ponies.

Maternal size is affected by race, health, nutrition and socioeconomic factors which date back to the mother's own childhood. There are growth charts which allow for the mother's height and weight when assessing the baby's weight. Small-for-dates babies are born more frequently into low social class families where smoking, pre-eclampsia and short stature are more common.

Maternal health in pregnancy is important. Most problems such as hypertension and pre-eclampsia result in slow growth because they impair the supply of nutrients to the fetus; poorly controlled maternal diabetes, however, results in overweight babies because the baby responds to the high maternal blood sugar levels transmitted across the placenta by secreting extra insulin which, in turn, promotes the deposition of fat.

The commonest fetal factor affecting growth is sex, male babies are heavier than female babies. Intrauterine infection, chromosomal, genetic and congenital malformations usually slow fetal growth. Transposition of the great arteries is a notable exception, these babies are often heavier than expected at birth. Multiple pregnancy also affects fetal growth because the nutrients must be shared, in twin pregnancy, slowing of growth starts around 33 weeks gestation.

Postnatal growth

After birth the growth velocity of the majority of body tissues tends to follow a general curve similar to that of height and weight (Fig. 3.1). Growth of the brain and head, however, continues as rapidly as before birth, only slowing at about 4 years, and then halting long before other tissues stop growing. Reproductive tissue starts its growth spurt much later, coinciding with the pubertal increase in height.

The general growth curve is rapid in the first 2 years of life, and during this period the child moves onto his genetically inherited growth curve, catching up from any constraint on fetal growth

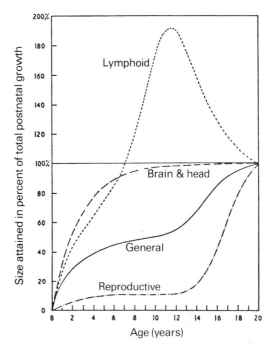

Fig. 3.1 Growth curves showing how the growth patterns of the brain and head, reproductive and lymphatic tissues vary from the general growth curve of the rest of the body (from Tanner 1962)

such as small maternal size. From 2 years, growth continues steadily until puberty. Most children have growth curves which follow the centile curves on the growth chart. During this period it is important to allow for parental height when considering whether a child is growing normally.

At puberty there is a sudden increase in growth velocity, the boys start their growth spurt about 18 months later than girls and ultimately achieve a greater height. There is a very wide variation in the time of onset of puberty, and to a lesser extent in the sequence of events. In girls, the first event is usually breast enlargement (range 8–13 years), followed closely by growth of pubic hair and approximately 2 years later by menarche. By this time the growth spurt is usually completed. In girls, puberty is defined as precocius if the onset is before 8.5 years and is regarded as delayed if there are no signs of puberty by 13.5 years, or menarche has not occurred by 16.5 years. In boys, the first sign of puberty is enlargement of the testes accompanied by changes in the skin of the scrotum which reddens and alters in texture (range 9.5–13.5 years). The growth spurt and changes in body dimensions, including growth of the penis and development of pubic hair, start about one year later and reach a peak over a 12-month period coinciding with the first seminal emissions. Breaking of the voice occurs relatively late in puberty and is due to lengthening of the vocal cords with the sudden growth spurt of the larynx. Puberty in boys is said to be precocious if it occurs before 10 years, and delayed if there are no signs by 14 years.

Measurement and use of growth charts

Growth is always assessed by measuring height (length in children under 2 years), (Figs. 3.2 & 3.3), weight and head circumference, and also on the stage of pubertal development where appropriate (Table 3.1). Sometimes where body proportions are disturbed, measurements of sitting height and limb length are made, e.g. in achondroplasia where the limbs are short. Special equipment is needed to measure height, but if it is not available a rough measurement is still useful for screening purposes.

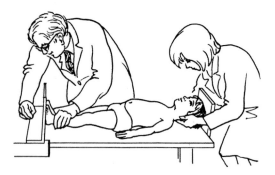

Fig. 3.3 Measuring a baby's length (length should be measured in children under 2 years). The baby lies on his back. One person holds his head in the Frankfort plane, and gently pulls to extend the baby to his full length. A second person straightens the baby's legs, so they lie flat on the table, and then brings a moveable footboard up against the heels. Length is often difficult to measure because babies prefer to lie curled up

Table 3.1 Stages of pubertal development

Boys: Genital development
Stage 1 Preadolescent; the testes, scrotum and penis are the same size and proportions as in early childhood
Stage 2 The scrotum and testes grow, and the skin of the scrotum reddens and changes in texture
Stage 3 The penis begins to grow longer
Stage 4 Growth continues; the penis broadens and the glans develops, the testes and scrotum enlarge and the scrotal skin darkens
Stage 5 The genitalia are adult in size and shape

Girls: Breast development
Stage 1 Preadolescent; only the papillae are raised
Stage 2 Formation of the breast bud; the breast and papilla become elevated into a small mound, and the areola enlarges
Stage 3 Further enlargement and elevation of breast and areola
Stage 4 The areola and papilla project to form a secondary mound above the level of the breast
Stage 5 Mature stage, only the papilla projects, the areola recedes to the general contour of the breast

Both Sexes: Pubic hair
Stage 1 Preadolescent; no pubic hair
Stage 2 Sparse growth of long pigmented downy hair, sometimes curly, at the base of the penis or along the labia
Stage 3 Hair spreads sparsely over the junction of the pubes and is coarser, darker and more curled
Stage 4 Hair is now adult in type, but has not spread to the medial surface of the thighs
Stage 5 Hair is adult in type and in distribution, having spread to the medial surface of the thighs. Spread up the linea alba occurs much later

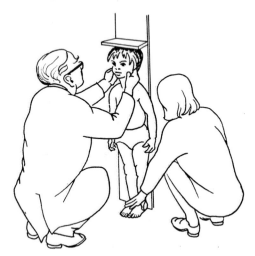

Fig. 3.2 Measuring the child's height. Make sure the child stands with the feet together, heels touching the ground and the heel plate. Young children tend to stand with their feet apart and to go up on tiptoe, they may need to have their feet held. The head should be in the Frankfort plane (so that a line drawn from the lower border of the eye to the upper margin of the external auditory meatus is horizontal) this avoids flexion of the neck. Encourage the child to stretch up to maximum height by gentle upward pressure on the bony mastoid processes, just behind the ears

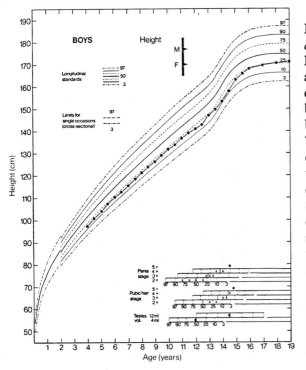

Fig. 3.4 Growth charts showing centiles for height and pubertal development (Tanner & Whitehouse 19). There are separate charts for boys (a) and girls (b)

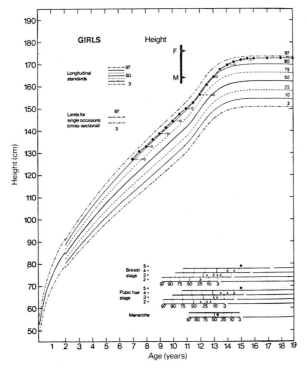

The best standards for assessing growth of British children are those designed by Tanner *et al* (1978) from measurements of many hundreds of British children at different ages. Charts are available for plotting height, weight, head circumference and growth velocity. The height charts for boys and girls are illustrated in Figures 3.4a and b. Each chart shows a series of centile curves. The 50th centile gives the median value for height of children at each age, that is half the children in the sample measured were taller than the 50th centile at each age, and half the children shorter. Similarly for the third centile, 97 per cent of children were taller at each age and 3 per cent were shorter. The third and 97th centile curves, or the two standard deviation lines, are regarded as the limits of normal, and children whose measurements fall outside this range may need to be studied. It is important to remember, however, that three normal children out of every 100 will have measurements below the third centile, and a further three normal children will be above the 97th centile.

When assessing height it is important to allow for parental height, tall parents tend to have tall children, and short parents have short children. There are special charts which allow for midparental height, or as a quick check the parents' heights can be plotted on the child's growth chart as if they were aged 19 years. When plotting maternal height on a boy's chart, add 13 cm (the average difference between men and women's height) or subtract 13 cm from the father's height for the girl's chart. The midpoint between the parental heights is then found on the chart, this is the midparental height centile, and a line extending 8.5 cm up and down from it will indicate the range of heights within which 95 per cent of their children should come. If parental height is allowed for in this way, a short child with short parents may move from below the third to the 50th centile, whereas a child of average height with tall parents may move from the 50th to below the third centile.

Single measurements of height, weight and head circumference give limited and, often misleading, information; it is much more useful to plot a series of measurements on the growth chart to ascertain the pattern of growth. Most children's growth curves tend to follow centile curves without crossing them, except in the first months of life, and at puberty. An individual child's curves for height, weight and head circumference also follow similar centiles. Children who are exceptionally large or small, taking into account parental size, or who have one growth parameter which differs greatly from the others, such as a large head circumference or short stature, or whose growth curves cross centile lines, may need investigation.

DEVELOPMENT

The study of child development is rather like looking down a series of increasingly powerful microscopes, the closer one looks the more detail emerges. Knowledge of detail is essential in order to help the handicapped child achieve various skills despite his handicap; for instance, helping the blind child learn to reach towards the sound made by a toy which he cannot see. The sooner difficulties are recognised, the sooner appropriate help can be given. Many argue, however, about the value of a therapy which is difficult to prove statistically and, therefore, question the cost-effectiveness of screening for delayed development.

In 1976 the Committee on Child Health Services chaired by Professor Court concluded that there were considerable advantages to be gained from surveying the health of all children, and suggested that children were seen at 6 weeks, around 2.5–3 years and 4.5–5 years (school entry) by a doctor, and at 7–8 months and 18 months by a health visitor. The following charts and notes outline development at these ages, and give the age range at which skills normally develop; only a percentage of children can be expected to come for assessment close to a given age. In the Denver Developmental Screening Test, a child failing several items at an age where 90 per cent of other children pass should be suspected of delay and referred for further examination. This American test has recently been restandardised for a UK population in the Cardiff area.

The developmental assessment should be brief as young children can and will only concentrate for short periods, 15 minutes or less is usually recom-

mended. Severe delay in motor development should become obvious in the first year, while most cases of cerebral palsy are detected by 18 months. It is hoped to identify the deaf child early, but many are only recognised because of poor speech development, by which time they are usually 2 or 3 years old. Parents are often aware that something is wrong and their anxieties should be taken seriously. The milder forms of mental handicap also become apparent around 2–3 years, with immature patterns of play and poor language skills being present. Special help at home, or in a nursery group should be made available, starting soon after the handicap is recognised.

The school entry examination is important and is, therefore, more detailed and slightly longer. In some areas it is carried out shortly after school entry. The doctor hopes to recognise those children with less obvious neurodevelopmental disorders who will need special help at school. About 5 per cent of children in normal schools have significant learning difficulties and up to 20 per cent are said to need extra help at some stage of their schooling.

Notes on development

6 weeks

Motor

Supine. lies with head to one side and arm and leg on that side more extended (asymmetric tonic neck reflex or ATNR).

Prone. less flexed than at birth, when awake hips are extended and pelvis is low on the couch, the sleeping baby often reverts to newborn flexed posture.

Head control is beginning to develop. When prone, the baby briefly lifts head and turns face to side. On pull to sit he momentarily lifts head as body reaches an angle of 45° to the couch, then head flops forward. Marked hip flexion when prone, and excessive head lag are abnormal.

Ventral suspension. If infant is suspended with a hand under his abdomen, he momentarily holds his head level with his body, and his hips, knees and elbows are partially flexed. In hypertonia, the head is held above the line of the trunk and cannot be flexed, and the hips and knees are fully extended in line with the trunk. The hypotonic infant limply hangs over the hand and is unable to lift head or limbs.

Neonatal reflexes should be present and symmetrical, but obligatory responses are abnormal.

Vision

Mothers usually know whether their babies look at them intently during feeds. Nevertheless, always test vision; it is important to recognise severe visual defects quickly as some benefit from early surgery, e.g. removal of cataracts, congenital glaucoma. Visual information is important for early learning and early developmental guidance is thought to help if there is poor vision.

Hearing

Hearing is difficult to test in the young infant. Loud sounds, at least 60 dB are often needed to elicit a response at this age. A special cradle designed to pick up a baby's response to sound is currently on trial, evidence so far suggests it allows recognition of severe hearing loss in the first weeks of life.

Social

A baby's alertness and interest is shown by his ability to imitate and his responses to social stimuli. No smile by 8 weeks is cause for serious concern, unless the baby was preterm. Sometimes

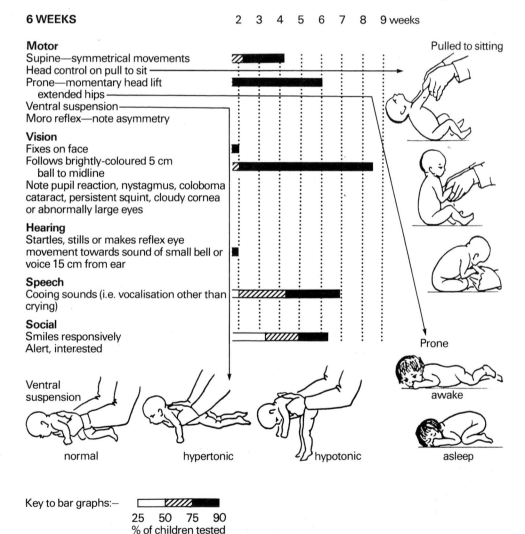

6 WEEKS   2 3 4 5 6 7 8 9 weeks

Motor
Supine—symmetrical movements
Head control on pull to sit
Prone—momentary head lift
    extended hips
Ventral suspension
Moro reflex—note asymmetry

Vision
Fixes on face
Follows brightly-coloured 5 cm
    ball to midline
Note pupil reaction, nystagmus, coloboma
cataract, persistent squint, cloudy cornea
or abnormally large eyes

Hearing
Startles, stills or makes reflex eye
movement towards sound of small bell or
voice 15 cm from ear

Speech
Cooing sounds (i.e. vocalisation other than
crying)

Social
Smiles responsively
Alert, interested

Pulled to sitting

Prone

awake

asleep

Ventral
suspension

normal   hypertonic   hypotonic

Key to bar graphs:—
25   50   75   90
% of children tested

babies of this age are hungry or uncomfortable at the time of testing, and are not very responsive. If you have to rely on the history, ensure that the mother understands you are referring to a smile in response to a social overture, rather than a smiling expression during sleep.

7–8 months

Motor

Head control is achieved by 4 months. In prone, head and chest should be lifted off the bed. In supine, the baby is starting to lift the head off the pillow and by 7–8 months there should be no head lag, shoulders should be braced and elbows flexed on pull to sit. Hypotonia is obvious, but if there is increased extensor tone, the child may rise to his feet when pulled to sit.

Sits alone for a few seconds with a straight back. Control of trunk muscles develops from above downwards, initially the back is C-shaped when sitting, then the thoracic spine straightens and finally the lumbar curve is lost.

Sitting balance. two responses develop; tilting of the trunk and head to correct the loss of upright position, and protective responses where the hands are put out to prevent falling over. Forward balance develops first, then sideways and finally backwards balance which is usually achieved by 12 months. A child cannot sit or walk alone until he has both balancing and protective reactions, they are often slow to develop in cerebral palsy.

Mobility. The infant is starting to move around usually by rolling, some are already pivoting or creeping on their stomachs, the average age for crawling on hands and knees is 10 months.

Neonatal reflexes should have disappeared, persistence is a serious sign of delay.

Manipulative and adaptive skills

Reaching develops in several stages. Initially there is a phase of hand regard, when the infant waves his hands in front of his eyes, pronating and supinating them at the wrists; this should have stopped by 5 months. During the next stage the infant looks excitedly at an object, moulding his hand as if to grasp it. Initially, reaching and touching the object occurs by accident, and is probably helped by the ATNR where the arm is extended in the direction the child is looking. Gradually, voluntary reaching occurs but is very ataxic to begin with. By 8 months the infant should have a steady accurate reach with either hand, good head and shoulder control is essential. Use of only one hand may indicate hemiplegia.

Grasp. The grasp reflex should have gone, so that the hands lie open and can be used to grasp objects. Initially objects are grasped in the palm for a few moments, but by 8 months there is a secure radial palmar grasp. There is also an awareness of holding an object, so it is briefly looked at, transferred from hand to hand, then explored in the mouth. The interest in objects may extend to looking for them when they disappear from view — concept of permanence of objects. One inch (2.5 cm) cubes are the correct size of a toy for the infant to grasp in his palm, smaller toys will be lost, and the hand is not big enough for larger toys.

Vision

Note visual interest for near and distant objects. Good head control leads to macular fixation and binocular vision, that is both eyes move together in all directions — test by moving a light from side to side and watching reflections of light in the eyes. Demonstrate convergence by persuading the child to look at a small sweet. Squint is abnormal. Obvious squints are detected by asymmetrical reflections of the light in the pupils. Less obvious squints are detected with the cover test, the infant is persuaded to look at a small toy (not a light), and then one eye is covered by moving a hand in front of the eye. A squint is present if the *uncovered* eye then moves to take up fixation on the toy.

Hearing

Parental anxiety should always be taken seriously. Ask parents for examples of sounds their child responds to, such as smiling in response to a quiet voice, looking towards the door when he hears it opened quietly, or excitement when he hears food being prepared or a bath run. Hearing tests are difficult to carry out accurately in a clinic. Distraction-type tests are used, where the child is only scored as passing if he turns and localises the sound. Localisation skills develop from reflex eye movements, where the eyes move towards the ear in which the sound is heard loudest. Sounds are first localised at ear level, then below and finally above ear level (localisation behind or above the head is very difficult and not achieved until much later). By 8 months the majority of children can localise sound at ear level, whereas a number fail at 6 months. After 10 months they are less easily distracted and may fail to turn to the test

sounds in spite of normal hearing. Success is more likely if interesting test sounds are used, particularly those familiar to the child, they should not be louder than 35–40 dB.

Speech

The sounds a baby makes are an indication of the sounds he hears and is trying to imitate. At 8 months babble should be tuneful and include consonants, for example 'adadadada' and 'umumum'. Parents deaf children often comment

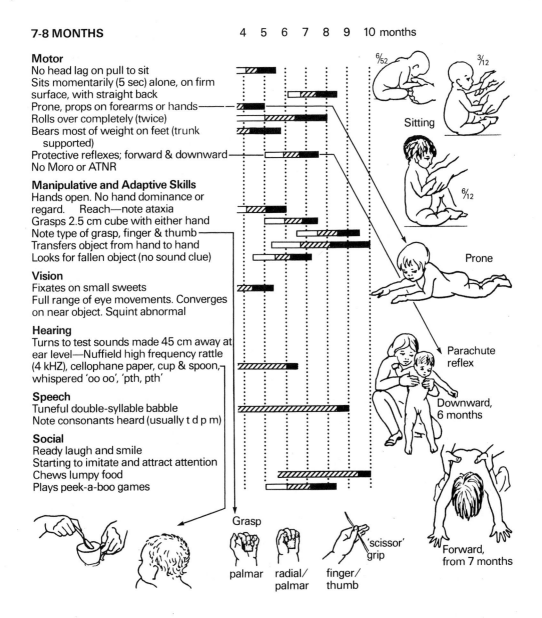

7-8 MONTHS 4 5 6 7 8 9 10 months

Motor
No head lag on pull to sit
Sits momentarily (5 sec) alone, on firm surface, with straight back
Prone, props on forearms or hands
Rolls over completely (twice)
Bears most of weight on feet (trunk supported)
Protective reflexes; forward & downward
No Moro or ATNR

Manipulative and Adaptive Skills
Hands open. No hand dominance or regard. Reach—note ataxia
Grasps 2.5 cm cube with either hand
Note type of grasp, finger & thumb
Transfers object from hand to hand
Looks for fallen object (no sound clue)

Vision
Fixates on small sweets
Full range of eye movements. Converges on near object. Squint abnormal

Hearing
Turns to test sounds made 45 cm away at ear level—Nuffield high frequency rattle (4 kHZ), cellophane paper, cup & spoon, whispered 'oo oo', 'pth, pth'

Speech
Tuneful double-syllable babble
Note consonants heard (usually t d p m)

Social
Ready laugh and smile
Starting to imitate and attract attention
Chews lumpy food
Plays peek-a-boo games

Sitting

6/52 3/12 6/12

Prone

Parachute reflex

Downward, 6 months

Forward, from 7 months

Grasp
palmar
radial/palmar
finger/thumb
'scissor' grip

on the striking lack of baby sounds made by their deaf child, compared with his normally hearing siblings.

Social

Lack of interest in surroundings, infrequent smiles and failure to imitate are cause for serious concern, and may indicate intellectual delay or sometimes social deprivation.

18 Months

Motor

During the second year children become increasingly adept at motor skills. The majority can walk alone, balance momentarily on one leg to kick a ball, or walk upstairs, but they crawl downstairs backwards. Children who cannot walk alone, must be examined carefully for signs of cerebral palsy, muscle disorder or intellectual delay. Some, who are not walking, may be moving around in other ways, such as rolling, creeping, or bottom shuffling. There is often a family history of moving in the same way. These children are slow to sit alone, although most do so by 15 months; and are slow to walk alone, this is usually achieved by 26–28 months.

Manipulative and adaptive skills

By 18 months a child should have developed accurate reach and a mature voluntary grasp and release. Stacking bricks test the accuracy of reach, grasp and release; the use of a raisin or tiny sweet demonstrates index pointing and fine pincer grasp between the tip of the thumb and first finger. During the second year children can concentrate on tasks of their own choice, but cannot use, or tolerate any intervention, or attempts to modify the task. The child's attention and understanding is shown by his attempts to stack bricks, dump the raisin from a narrow-necked bottle after being shown, and his interest in books and pictures. Ataxia or tremor when reaching, immature grasp, and obvious hand preference are abnormal, and suggestive of cerebral palsy. The mouthing of toys and drooling seen in the first year should have

disappeared; so should casting, which is the deliberate throwing of toys onto the floor in a repetitive manner normally seen between 12 and 15 months — persistence of any of these suggests intellectual delay.

Vision

Visual acuity is tested using Stycar tests designed by Mary Sheridan.

Near vision is crudely assessed using hundreds and thousands, small round coloured cake decorations, which are about 1 mm in diameter. One or two sweets are discretely dropped onto a felt covered table top of contrasting colour, taking care not to indicate the position of the sweets with the hand or eye. To pass, the child should point to a sweet or try to pick it up.

Distance vision is assessed using white balls of graded sizes from 6 cm down to 3 mm in diameter. These balls are either rolled along the ground, or mounted on sticks and shown from behind a screen 3 (or 6) m from the child. The balls should always be shown against a plain, black background. By watching the child's eyes, one can detect whether he has seen the balls. He should see a 3 mm ball at 3 m, which is approximately equivalent to Snellen 6/18.

Cover test should always be done, as squints can appear at any time during the pre-school years. They are sometimes more obvious on distance vision tests, particularly when there is a defect of distance vision in one eye.

Hearing and language

Hearing tests are difficult to carry out accurately at this age, so reliance is placed on the child's response to commands spoken quietly, with head dropped, and hand covering the mouth, so as to avoid lip reading. Parental concern about hearing, failure to respond to spoken commands or poor vocalisation, are indications for a formal hearing test. By 18 months most children recognise life-size objects, and indicate an understanding of their use by appropriate gesture, e.g. brushing hair, putting a spoon in the cup, and sometimes they name the objects.

Comprehension of spoken language can be tested by asking the child to select the appropriate life-size object on naming, e.g. 'give Mummy the shoe', or asking him to point to different parts of the body. Differentiation of the sounds in the words 'sock' and 'shoe', or 'feet' and 'teeth', demonstrate not only the ability to hear high frequency sounds, but also to subtly discriminate between them.

Expressive language is less easy to elicit in a strange place. Toddlers often chatter when they are happily playing and this should be listened for. There is usually a lot of tuneful jargon, with some words said clearly with meaning, and occasionally two words put together, e.g. 'Daddy car' or 'Sara bikit' (= biscuit). Phrases such as 'all gone' do not count as they are learnt as a single word.

Social

Social skills such as drinking from a cup, or using a spoon depend on whether the child has been allowed to try and feed himself. Most toddlers want to imitate adults and are keen to test their independence. They sometimes refuse to feed if parents insist on helping them to ensure a good food intake or to avoid mess. As a result temper tantrums, and feeding, sleeping, or bowel problems are particularly common amongst toddlers.

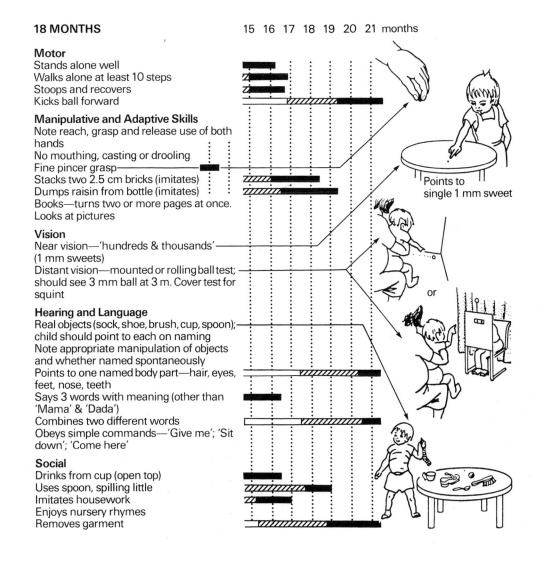

18 MONTHS

15 16 17 18 19 20 21 months

Motor
Stands alone well
Walks alone at least 10 steps
Stoops and recovers
Kicks ball forward

Manipulative and Adaptive Skills
Note reach, grasp and release use of both hands
No mouthing, casting or drooling
Fine pincer grasp
Stacks two 2.5 cm bricks (imitates)
Dumps raisin from bottle (imitates)
Books—turns two or more pages at once.
Looks at pictures

Vision
Near vision—'hundreds & thousands' (1 mm sweets)
Distant vision—mounted or rolling ball test; should see 3 mm ball at 3 m. Cover test for squint

Hearing and Language
Real objects (sock, shoe, brush, cup, spoon); child should point to each on naming
Note appropriate manipulation of objects and whether named spontaneously
Points to one named body part—hair, eyes, feet, nose, teeth
Says 3 words with meaning (other than 'Mama' & 'Dada')
Combines two different words
Obeys simple commands—'Give me'; 'Sit down'; 'Come here'

Social
Drinks from cup (open top)
Uses spoon, spilling little
Imitates housework
Enjoys nursery rhymes
Removes garment

Points to single 1 mm sweet

or

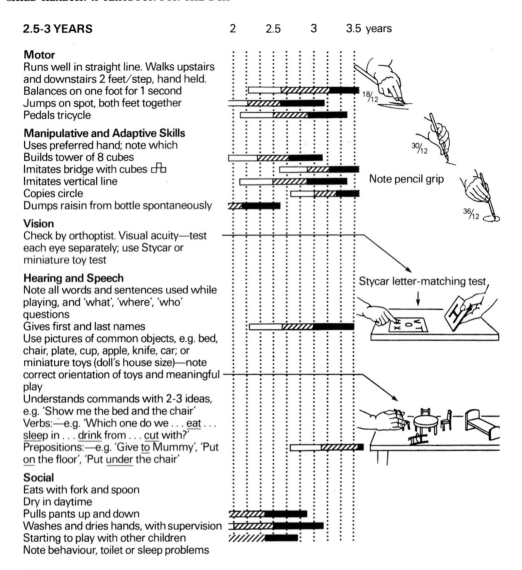

2.5-3 YEARS

2   2.5   3   3.5 years

Motor
Runs well in straight line. Walks upstairs and downstairs 2 feet/step, hand held.
Balances on one foot for 1 second
Jumps on spot, both feet together
Pedals tricycle

Manipulative and Adaptive Skills
Uses preferred hand; note which
Builds tower of 8 cubes
Imitates bridge with cubes
Imitates vertical line
Copies circle
Dumps raisin from bottle spontaneously

Note pencil grip

Vision
Check by orthoptist. Visual acuity—test each eye separately; use Stycar or miniature toy test

Stycar letter-matching test

Hearing and Speech
Note all words and sentences used while playing, and 'what', 'where', 'who' questions
Gives first and last names
Use pictures of common objects, e.g. bed, chair, plate, cup, apple, knife, car; or miniature toys (doll's house size)—note correct orientation of toys and meaningful play
Understands commands with 2-3 ideas, e.g. 'Show me the bed and the chair'
Verbs:—e.g. 'Which one do we . . . eat . . . sleep in . . . drink from . . . cut with?'
Prepositions:—e.g. 'Give to Mummy', 'Put on the floor', 'Put under the chair'

Social
Eats with fork and spoon
Dry in daytime
Pulls pants up and down
Washes and dries hands, with supervision
Starting to play with other children
Note behaviour, toilet or sleep problems

2.5–3 Years

Motor

The 2.5-year-old child walks well with a steady even stride, feet fairly close together; he goes up and down stairs, two feet per step holding the bannister, and by 3 years many go upstairs alternate feet to each step. Balance and running skills have improved. Initially the child runs well indoors in a straight line, and later, develops the ability to negotiate objects whilst running. Jumping and climbing are practised in play, and peddling a tricycle, shows the ability to coordinate alternate leg movements.

Manipulative and adaptive skills

From 18 months children start to demonstrate hand preference, but the other hand is frequently used for additional help. Exclusive use of one hand is suggestive of hemiplegia. The pencil grip matures from the initial palmar grasp in the midshaft of the pencil, with a movement of the whole arm at 18 months, to an early tripod grip by 2.5–3 years. The pencil is held near the point between the thumb and first two fingers permitting finer movements of the hand and forearm.

In the third year a child's attention is still single channelled, but much more flexible; so that once his full attention has been obtained he can be given directions to carry out a task, and then must be encouraged to transfer his interest back to the task. The child's ability to carry out some of the manipulative, and linguistic test items, will give a measure of his attention level. When he is asked to imitate a bridge made of cubes, the bridge is built in front of him, and then he is asked to make another. Copying is more difficult, for example the circle is drawn out of his sight, he is then shown the circle and asked to copy it.

Vision

In some parts of the UK, orthoptists routinely see children to check for less obvious squints and refractive errors. By 3 years the majority of children are able to cooperate with their tests, and this is thought to be a good age for screening.

In the Stycar letter matching tests the children are shown single letters at a distance of 3 m, and asked to point to the matching letter on the card in front of them. It is important to check that they are able to match the letters correctly close-up, before testing at a distance — 50–80 per cent of 2.5–3-year-olds can do this. Children who fail to match the letter size 4 (equivalent to Snellen 6/9) with each eye separately, should be referred to an ophthalmologist. If the child cannot match letters, he can be asked to match special miniature toys, which test his ability to discriminate between knives, forks and spoons from a distance of 3 m.

Hearing and language

It is important to check language skills carefully as delay may be the first indication of poor hearing, intellectual retardation, or less commonly a specific language disorder. Inability to communicate in the presence of normal intelligence leads to great frustration, and the children often resort to gesture and mime. If any abnormalities are found formal hearing tests should be carried out.

The child of 2.5–3 years should understand pictures and that doll's-house-size miniature toys represent real objects and play meaningfully with them; failure to do so suggests intellectual delay. Comprehension can be tested with pictures or miniature toys; at 2 years most children can relate

two ideas together and by 3 years, four ideas together, for example 'put the cup on the table and put the baby in the bath'. Most children chatter continuously whilst playing and have a vocabulary of at least 200 words. Sentences consist of subject — verb — object, for instance, 'Sara eat cake'. The pronouns 'I', 'me' and 'you' are used correctly by 3 years, as are most prepositions. Persistent and frequent 'what', 'where', 'who' questions are a feature of this age.

Social

Feeding, washing and dressing are carried out increasingly skilfully, and most children like to do everything without help. The majority of children are dry in the daytime, and some are also dry at night. It is again important to enquire about behaviour problems, one study found they occurred in 18 per cent of children over 2-years-old and were frequently associated with maternal depression.

4.5–5 years (school entrance examination

Motor

There is a wide variation of normal motor skills, but a number of children, particularly boys, are significantly slow in motor development and appear clumsy compared with their more agile peers. If clumsiness is severe, or is associated with poor skills in other areas, educational difficulties are likely; otherwise the majority of clumsy children seem to cope. A number of physiotherapists have developed therapy programmes to help these children become more aware of their body images, and the position of their joints and limbs. At present it only seems practicable to refer the most severely affected children for this type of help.

Manipulative and adaptive skills

In order to cope at school a child must be able to control his focus of attention and integrate information from several sources at once. For instance, the teacher may be speaking about an object and the child needs to be able to look at it and listen to the teacher at the same time. He should be able

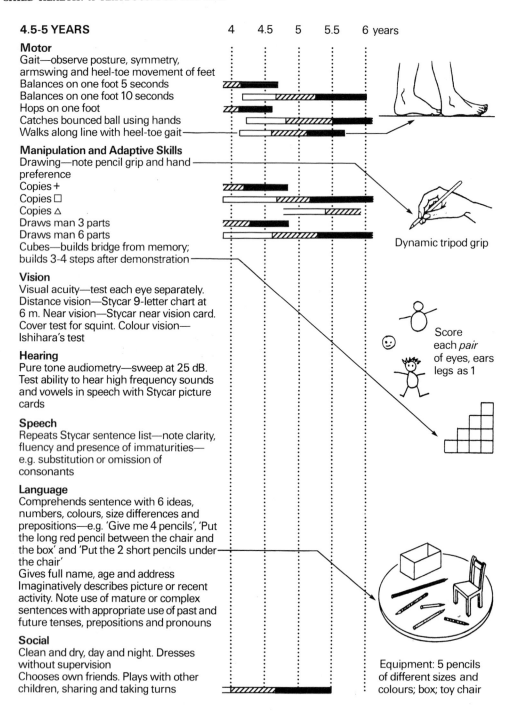

4.5-5 YEARS

| | 4 | 4.5 | 5 | 5.5 | 6 years |

Motor
Gait—observe posture, symmetry, armswing and heel-toe movement of feet
Balances on one foot 5 seconds
Balances on one foot 10 seconds
Hops on one foot
Catches bounced ball using hands
Walks along line with heel-toe gait

Manipulation and Adaptive Skills
Drawing—note pencil grip and hand preference
Copies +
Copies □
Copies △
Draws man 3 parts
Draws man 6 parts
Cubes—builds bridge from memory; builds 3-4 steps after demonstration

Dynamic tripod grip

Vision
Visual acuity—test each eye separately. Distance vision—Stycar 9-letter chart at 6 m. Near vision—Stycar near vision card. Cover test for squint. Colour vision—Ishihara's test

Score each *pair* of eyes, ears legs as 1

Hearing
Pure tone audiometry—sweep at 25 dB. Test ability to hear high frequency sounds and vowels in speech with Stycar picture cards

Speech
Repeats Stycar sentence list—note clarity, fluency and presence of immaturities—e.g. substitution or omission of consonants

Language
Comprehends sentence with 6 ideas, numbers, colours, size differences and prepositions—e.g. 'Give me 4 pencils', 'Put the long red pencil between the chair and the box' and 'Put the 2 short pencils under the chair'
Gives full name, age and address
Imaginatively describes picture or recent activity. Note use of mature or complex sentences with appropriate use of past and future tenses, prepositions and pronouns

Social
Clean and dry, day and night. Dresses without supervision
Chooses own friends. Plays with other children, sharing and taking turns

Equipment: 5 pencils of different sizes and colours; box; toy chair

to hold a pencil in a mature tripod grip, thus enabling him to make small controlled movements of his hand, and to put even pressure on the pencil. He should also be able to copy shapes as a preliminary to writing, and demonstrate his visual perception of people in a drawing. Construction of three-dimensional shapes from a model is tested.

Vision

Visual defects can appear at any stage of childhood due to growth of the eyeball, this usually causes shortsightedness (myopia) and therefore visual acuity should be checked every couple of years at school. A number of 5-year-olds are found to have previously unrecognised squints, a tendency to tilt the head to one side should raise suspicions. Colour vision should also be checked, defects are much more common amongst boys.

Hearing

Hearing is tested in two ways. First, the ability to hear quiet sounds at different frequencies is tested with an audiogram. Second the ability to listen to sounds and discriminate between them, is tested with the Stycar picture cards for high and low frequency sounds. The latter test is more likely to be failed by children with poor ability to attend, in spite of normal hearing.

Speech and language

Speech should be clear, fluent and easily understood by persons other than members of the family. Some minor immaturities such as substitution of the consonants R, L, W or Y and S, F or Th are still common and usually disappear by 7 years. Encourage the child to talk by asking him about a recent outing, or to describe a picture. Write down some examples of what he says. He should speak imaginatively using mature sentences, containing two clauses joined by 'and', for example, 'I went shopping and Mummy stayed at home'; or complex sentences containing two verbs such as 'I didn't go shopping because I was ill'. Past, present and future tenses of verbs, prepositions and pronouns should be used appropriately. Children who have poor linguistic skills at school entry, frequently have difficulty with learning, in particular with learning to read. They urgently need assessment of hearing and speech therapy. Ideally these problems should be recognised at the 2.5–3-year examination, so the children can be helped before starting at school.

Social

A child needs to be independent in daily living skills, feeding, dressing, washing and toileting, to manage at school. In addition, he should separate easily from his family, and make friends with other children, understanding the need to share and take turns in games.

FURTHER READING

Bryant G J, Davies K J Newcombe R G 1979 Standardisation of the Denver developmental screening test for Cardiff children. Developmental Medicine and Child Neurology 21: 353–364

DHSS Fit for the Future. DHSS, London

Drillien C M Drummond M B (ed) 1977 Neurodevelopmental problems in early childhood. Blackwell Scientific Publications, Oxford

Egan D F, Illingworth R S MacKeith R C 1969 Developmental screening 0–5 years. Spastics International Medical Publications, London

Holt K S 1977 Developmental paediatrics, postgraduate paediatric series. Butterworths, London

Sheridan M D 1968 Manual for the Stycar hearing tests. NFER Publishing Company Ltd, Windsor

Sheridan M D 1973 Manual for the Stycar vision tests. NFER Publishing Company Ltd, Windsor

Tanner J M 1978 Foetus into man. Open Books Publishing Ltd, London

4

Prevention of illness and the care of the normal child

The health of the population of the UK has improved markedly over the last 60 years. This is related to higher standards of living; the incidence of severe poverty has fallen, undernutrition of mothers and children is rarely encountered, many more people live in dry, warm housing and the control of environmental hazards, such as air pollution, has reduced the incidence of chronic lung disease. The medical profession has made some contribution to this improvement by the recognition of disease at an early stage when treatment may be undertaken and complications prevented. Health education aims to modify people's behaviour so that they can avoid activities which are likely to produce injury or disease, and encourages them to adopt life-styles that promote good health.

Classification of preventive measures

Primary prevention aims to prevent the occurrence of a disease

Secondary prevention aims to detect a disease early or at a pre-symptomatic stage when its effects can sometimes be reversed and its progress halted.

Tertiary prevention aims to halt the development of complication in a previously recognised disease.

Screening

Secondary prevention of a disease can be undertaken by screening a population. For this to be effective the disease must satisfy the following criteria:

1. Untreated it must have serious consequences

2. It must be easily and reliably recognisable at an early or pre-symptomatic stage
3. Effective treatment must be readily and economically available.

Examples of preventive measures and conditions for which they are used are shown in Table 4.1.

OTHER PREVENTIVE ACTIVITIES

The National Health Service has sometimes separated the preventive service from those designed to treat a sick child. Indeed, the two services are often carried out in different buildings by different people. This is unfortunate; ideally one doctor should be responsible for both the preventive and therapeutic services. Where more than one doctor is involved, each should be in close contact with the other.

Traditionally, the general practitioner (GP) was seen as the doctor responsible for treating episodic illness in children: this is still one of his important roles. However, he is also ideally placed to undertake prevention. He should be able to provide *comprehensive* child care for all the children on his list.

Preventive child health should not be practised only in well-baby clinics or immunisation sessions; the GP has an opportunity to prevent illness and to educate parents and patients on each occasion that he sees them.

Thus, a check on a child's immunisation status can be made when he is brought for treatment of otitis media; teeth can be checked when the throat is examined; obesity noted and appropriate dietary advice given at the same time as treatment for a

Table 4.1 Preventive measures and conditions for which they are used

Type of prevention	Definition	Conditions against which these measures are used
Primary prevention	Primary prevention prevents a disease from occurring and reduces its incidence	Immunisation: against infectious diseases such as tetanus, diphtheria, pertussis, poliomyelitis, measles, rubella, tuberculosis Immunisation: with anti-D globulin to Rhesus-negative mothers to prevent Rhesus disease in future pregnancies Contraception: to prevent conception in those at increased risk of genetic disorders such as haemophilia, Duchenne muscular dystrophy or serious haemoglobinopathy. Also in those at greater risk of conceiving a baby with Down's syndrome or spine bifida Health education: to prevent the use of teratogenic drugs in pregnancy, to reduce smoking and excessive alcohol drinking in pregnancy, advice designed to reduce the incidence of accident hazards at home and on the roads
Secondary prevention	Secondary prevention detects previously unrecognised disease at a time when deterioration and complications can be prevented	Early antenatal detection and termination of pregnancy for conditions such as Down's syndrome, spina bifida, haemoglobinopathy, and X-linked disorders such as haemophilia and Duchenne muscular dystrophy. Screening by blood tests in the newborn period for phenylketonuria and hypothyroidism Physical examination in the newborn period and in developmental clinics for such disorders as congenital dislocation of the hip, undescended testes, squint, deafness, and inguinal hernias
Tertiary prevention	Tertiary prevention halts the progress of a previously recognised disease	Effective treatment for diabetes mellitus and hypertension

planter wart; the house-call for measles may reveal the unguarded fire or stairs and the need for appropriate advice on accident prevention.

Many GPs' arrange special sessions that are mainly preventive in content and to which more time can be devoted outside the hurly-burly of surgery hours. Theses include sessions for immunisation against infectious disease; developmental surveillance, and health visitors' clinics for mothers of small babies to discuss infant feeding and general management.

The prevention of illness in childhood can be considered under the following headings:

1. The prevention of genetic and congenital disease

Prevention is based mainly on the genetic counselling of parents who may have already had one child with a genetic disorder or one of the parents, or a near relative, may have suffered from such a condition. After genetic counselling, a couple may decide against future pregnancies (primary prevention); others may feel that the risk of having an affected baby is low enough to be worth taking, especially if the disorder can be detected in utero at a stage of pregnancy when termination is possible (secondary prevention). Such disorders include Down's syndrome, which can be diagnosed by the tissue culture and cytological examination of fetal cells obtained by amniocentesis, or neural tube defects which can be detected by the finding of a raised alphafetoprotein concentration in the mother's blood or the amniotic fluid.

The prevention of illness in the newborn baby is one of the aims of antenatal care. Thus, prompt detection and proper care in pregnancy of disorders such as pre-eclampsia, diabetes mellitus, placental insufficiency or premature labour contribute to lessening ill health of the newborn. The administration of anti-D gamma globulin to the rhesus-negative mother of a rhesus-positive baby within 24 hours of birth prevents the development of rhesus disease in future pregnancies with rhesus-positive children.

2. Prevention of metabolic and nutritional disorders

The detection of raised blood levels of phenylalanine within the first few days of birth in the baby with phenylketonuria by the Guthrie test is an example of secondary prevention. The affected child must then be maintained on a phenylalanine-free diet to ensure normal future development. Untreated, high blood levels of phenylalanine will cause brain damage and mental retardation. Similarly, the detection of cretinism shortly after birth by blood tests means that effective therapy is possible with thyroxine to prevent mental handicap.

The commonest nutritional disorder of childhood is obesity. Appropriate health education to mothers may help to prevent it, in particular, the early weaning of babies onto solid foods and the use of carbohydrate-rich cereals should be discouraged. Restriction of sugar-containing foods also has the advantage of preventing dental caries.

Nutritional deficiency disorders are rare, but occur in at-risk groups. Babies of Asian origin are more likely to develop iron-deficiency anaemia in the first 3 years of life. This is probably related to prolonged milk feeding and late weaning. Dietary advice should be directed to earlier weaning with meals containing meat, vegetables and cereals. These children also have a greater incidence of rickets. The peak incidence is in the second and third years of life at a stage when they have been weaned from vitamin-D fortified artificial milk preparations to cow's milk. Older Asian children also show an increased incidence of rickets and it has been postulated that the whole-wheat flour used in the preparation of chapatis interferes with the absorption of vitamin D and calcium from the diet. This flour is rich in phytic acid which forms insoluble calcium phytate in the gut. Vitamin D drops given regularly to Asian babies should prevent the development of rickets, and the use of chapati flour which has been fortified with vitamin D and calcium is an effective preventive measure.

3. The prevention of handicap

Effective antenatal and intrapartum care contributes much to the primary prevention of mentally and physically handicapped children.

Secondary prevention aims to detect problems as early as possible, ideally at a stage when a potentially handicapping condition can be reversed. Such reversible disorders include squint, congenital dislocation of the hip, undescended testes and deafness. These are sought at regular intervals in well-baby and developmental assessment clinics.

Regular developmental assessment (see Chapter 3) may reveal the child whose development is not progressing normally and further investigation may be necessary to determine the reason. Rarely, a potentially reversible condition may be discovered, such as conductive deafness from a glue ear. More usually, the cause is irreversible and a programme of special care and schooling has to be devised to facilitate the child's future development to his greatest potential.

4. The prevention of accidents

In England and Wales accidents account for almost 30 per cent of the deaths of children aged between one and 14 years; they are the commonest cause of death in this age group. In 1978, 1310 children died from accidents; 610 of these were road traffic accidents and 324 were accidents in the home.

The doctor should educate parents about the hazards of life in modern society: the dangers of modern transport, including the banning of children from sitting in the front seat of a car; and the dangers that are present in the home, from heaters and cookers, electricity, unguarded stairs, drugs and chemicals in the garden and kitchen. The proper supervision of recreational activities should also be emphasised, in children's playgrounds, on bicycles and ponies, and in swimming pools. The GP on a house call should always be alert to accident hazards in the home and must be prepared to offer appropriate constructive advice.

The balance between over-protection and carelessness can often be difficult for parents to achieve, but they must be encouraged to identify for themselves the potential hazards in their children's environment.

5. The prevention of emotional illness

Serious psychiatric illness in childhood is rare; but behaviour disorders are common and include tearfulness, unreasonable timidity and disruptive or aggressive behaviour. The incidence of these disorders is higher in certain groups of children: those from broken families; those with repeated hospital admissions in the pre-school years; those with a mentally-ill parent; and those from over-crowded unhappy homes.

The recognition of vulnerable children and emotional support for them and their parents may help prevent the development of behaviour disorder in·the future. The doctor, working with the local social services department, may be able to help in material ways to relieve the pressure on overtaxed parents; they may need guidance on housing or finance, support for the provision of a nursery school place or contraceptive advice. Such help lessens the uncertainty and hostility in the home and allows parents and their children to live more harmoniously.

6. The prevention of infectious diseases

The control of infectious diseases is based upon four principles:

   a. Isolation of infected patients from those at risk of the disease
   b. Eradication of factors that transmit the infection
   c. The elimination of infecting organisms
   d. Increasing the resistance of the possible host.

The isolation of infected patients is a method for limiting the spread of a disease that has been used for centuries (quarantine); it is still employed today and patients are isolated until their known period of infectivity is over (see also Chapter 12).

Transmission agents, when recognised, can be controlled, for example clean water supplies have eradicated cholera and typhoid; the elimination of mosquitoes has limited the spread of yellow fever.

It is not always possible to eliminate an infecting organism, especially if it is a virus. However, most bacteria have an antibiotic to which they are sensitive. The earlier that patients with infectious

diseases are detected, the sooner they can be isolated and appropriate treatment instituted. Prompt correct management does limit the spread of such diseases.

The resistance of the potential host can be increased by general measures such as proper nutrition and warm, dry housing. The resistance to a specific infection is increased by immunisation and this, together with the improvement in general living conditions, has contributed dramatically to the declining incidence of many infectious diseases.

IMMUNISATION AGAINST INFECTIOUS DISEASE

General Principles

Resistance to infection can be increased by raising the concentration of specific serum antibodies in the individual who would otherwise be susceptible to that infection; this is known as acquired immunity.

Acquired immunity arises naturally following clinical or subclinical infection, so that it is unusual for an individual to be infected more than once by specific organisms such as the measles virus or the rubella virus. Acquired immunity can also be produced artificially either by the injection of a preparation that is known to contain antibodies, such as gamma globulin (passive immunity), or by injecting a preparation (vaccine) that will stimulate a previously susceptible individual to produce antibodies without developing symptoms or signs of disease (active immunity).

Passive immunisation

The injection of antibodies into a susceptible individual is a less efficient method of immunisation than is the stimulation of active immunity, since passively transferred antibodies are eliminated from the body within a few weeks; the immunity provided is only temporary. However, the increase in resistance to infection is immediate, unlike that produced by active immunity which may take up to 2 weeks.

Passive immunity can be provided by animal sera or by human immunoglobulin prepared from pooled donor blood. The latter preparation is usually preferred as the immunity it produces lasts longer and the incidence of allergic reactions is less. However, some antitoxins are not readily available in donor blood so that horse antitoxin continues to be needed in the treatment of gas gangrene and botulism. Donor blood does contain antitoxins to diphtheria and tetanus and human antitoxin is therefore available in the treatment of these conditions.

Human immunoglobulin is also used to provide immediate passive immunity to viral infections, for example in the non-immune pregnant mother who has come into contact with rubella in the first trimester, the non-immune chronically ill child with coeliac disease who has been in contact with measles, or the leukaemic in contact with chickenpox. Human immunoglobulin is also given prophylactically to travellers in areas where they may be at risk of contracting hepatitis.

Active immunisation

The increase in resistance to infection after active immunisation is longer lasting than that produced by passive immunisation, and this is especially so if a course of vaccination is given. Such immunisation may last for years and reinforcing doses of vaccine at intervals can produce life-long immunity. Active immunity is acquired over a period of time and it may take 2 weeks from the first dose of vaccine for the increase in host resistance to be detected. If an immediate increase in resistance to infection is required, then passive immunisation is necessary.

There are many different methods for artificially stimulating acquired active immunity. Living organisms can be used — such preparations may include an organism closely related to the one that causes the disease (for example vaccinia virus for immunisation against smallpox), or the disease-producing organism itself that has been attenuated to reduce its virulence, for example BCG vaccine against tuberculosis, oral poliomyelitis vaccine (Sabin), measles vaccine and rubella vaccine. Alternatively, some preparations contain killed organisms which although still antigenic and capable of producing acquired immunity are incapable of infection. Such inactivated vaccines include typhoid monovalent and TAB vaccines, pertusis vaccine and inactivated poliomyelitis vaccine (Salk). Vaccines that contain live and killed organisms are listed in Table 4.2.

Toxoids are bacterial toxins whose harmful effects have been neutralised with formaldehyde. They are present in diphtheria and tetanus vaccines, neither of which contains bacteria.

All the vaccines in common use, except BCG vaccine, principally produce active immunity to infection by stimulating the production of circulating antibodies which are specific against the antigens contained in the vaccine. The immunity produced by BCG vaccine is thought to depend on a cell-bound mechanism.

Some vaccines contain adjuvants whose presence enhances the production of antibodies. Aluminium salts have this property and in some preparations diphtheria and tetanus toxoid is adsorbed onto either aluminium phosphate or aluminium hydroxide.

The first administration of a vaccine produces a primary response in which the production of antibodies is slow and their concentration low. The second dose causes a secondary response in which the concentration of antibodies produced is higher and attained more quickly. This higher concen-

Table 4.2 Vaccines that contain live attenuated organisms, those that contain inactive killed organisms and those that contain toxoid

Live vaccines	Vaccines containing killed organisms	Toxoid-containing preparations
Measles	Cholera	Diphtheria
Oral poliomyelitis (Sabin)	Pertussis	Tetanus
Rubella	Parenteral poliomyelitis (Salk)	
Smallpox	Typhoid monovalent	
Tuberculosis (BCG)		
Yellow fever		

tration may be maintained for some months or years and, even if it decreases, can be quickly increased by a further reinforcing dose of vaccine.

Storage of vaccines

Measles and rubella vaccines are live, freeze-dried preparations which have to be reconstituted with water for injection or special diluent immediately before use. They must be stored in the dark at between 2° and 8° C and should be used as soon as possible after they have been reconstituted, and certainly within one hour. Such live vaccines can be killed by high temperatures. Inactivated vaccines should be stored in the dark between 2° and 8° C and should never be frozen.

Immunisation in infancy

Immunisation in infancy has contributed markedly to the decreased incidence of infectious disease in the UK. Some of these disorders are now so rare, for example diphtheria, that there is a danger of complacency amongst both doctors and parents so that immunisation rates may fall to a level where many of these fatal and disabling conditions could return in large numbers.

Doctors responsible for immunisation in infancy must understand the immunological concepts involved, for they must be able to explain them in simple terms to parents, many of whom are, at the least, anxious and often sceptical of the value of what they see as unnecessary and unpleasant procedures. As well as providing the opportunities for children to attend for immunisation, doctors must develop effective systems of follow-up to identify those children who have not been immunised in order to ascertain why this has been so and to persuade the parents of the necessity of such protection against infection. Age/sex registers in many general practices make such follow-up easy, and the recent development of district-based computer systems also contributes to the identification of defaulters.

General practitioners, clinical medical officers, district community physicians and health visitors all have important roles in ensuring that as many children as possible take advantage of the immunisation sessions that are available, and local

immunisation uptake rates should be disseminated at regular intervals to these personnel in order to maintain their interest and motivation in this important task.

To be suitable for prevention by immunisation an infectious disease should satisfy the following criteria:

1. must cause serious and severe illness
2. must occur at a significant frequency in the community
3. must not be readily treatable
4. must have an effective safe vaccine available against it
5. the hazards of the disease must be greater than those of immunisation.

A population's immunisation requirements do not remain static and must be modified by advances in therapy and the disappearance of certain infectious diseases. Thus, effective treatment for measles might make immunisation against this disease unnecessary, although this has not happened to date. The World Health Organisation has declared the world free from smallpox, so that immunisation against this disease is no longer required and it has been removed from the immunisation schedule for infants.

Immunisation schedule

The ideal schedule provides a basic course of immunisation against diphtheria, tetanus, pertussis (whooping cough) and poliomyelitis in the first year of life. Reinforcing doses of diphtheria, tetanus and poliomyelitis vaccine are then given at school entry. Measles immunisation is best performed sometime during the second year and rubella is given to all schoolgirls between 10 and 13 years of age. BCG vaccine should be administered to all tuberculin-negative children sometime between 11 and 13 years of age.

Triple vaccine is a preparation containing diphtheria toxoid, tetanus toxoid and inactivated pertussis organisms; it is given as a single injection into the deltoid or triceps muscle. Poliomyelitis vaccine is an oral preparation containing live organisms, it is given by mouth in the dosage of three drops.

In order to induce immunity as young as possible, the basic course of immunisation with triple vaccine and oral polio should be given early. However, early immunisation is not ideal since there is a greater incidence of reactions to immunisation in young babies. Early immunisation also results in poorer antibody responses — possibly because the antibody producing system is not fully developed and possibly also because maternal antibodies which persist for up to 9 months may bring about the rapid elimination of antigens before a satisfactory antibody response can be evoked. Some immunologists state that the initial immunisation against diphtheria, tetanus, pertussis and poliomyelitis should be delayed until the second half of the first year; others believe that there is a need to protect small babies against pertussis as early as possible and they recommend that immunisation with triple vaccine and oral poliomyelitis begin at 3 months of age. This latter approach is recommended by the Department of Health and Social Security's Joint Committee on Vaccination and Immunisation (Table 4.3).

Measles vaccine should not be given until the second year of life to avoid interference from maternally-transmitted antibodies. There should be an interval of at least 3 weeks before the last dose of oral poliomyelitis vaccine and immunisation against measles. Such an interval is recommended between the administration of any 2 vaccines containing live organisms.

Reactions and contra-indications to immunisation

Minor reactions to immunisation are common but are usually mild. Parents are best advised to anticipate them in advance. Such reactions include irritability or a low grade fever in the evening following immunisation. Redness and swelling may develop at the site of injection but this usually subsides within 48 hours. No treatment is usually

Table 4.3 Immunisation schedule for infancy and childhood (based on the recommendations of the Joint Committee on Vaccination and Immunisation — revised 1978)

Age	Interval between injections	Immunisation against
At birth		Tuberculosis with BCG vaccine to children at risk.
3 months		Diphtheria, tetanus and pertussis (triple vaccine). Poliomyelitis
4.5–5 months	6–8 weeks after first dose	Diphtheria, tetanus and pertussis. Poliomyelitis
8.5–11 months	4–6 months after the second dose	Diphtheria, tetanus and pertussis. Poliomyelitis
12–15 months	At least 3 weeks after third dose of polio	Measles
School entry (5 years)	At least 3 years after completion of basic course	Diphtheria and tetanus Poliomyelitis
10–13 years (girls only)	There should be an interval of at least 3 weeks between these	Tuberculosis (with BCG vaccine)
11–13 years (if tuberculin-negative).		Rubella
School leaving (15–19 years)		Tetanus Poliomyelitis

Vaccination against smallpox is not now part of the normal routine immunisation programme required but a mild analgesic such as paracetamol may make the baby less irritable. Serious reactions such as persistent screaming, signs of cerebral irritation and convulsions are very rare but present in the first 24 hours. Their incidence is probably less than one for every 300 000 injections.

Sometimes an injection of triple vaccine will produce a firm subcutaneous nodule that may persist for some weeks. Parents can be reassured that it is harmless and will disappear in due course.

Contra-indications to immunisation include a severe general or local reaction to a previous dose of vaccine. No vaccine should be given to a child who is ill or febrile, and a previous history of seizures, convulsions or cerebral irritation in the neonatal period are contra-indications to some vaccines and to pertussis vaccine in particular. Live vaccines should be avoided in those with hypogammaglobulinaemia, reticuloendothelial system disease or those taking corticosteroid or immunosuppressive drugs. Further contra-indications against immunisation for specific diseases are considered under the appropriate individual headings.

Diphtheria

Mass immunisation against diphtheria was introduced in 1940 and since then the notifications of this disease in England and Wales has rapidly declined. In 1940 there were 50 000 notifications; in 1950 there were less than 1000 cases and in 1960, 48. In 1979 no cases were notified.

Although this disease is now rare in the UK it persists in other countries. Diphtheria toxoid rarely causes reactions so that it is reasonable at the present time to include it in the basic immunisation schedule for infants. National immunisation acceptance rates for diphtheria have varied between 70 per cent and 80 per cent and this seems to be high enough to prevent the re-emergence of this infectious disease. However, such acceptance rates must be maintained and the constant encouragement to parents to bring their children for immunisation must continue. Routinely, diphtheria toxoid is given in triple vaccine in three doses during the first year of life.

Diphtheria vaccine contains a toxoid which is adsorbed onto an aluminium salt, phosphate or hydroxide, which acts as an adjuvant and promotes antibody production. Diphtheria toxoid is also a component of triple vaccine (together with pertussis and tetanus toxoid), and the pertussis component of this preparation also has adjuvant properties.

The first vaccination is given when the infant is aged about 3 months, the second 6–8 weeks later and the third 4–6 months after the second dose.

Diphtheria toxoid can cause a severe reaction in the person who has been previously immunised so that it must not be given routinely to older children or adults. If a reinforcing dose is contemplated or if a primary course of immunisation is considered neccessary after the age of 10 years, then the patient must undergo a Schick test.

The Schick test is a skin test in which 0.2 ml of diphtheria toxin is injected intradermally. A positive result develops in the non-immune subject, the site of the injection becomes swollen and inflamed within 2 days and this may persist for a couple of weeks. Such a person is susceptible to infection and should be immunised against diphtheria. If no such response develops, a negative result, then the subject has adequate circulating antitoxin and would be at risk to a generalised reaction from immunisation with diphtheria toxoid.

Pertussis (whooping cough)

Immunisation against pertussis was introduced nationally, in the UK in 1957. The notification rate for pertussis in the early 1950s was around 160 000 per year; by 1962 this had fallen to less than 10 000 and until 1976 was rarely above 20 000 cases per year.

In the 1970s neurological complications after immunisation were reported with varying frequency, but no reliable estimate of the incidence of these was possible. The Joint Committee on Vaccination and Immunisation reviewed these reports and concluded that the risk of severe complications from immunisation against pertussis was slight and was far outweighed by the advantages of immunisation. The controversy engendered by the reports of neurological complications resulted in a marked fall in national acceptance rates for pertussis vaccine. This fell from between 70 and 80 per cent in the years 1965/74 to 30 per cent in 1978. In consequence, in 1977/79 there was the largest outbreak of whooping cough since the 1950s, and in 1978 over 60 000 cases were notified. There was an even bigger outbreak in 1982/3.

Whooping cough is an unpleasant disease and, especially in infancy, it is associated with serious complications. Immunisation against it must be encouraged and the previous high acceptance rates must be sought.

Whooping cough vaccine contains killed organisms of *Bordetella pertussis* and it is usually given in the first year of life, together with diphtheria and tetanus toxoids, as part of the triple vaccine.

Pertussis vaccine is contra-indicated in babies with a previous history of fits or evidence of abnormality in the central nervous system. Neonatal asphyxia or hypoglycaemia are also contra-indications to this vaccine. It should not be given to children with a close family history of epilepsy.

If a previous dose of the vaccine is associated with convulsions or with a severe local reaction, a further dose should not be given and the immunisation programme should be completed with a mixture of diphtheria and tetanus toxoids only. A history of allergy or asthma in a child or the members of his family is not a contra-indication to pertussis vaccination.

Tetanus

This disease was not made notifiable in the UK until 1968; immunisation against it was not introduced into the routine childhood immunisation schedule until the early 1960s. Although rare in the UK its case fatality rate is about 20 per cent. The vaccine is effective and safe.

Tetanus is much more common in rural tropical Africa, Asia and South America where 30 per cent of cases arise in the newborn from contamination of the umbilical stump. These deaths are preventable by immunising mothers.

Deaths from tetanus in the UK, fell from 18 in 1960 to 2 in 1978; in the 5-year period 1969/73 there were 107 notifications, and in the 5-year period 1974/78 there were 86. In children under 15 years there were 22 notifications for the years 1969/73 and only 5 for the years 1974/78; immunisation probably accounts for this fall.

The basic course of immunisation against tetanus consists of three injections with an interval of 6–8 weeks between the first and second, and 4–6 months between the second and third. This course is best given in the first year of life. A reinforcing dose is administered at school entry and another between 10 and 15 years later.

Tetanus antitoxin acquired by active immunisation persists for a long time and it has been suggested that the basic immunisation course of infancy, together with a dose at school entry, may give adequate levels, the reinforcing dose at school leaving may be unnecessary. However, if a person who has been previously immunised is in any danger of tetanus, then the circulating levels of antibody can be quickly raised by a further dose of toxoid as the need arises.

Tetanus toxoid can be given plain or with an aluminium adjuvant. It is contained in triple vaccine and also in some preparations that contain typhoid and paratyphoid inactivated organisms.

Triple Vaccine

Triple vaccine is the preparation that most babies are given as part of their basic immunisation programme in the first year of life. It contains purified tetanus toxoid, purified diphtheria toxoid and killed whole *Bordetella pertussis* organisms. Aluminium hydroxide may be present as an adjuvant. Its use is not recommended after the age of 5 years; only preparations containing diphtheria and tetanus toxoids should be used, since pertussis is rarely a problem in older children.

Triple vaccine is usually administered in a dose of 0.5 ml given by deep subcutaneous or intramuscular injection into the deltoid muscle. Contra-indications to triple vaccine are those for any preparation containing pertussis organisms. Any child who has had a severe local or general reaction to triple vaccine should continue his immunisation programme with a preparation that contains diphtheria and tetanus toxoid only. Severe reactions to the vaccine should be reported to the Committee on the Safety of Medicines at Market

Towers, 1 Nine Elms Lane, London, SW8 5NQ.

Poliomyelitis

Immunisation has contributed markedly to the decreasing incidence of this disabling condition. In 1947 there were over 7000 notifications of paralytic poliomyelitis in England and Wales; in 1955 there were almost 4000 notifications and in 1960 there were 257. In 1979, six cases were reported and only two of these had been infected in the UK.

Immunisation by injection with the inactivated Salk vaccine was begun in England and Wales in 1956, and in 1962 this was replaced for routine use by the live, attenuated Sabin vaccine which is administered orally. This mode of administration has an advantage in that it avoids an injection and is more acceptable to children. Oral administration also allows the attenuated virus to become established in the intestine so that local resistance to infection with poliovirus with IgA antibodies is possible at this site as well as by the induction of blood-borne (IgM and IgG) antibodies.

Sabin vaccine contains live polioviruses of types 1, 2 and 3 which have been cultured in monkey kidney tissue and attenuated by formaldehyde.

Poliomyelitis oral vaccine is best administered as part of the basic immunisation programme of infancy. The dose is three drops, and three doses are given with 6–8 weeks between the first and second doses and 4–6 months between the second and third. A booster dose should be given at school entry and a further reinforcing dose between 15 and 19 years of age. Reinforcing doses are not necessary for adults, although the occurrence of a single case of paralytic polio is an indication for oral poliomyelitis vaccine to be given to all persons in the area, regardless of their immunisation status. The Joint Committee on Vaccination and Immunisation also recommends that whenever infants are given oral poliomyelitis vaccine, it should also be administered to their parents if they are unimmunised. It must be remembered, however, that this vaccine contains live organisms and it should not be given to mothers in the first 4 months of pregnancy.

Poliomyelitis vaccine should not be given to those who have received another live vaccine within the previous 3 weeks. It should be avoided in those who are generally ill and especially those with diarrhoea or chronic bowel disease.

Poliomyelitis is still endemic in many countries and it is occasionally imported into the UK from abroad. For this reason, high levels of immunisation of infants must be maintained. Also, travellers to endemic areas should be immunised prior to their proposed visits. Many are aware of the risks of typhoid, malaria and cholera, but few consider protection against this crippling disease. They should therefore be offered poliomyelitis vaccine when attending for pre-travel immunisation against these other infectious diseases.

Poliomyelitis vaccine should be stored at 4°C. Opened containers should be discarded after use as, once opened, the vaccine may lose its potency however it is stored.

Measles

Measles is often mistakenly considered to be a mild disorder. However, potentially serious complications such as encephalitis, can occur. Immunisation against this condition is therefore still worthwhile.

Measles was made notifiable in England and Wales in 1940 and its prevalence has had a biennial pattern of peaks and troughs. In 1961 almost 800 000 cases were notified in England and Wales. The national immunisation programme began in 1968 and the expected epidemic in 1969 did not occur. Notification rates for the 9 years following the introduction of immunisation was 60 per cent less than those for the previous 9 year period, and in 1979, less than 80 000 cases were notified. However, vaccination rates have always been low, about 50 per cent, and a biennial pattern of measles notification has re-emerged, although at a lower level than previously. Vaccination rates of 80–90 per cent are probably necessary to eliminate this disease.

Immunisation against measles is especially recommended for those who are malnourished or who suffer from chronic conditions such as congenital heart disease or cystic fibrosis. Those living in residential accommodation should also be immunised against measles. Possible reactions to the vaccine can be modified by giving human gamma globulin, at the same time as the vaccine, into the opposite arm.

Measles vaccine is a freeze-dried preparation containing attenuated virus. It is reconstituted immediately before use and given by subcutaneous or intramuscular injection into the triceps or deltoid muscle. It is best given in the second year of life and should not be administered to children below the age of 9 months since the presence of maternally-transmitted antibodies results in a poor antibody response in this age group. The vaccine should not be administered within 3 weeks of another vaccine containing live organisms.

Measles vaccines may occasionally cause a febrile reaction and transient rashes between 5 and 10 days after administration. It is contra-indicated in children with leukaemia, Hodgkin's disease, hypogammaglobulinaemia and those on cortico-steroid or immunosuppressive therapy.

There is no upper age limit for measles vaccination.

Rubella

Rubella contracted in the first trimester of pregnancy may result in the birth of a baby severely affected with congenital defects. Thus, although rubella in itself is a mild infectious disease in which serious complications are rare, there is a need to protect pregnant women from contracting this infection. The best way of doing this is by ensuring that they begin pregnancy immune to it. Active immunisation against rubella makes this possible.

Rubella vaccine is a freeze-dried preparation containing attenuated live virus. It must be reconstituted with diluent immediately before use and is given by subcutaneous injection into the deltoid muscle.

The vaccine is offered to all girls from the age of 10 years irrespective of whether they report previous infection with rubella since this disease is very difficult to diagnose clinically. The vaccine can also be offered to any woman of child-bearing age who requests it and whose blood contains no antibodies against rubella virus. However, such a woman should avoid pregnancy for at least 2 months after immunisation. The

determination of rubella antibody status is now part of routine antenatal care so that seronegative women can be offered the vaccine early in the postpartum period. Certain groups of women are at particular risk of contracting rubella and their rubella antibody status should be determined and the vaccine offered to those who are seronegative. These groups include school teachers, nurses and doctors.

Mild reactions may follow immunisation with rubella virus, symptoms include a slight fever and sore throat together with lymphadenopathy, rashes or mild arthralgia.

Rubella virus must not be given to anybody who is pregnant and should be avoided in those who have been immunised with a vaccine containing live organisms within the preceeding 3 weeks.

Tuberculosis

The notification of tuberculosis began in 1913 when over 117 000 notifications were made and almost 50 000 deaths were reported. Improved living standards resulted in a considerable decrease in these figures. By 1950 there were about 50 000 notifications per year and 16 000 deaths. Effective chemotherapy was then developed and introduced in the 1950s as was mass miniature radiography and BCG vaccination. By 1960, the annual notification rate was less than 24 000 per year and less than 3500 deaths had been reported; in 1978 notifications had fallen to less than 10 000 a year, and deaths to less than 1000.

The role of mass BCG vaccination in the declining incidence of this infectious disease is not clear. A marked decline in notification and deaths had occurred prior to its institution. Nevertheless, the routine BCG vaccination of all children should continue until the infectious pool of sputum-smear positive pulmonary tuberculosis has been greatly reduced. Tuberculosis has a much higher incidence in immigrants of Asian origin in whom non-pulmonary forms of the disease are also more likely to occur.

Tuberculosis vaccine contains attenuated, live tubercle bacilli of a bovine strain of *Mycobacterium tuberculosis*. This vaccine was developed by Calmette and Guérin and bears their name, Bacillus Calmette Guérin (BCG). The vaccine is a freeze-dried preparation that must be stored at 4°C and which must be reconstituted at the time of injection. It is administered by the intradermal innoculation of 0.1 ml into the region of the deltoid muscle. Such injection is said to protect against tuberculosis for at least 15 years. About one week after injection a red papule develops and this progresses to a nodule 2–3 weeks later. This may ulcerate and subsequent healing may take up to 6 months. The conversion to a Mantoux positive reaction 3–4 weeks after BCG vaccination indicates that the procedure has been successful; this should occur in all persons who have been so immunised.

This vaccine is administered in the UK to children aged 11–13 years who previously have been shown to be tuberculin negative on Mantoux or Heaf testing. It may also be given to newborn babies who may be at risk of contracting this infection from other members of their family. Children of those immigrant groups in which there is a high incidence of tuberculosis should also be considered for BCG vaccination in the newborn period. The dose for babies is 0.05 ml given intradermally.

PREVENTION OF RARER INFECTIOUS DISEASES

The development of efficient worldwide systems of transportation has meant that all doctors in the UK must be alert to the possibility of what were formerly regarded as rare infectious diseases. Thus, travellers from endemic areas may bring typhoid fever, malaria or cholera into the UK; of the six cases of poliomyelitis notified in 1979, four had acquired infection abroad. These conditions can be prevented by immunisation or by prophylactic chemotherapy thus, travellers who may be at risk must be given the appropriate proper advice before their journeys. They must also be advised on simple hygienic measures that diminish the likelihood of contracting infection overseas.

General measures

The usual sources of many infectious diseases in warm countries are food and water. To be safe, water should be boiled or sterilised chemically before drinking or used to clean teeth. Salads and raw vegetables may have been irrigated with sewage and should be avoided; so, too, should uncooked shellfish, ice-cream, cream and unpasteurised milk. Under-cooked meat, including poultry, fish and the products of street stalls, should not be eaten. Doubts about the reliability of any item of food should lead to its avoidance, or where possible, its sterilisation by boiling.

Immunisation

Immunisation should be recommended to all those travelling to areas where the following diseases are endemic.

Yellow Fever

This disease is endemic in the countries of West, Central and East Africa and in Central and South America. The vaccine contains live attenuated virus and, since it is prepared in chick embryos, it should not be given to people who are allergic to eggs.

Immunisation against yellow fever is only possible at one of the yellow fever vaccination centres in the UK. A single injection confers immunity for a prolonged period and re-immunisation is not recommended before 10 years. The vaccine should not be given to children under 9 months of age and should be administered first in any vaccination programme. As it is a live vaccine it should preceed smallpox vaccination by at least 3 weeks. The vaccine is contra-indicated in pregnant women.

Many countries require travellers from areas in which yellow fever is endemic to have a valid certificate of vaccination against this disease.

Smallpox

The World Health Organisation has declared the world free from smallpox and only four countries now require international certificates of vaccination for this disease.

Formerly, vaccination against smallpox was undertaken using vaccinia virus, a virus closely related to the smallpox virus (variola). Modern vaccines are extremely potent and must be used and disposed of carefully to avoid cross-infection. For this reason, on those rare occasions when vaccination against smallpox is necessary, it is best undertaken at a vaccination centre at which staff are used to working with this highly infectious preparation.

Smallpox vaccine is introduced intradermally using a multiple puncture or scratch technique on the skin overlying the deltoid muscle. Such immunisation is contra-indicated in those who are pregnant, those with disease of the reticuloendothelial system or those who are on treatment with corticosteroids or immunosuppressive drugs. Eczema, either in the patient or a close member of his family, is an outright contra-indication because of the serious risk of the development of a potentially fatal generalised vaccinia infection.

International certificates of vaccination against smallpox are valid for 3 years. Such vaccination is now no longer part of the basic immunisation programme of infancy.

Typhoid fever

Typhoid vaccine contains bacilli of *Salmonella typhi* that have been killed by heat.

A course of immunisation comprises two injections with between 4 and 6 weeks between each one. Reinforcing doses are given when required at intervals of 3 years. Subcutaneous injections may be associated with a generalised reaction which occurs within a few hours and which produces a fever, headache, malaise and nausea. The incidence of such reactions can be diminished by using the intradermal route. However, the first dose

requires a larger volume and should always be given subcutaneously. The intradermal route can then be used for second and reinforcing doses. The dosage schedule for typhoid vaccine is shown in Table 4.4.

Typhoid vaccine should not be given to children under the age of 12 months.

Cholera

Cholera vaccine contains killed organisms of *Vibrio cholerae*. The dosage schedule for cholera immunisation is shown in Table 4.5. For primary vaccination two doses of vaccine must be given subcutaneously or intramuscularly with a period of at least 4 weeks between each injection. First doses must always be given by the subcutaneous or intramuscular route but subsequent doses can be given intradermally.

Immunity from cholera vaccination is short-lived and booster doses when required must be given every 6 months. Some countries still require international certificates of vaccination against cholera from travellers from endemic areas.

Table 4.5 Schedule for immunisation against cholera

Age (years)	First dose (ml)	Subsequent doses (ml)	
	Subcutaneous or intramuscular	Subcutaneous or intramuscular	Intradermal
1–5	0.1	0.3	0.1
5–10	0.3	0.5	0.1
10 and over	0.5	1.0	0.2

Poliomyelitis

(See above).

Rabies

Rabies may develop after a bite or lick from a rabid animal. A person who is suspected of having acquired such an infection is treated with human rabies immunoglobulin (passive immunisation) as soon as possible after the infecting episode, and

Table 4.4 Schedules for immunisation against typhoid fever

Adults and children over 10 years		Children aged 1–10 years	
Subcutaneous	Intradermal	Subcutaneous	Intradermal
1st dose 0.5 ml	—	0.25 ml	—
2nd dose 0.5 ml	0.1 ml	0.25 ml	0.1 ml
Subsequent doses 0.5 ml	0.1 ml	0.25 ml	0.1 ml

concomitantly, a course of anti-rabies vaccine containing killed virus is begun (active immunisation).

Infectious Hepatitis

Infectious hepatitis can be prevented in travellers to endemic areas by passive immunisation using human gamma globulin prepared from pooled donor serum.

PROPHYLACTIC CHEMOTHERAPY

Malaria

In 1979, 1053 cases of malaria were imported into Britain; around 30 per cent had been infected in Africa and 65 per cent in the Indian subcontinent. *Plasmodium vivax* was the commonest species responsible and was usually acquired in the Indian subcontinent. *Plasmodium falciparum*, the species responsible for the potentially fatal malignant malaria, was the next most common and most patients acquired this infection in Africa. In 1979 5 people died in the UK from *Plasmodium falciparum* malaria after visits to endemic areas in Africa.

Two factors are responsible for the dramatic increase in malaria in the UK; these are the greater ease of fast worldwide travel together with the increasing number of New Commonwealth immigrants who now live here. Malaria occurs in those who have travelled or stopped off, even momentarily, in an endemic area and so should be suspected in air crews, businessmen on visits overseas, tourists and children who have been living abroad with their parents.

Although malaria may present in immigrants who have not recently revisited their country of origin, it is more common in those who have made such a trip, for their resistance to endemic malaria may have waned after living in the UK for some years. In 1979, 92 British born children of immigrants acquired infection while visiting their parents' country of origin.

To date, there is no effective vaccine in clinical use for immunising against malaria. Prophylaxis is by chemotherapy and drugs must be taken which destroy the malarial parasites at an early stage in their life cycle. Proguanil, pyrimethamine and chloroquine are effective in this and give reliable protection against malarial infection. These drugs must be taken before entering an endemic area and for at least 6 weeks after leaving it.

Proguanil must be taken daily, the dose for adults and children over the age of 9 years is 100 mg, but this should be doubled in a highly endemic area. The dose for children under one year is 25 mg daily, for those between one and 4 years, 50 mg daily and for those between 5 and 8 years, 75 mg daily. This drug has not been shown to be teratogenic, but in any case, anti-malarial drugs are safer in pregnancy than malaria.

Pyrimethamine must be taken as a weekly dose, 25 mg for adults, 6.25 mg for children up to the age of 5 years and 12.5 mg for children between 5 and 10 years. Chloroquine also is taken weekly, the adult dose is 300 mg.

In some areas, such as Eastern India, Bangladesh, South-East Asia and Central and South America, there may be strains of *Plasmodium* resistant to these drugs. When this is known, alternative preparations which contain two anti-malarials must be used. Examples of these include Fansidar, which contains 25 mg of pyrimethamine and 500 mg sulfadoxin and Maloprim which contains 12.5 mg of pyrimethamine and 100 mg dapsone. Fansidar should not be used during pregnancy.

CARE OF THE NORMAL CHILD

The normal child would normally be seen at least five times during his first year of life for formal preventive procedures, these include three visits for immunisation and two visits for developmental assessment. In his second year he will be seen at least twice, once for measles immunisation and possibly another time for further developmental assessment. He may be seen again once in his third year and once in his fourth year for developmental assessment, but the value of such checks is still a matter for debate. However, there is general agreement that such assessment is essential in the pre-school period and booster doses of diphtheria, tetanus and poliomyelitis vaccine must also be given then. Thus, in his first 5 years, the normal child will be seen at least 10 times for preventive procedures.

The normal child under the age of 5 consults his general practitioner between four and five times a year so that he will be seen by his doctor a further 20 times for episodes of illness that are commonly upper respiratory tract infections, otitis media and infectious fevers. Although the main purpose of these visits will be for the treatment of episodic illness, they also provide opportunities for preventive measures; opportunities to check on immunisation status, to monitor the progress of those who are at physical or social disadvantage or special risk, to offer advice on feeding and accident prevention and to identify and help those mothers who have difficulty in coping.

The progress of babies and small children will also be monitored by health visitors as well as by clinical medical officers and general practitioners. In a baby's first year his contact with his health visitor may be very great indeed, possibly 20 times. Ideally, these three professional advisers should be working closely together so that communication between them is easy and mothers can be given clear, non-conflicting advice.

It must never be forgotten that the care of normal children is best left to their parents. There will be times when parents will need advice and help from doctors and health visitors and they must be helped to recognise when such consultation is appropriate and how and where to seek it. Some will need more help than others in learning how to use the system of care that has evolved; sometimes, the parents of a child who needs our attention most, have the greatest difficulty in obtaining it. For this reason, doctors should be more active in seeking out those who need their attention, rather than waiting passively, as in previous years, for parents to seek their help. This may imply a system of surveillance that threatens to invade the privacy of an individual and his family, yet all that is required is a general practitioner with an up-to-date age/sex register, an enthusiastic health visitor and a belief in the prevention of illness. Nobody need be afraid of that.

FURTHER READING

Department of Health & Social security 1972 Immunisation against infectious disease. HMSO, London

Department of Health & Social Security 1978 Revised schedule on vaccination and immunisation procedures. Circular no CMO(78)15, CNO(78)12, HMSO, London

Dick G, 1978 Immunisation. Update Books, London & New Jersey

The Royal College of General Practitioners 1982 Healther Children — Thinking Prevention Reports from General Practice No 22

The Royal College of General Practitioners 1983 Promoting Prevention Occasional Paper 22

5

Caring for children in general practice

Effective care of illness depends upon an understanding and concern for the physical, emotional and social factors that lead to the development of symptoms. This whole-person approach is essential in looking after all patients, and especially in caring for children.

In the UK, the general practitioner in the National Health Service provides primary care to all the patients registered on his list. This means that he is the doctor of first contact and that his patients can see him on their own initiative without prior referral. He is directly accessible.

The care provided by the general practitioner is constantly available, every hour of every day of every year. Such a service cannot always be provided by the individual doctor himself if he is to have reasonable leisure time. Nevertheless, he is responsible for ensuring that a doctor is available to all his patients when he himself is not working. Usually, a group of doctors will organise a rota to cover each others practice for out of hours work and holidays, or a doctor may arrange for a commercial deputising service to do this. Whatever the arrangements, the individual general practitioner remains responsible for ensuring that his colleagues look after his patients while he himself is absent from his practice.

Another feature of general practitioner care is its continuing nature — a general practitioner may look after patients for periods extending over many years and in this time collects information about their health and way of living which he can apply to their future care. Usually, he looks after more than one member of the same family and he can observe their inter-relationships and how the tensions that may be created between them can lead to illness and even disease.

He is in a position to visit his patients in their own homes, this may help him obtain a clearer understanding of their behaviour by the observations he makes in their environment.

The general practitioner must recognise how emotional and social factors produce illness, for such illnesses present daily in his surgery. He must recognise the common diseases, understand their natural history and when it is appropriate *not* to intervene. He must diagnose as soon as possible those rare and unexpected disorders which untreated, may cause death or handicap yet, when treated promptly can be effectively overcome. As well as the treatment of episodic illness, his work involves such preventive activities as immunisation, screening and health education, and in this he will work closely with others, especially health visitors and clinical medical officers.

UK GENERAL PRACTICE STATISTICS

In the NHS the general practitioner is in contract with a Family Practitioner Committee (FPC) to provide general medical services to the patients registered on his list.

At present, there are over 29 000 general practitioners in the UK and the average number of patients on each practitioner's list is about 2100. Approximately 25 per cent of the population is under 15 years of age so that each general practitioner has about 500 children on his list.

Patients do not seek help for all their childrens' illnesses and about 40 per cent of illness is managed with advice from other members of the family or from the local chemist. Nevertheless, in one year, 3 out of every 4 children below the age of 15 years will see their general practitioner for the treatment of episodic illness, and on average, each will have about four consultations each year with the doctor. In the first year of life a child will be seen about eight times by his doctor, but this includes visits for such preventive measures as immunisation and developmental surveillance. In one year, 90 per cent of all children under the age of 5 see their doctor, the percentage for the whole population is 67 per cent. Socially-deprived families make more than average use of the general practitioner for episodic care, but they make less use of the preventive services.

The British general practitioner will have almost 2000 consultations with children each year, that is, about 40 per week. These will occupy almost one-third of his time. The commonest reasons for children consulting their doctors are shown in Table 5.1. Referral to a hospital outpatient department

Table 5.1 Commonest reasons for children consulting their general practitioner (Court report)

Reason	Percentage
Respiratory diseases including asthma	28
Ill-defined symptoms	13
Infectious diseases	11
Skin diseases	10
Preventive procedures	10
Accidents	10

occurs in less than 5 per cent of consultations with children in general practice and, in group practices, where one or more members of the group has greater experience in paediatrics, hospital referral rates are much lower. Less than 1 per cent of consultations result in referral for hospital admission.

There has been a considerable increase in the number of group practices in recent years (see Table 5.2); the number of single-handed and two-man practices has diminished and subsequently there has been an increase in practices with three or more partners. This, together with an increase in the number of health visitors attached to group practices, has promoted the development of a team approach to the provision of child health care in general practice. This has been especially valuable in developing the provision of preventive services and health education.

THE CONTENT OF CHILD CARE WORK IN GENERAL PRACTICE

Until recently, the work of the general practitioner was concerned solely with the recognition and treatment of episodic illness. This still remains an important activity and, as well as managing the common and often self-limiting diseases, the general practitioner must be able to treat life-threatening or incapacitating disorders such as pneumonia, asthma or otitis media without referral to specialist help. He must always remain sensitive to the diagnosis of the rare and unpredictable, the disease that untreated is fatal, yet for which prompt effective therapy is life-saving, for example, meningococcal meningitis, tuberculosis, diabetes mellitus or malaria.

Advances in knowledge have brought other changes in the general practitioner's work. Now, more than previously, he is concerned with the long-term effects of serious illness, with chronic disease and handicap and with the social and

Table 5.2 Percentage of general practitioners in partnership in England and Wales — 1948–1977

Year	1948	1954	1960	1965	1970	1974	1977
Number unrestricted principals		18 552	19 914	20 014	20 357	21 510	22 100
Percentage							
Single handed	83	38	31	24	21	18	16
2-man partnership		35	34	32	25	21	20
3-man partnership		16	21	24	26	25	24
4-man partnership		7	9	12	16	18	19
5-man partnership		3	3	5	7	10	11
6-man or more		1	2	3	5	8	10

emotional problems that are often associated with these conditions.

General practitioners are now more involved in the prevention of disease and many now provide immunisation and developmental surveillance services to their patients.

The practitioner is in a unique position, for he cares not only for children, but also for the families with whom they live, the mother, father and siblings and, sometimes, the grandparents, nannies and au pairs. He has knowledge of the social and emotional pressures that exist in such a unit and can assess the degree of stress and disadvantage to which its members are subjected. This enables him to predict those at risk to certain medical and behavioural disorders. Thus, in immigrant groups of Asian origin, there is a higher incidence of rickets and tuberculosis than in the indigenous population. The socially disadvantaged and emotionally stressed have a higher incidence of cot death and child abuse. A recognition of these groups enables the general practitioner to provide care and to direct practical help to those whose need is greatest.

A common way for family stress to present is by the repeated attendance at the general practitioner's surgery of a child whose parent describes a variety of symptoms. On examination, such a child will show no signs of disease for often he is the presentation of illness and stress within the mother or other members of the family. Prescription for him is unnecessary, for this will not relieve the underlying difficulty and tends to divert attention away from those who are in most need of help.

The content of the general practitioner's work with children can be considered best under the following headings:

1. Preventive services
2. Recognition and treatment of episodic illness
3. Management of chronic disease and handicap
4. Recognition and care for at risk groups.

1. Preventive Services

The prevention of illness in childhood has been described in detail in Chapter 4, and this aspect of child care forms an increasing proportion of the general practitioner's work. One-fifth of doctors organise their own child health clinics in which they undertake developmental and preventive surveillance; many more provide for immunisation against infectious diseases. Close liaison with health visitors improves the quality of this work and the attachment of health visitors to practices facilitates communication with them.

Ideally, the formal preventive services necessary in early childhood should be provided by the general practitioner and the health visitor who works closely with him. In practices where this is not possible, mothers must take their children to a health authority clinic, and this sometimes causes confusion amongst many parents who are not clear about the role of such clinics in relation to the general practitioner. Often they may consult the general practitioner and clinic doctor about the same problem and sometimes they are given conflicting advice. Where the preventive child care services are provided outside the practice, the general practitioner must ensure effective communication with clinical medical officers. Perhaps the best way for the general practitioner to arrange this is for him to invite clinical medical officers into his practice so that they can do their work from his premises.

The general practitioner's work in preventing ill health must not be limited solely to such formal preventive occasions as immunisation and well-baby clinics. Every contact with a patient provides the opportunity for education towards a healthier life. Thus, the prompt effective treatment of otitis media may prevent deafness from glue ear or chronic suppurative otitis media; the recognition of carious teeth during an ENT examination may prevent serious dental disease in later life; the identification of ill-fitting shoes may prevent irreversible deformity in the future; and in an age when one-half of all boys and one-third of all girls smoke cigarettes by the age of 17, auscultation of the chest may provide an opportunity to explore this problem.

The general practitioner must recognise that there are groups of patients who are more at risk to illness than others. These include the small-for-dates babies, children with feuding or mentally-ill parents, overcrowded families and the homeless, all of whom are more at risk to physical and emotional illness. They deserve more of the doctor's attention than they sometimes get, for often those most in need of medical care are the people who are most reluctant to seek it. It is these patients that the general practitioner and the health visitor must actively seek out in order to demonstrate the help they can offer.

Health education is another of the general practitioner's most important tasks, it can be undertaken on every occasion he meets a patient and need not be limited to formal preventive sessions. He can promote children's health in the antenatal months by advising the pregnant mother on diet, and the avoidance of unnecessary medication, alcohol and cigarette smoking. At this stage, he should promote breast feeding and will continue to advise on infant feeding and child nutrition in the pre-school years. Advice on immunisation will follow, as will opportunities to discuss accident prevention.

2. Recognition and treatment of episodic illness

Detecting the cause of a patient's symptoms and recommending appropriate therapy has been the doctor's function for centuries; it is the basis of most of our medical education. The prevention of illness is a much more recent, but no less important, responsibility.

The general practitioner as doctor of first contact is presented with symptoms at an undifferentiated and disorganised stage and his skill is using the information he collects to understand why his patient has come, or has been brought, to see him. The general practitioner does not limit his work to special types of disease or areas of the body; any problem is relevant to him. Daily, he faces social problems arising from factors such as poverty or inadequate housing; emotional problems from marital disharmony or stress at work and physical problems from infection or injury. All these problems may be present in the same patient at one time; the doctor's task is to determine the best form of help which he often must do before making a formal diagnosis.

Skill in the art of the consultation is essential if the doctor is to answer the fundamental questions: why does this patient need to see me, and why now? And in finding answers to these, more questions frequently arise — is the symptom presented really the problem in this patient's life or are there other difficulties which he himself has not even recognised? Is this the patient that really needs my help or are his symptoms a presentation of someone else's problem? Hence, the crying or sleepless baby is often a presenting sign of a depressed mother; the child with a behaviour problem is often an indicator of sickness elsewhere in the family.

Medical education is based on the traditional diagnosis and treatment of physical disease. The good general practitioner must be skilled in this; he must be able to cope with common diseases as well as recognise at an early stage those that are life-threatening. However, he must also be aware of how much social and physical factors contribute to ill health and as well as treating disease he must be skilled in helping his patient or parents to see how they can cope with their own difficulties.

A large proportion of physical illness seen by the general practitioner is not life-threatening but is self-limiting without treatment. He must educate patients and parents to recognise and manage these conditions for themselves. Caring for children demands a team approach, and there are no more important members of that team than a child's parents. The general practitioner must teach them how to recognise and manage minor illness and to determine when their child's condition requires his help. This is particularly important for minor symptoms that are potentially life-threatening and parents should be taught the significance of symptoms such as lethargy, and diarrhoea and vomiting in early infancy.

Infections of the respiratory tract account for almost one-third of the episodic illness in children seen by the general practitioner and such episodes are particularly common in infancy and in the first 2 years at school. Over one-half of children under the age of 5 years consult their doctors for respiratory illness in one year, and one-third of those aged from 5–15 years will see him for the same reason. About 15 per cent of children from birth to 5 years are seen in one year with acute otitis media and around 20 per cent of children in this age group are seen with specific infectious disease; 10 per cent of children under the age of 5 are seen in one year with diarrhoea and vomiting.

Emotional problems in children also form a moderate proportion of the general practitioner's work. Although less than 5 per cent of contacts with children are with behaviour disorders, about one-quarter of children seen with physical symptoms also have emotional difficulties. The recognition of children with emotional problems is an important part of the general practitioner's work — often they present with physical symptoms such as abdominal pain, vomiting, recurrent headache or limb pains. The practitioner is in an ideal position to care for these patients, for his relationship with them and their families is a continuing one and he will have first-hand knowledge of their home environment, the medical history of the members of the family and often the inter-personal stresses that exist in that family. By acquiring an understanding of these inter-personal dynamics and by counselling the members of the family in such a way that each member can see for himself how his behaviour affects that of the others, it is often possible to help parents understand the origins of their children's difficulties and, how, by modifying their own behaviour, they can help him. This can take a considerable time but in general practice it should be possible for a child or his parents to be seen together or alone for short periods and at frequent intervals.

Providing primary care for episodic illness in children requires a service that is readily accessible and constantly available. Serious illness in childhood can present suddenly and medical help is then required as soon as possible. The general practitioner is responsible for providing care for his patients for 24 hours a day; his practice organisation must ensure that children with serious illness can be seen promptly at any time of the day. In particular, appointments systems should be arranged so that emergency consultations with children can be fitted in and arrangements for out-of-hours work should be organised so that prompt attention is readily available when required.

Doctors must educate parents to recognise when their children are seriously ill and must encourage them to seek help when this arises. The general practitioner's staff must be sympathetic to the anxieties and needs of parents seeking medical help for their children.

3. Management of chronic disease and handicap

Any disability that adversely affects normal growth, development and learning ability can be classified as a handicap. Severe handicapping conditions may be physical and include blindness, cardiac abnormalities, deafness and neurological disorders such as spina bifida and cerebral palsy. Psychological causes of severe handicap include mental retardation (the commonest cause of which is Down' syndrome), educational backwardness and psychiatric disorders such as autism. About one-quarter of handicapped children have more than one handicap. Social disadvantage may also inhibit a child's normal growth and development and should also be considered a handicapping condition.

The prevalence of severe handicap in the UK is around 3 per cent, which means that each general practitioner has between 10 and 15 severely handicapped children on his list. However, lesser degrees of handicap are more common and must not be overlooked if a child's needs are to be fully met. These conditions include epilepsy, asthma, visual impairment, hearing loss and dyslexia; they may be present in a further 10–15 per cent of children on a doctor's list.

Care of the handicapped child requires a team approach; specialist medical help from general and specialist paediatricians is invariably needed together with skilled help from nursing staff and treatment from physiotherapists, occupational therapists, speech therapists, audiologists, social workers and teachers. Difficulties can arise in limiting the number dealing with any one family and it is important that effective communication is maintained between all those involved. The general practitioner's role is to ensure that his handicapped patients and their families acquire all the help possible from these agencies. Caring for a handicapped child inevitably produces stress on the other members of the family; marital disharmony and parental separation are more common in these families as is the incidence of behaviour disorders in brothers and sisters.

Parents must be kept fully informed about their child's disability and must be closely involved with any future planning. They must be helped to come to terms with their own feelings about their child's disability, their grief for the normal child they hoped they would have, their feelings of shame, guilt, anger and resentment. As soon as possible they must be given a clear explanation about the causes of their child's condition and the risks of recurrence in a future pregnancy. They must be given guidance as to whom they can turn should problems arise. Ideally, such a child is best cared for at home, but there will be occasions when more help than usual is required to ease the domestic burden. On such occasions, admission to hospital may be necessary or the aid of voluntary societies can be sought to provide holidays. Family financial resources are also inevitably stretched in looking after a handicapped child. An attendance allowance is paid by the DHSS to a parent who is committed to the full-time care of such a child and social services departments and voluntary societies such as The Spastics Society or the Family Fund of The Joseph Rowntree Memorial Trust can sometimes provide financial aid.

In caring for the handicapped child, the general practitioner is in an ideal position to monitor the progress of the other members of the family and to help those who seem to be under the most stress. Too often such families are reticent in seeking help; having recognised their need, it is the doctor's duty to offer practical support without being asked.

The prevention of handicap is possible by avoiding the birth of handicapped children. Improved diagnostic methods enable handicapping conditions to be diagnosed early in pregnancy when termination is possible. Such diagnostic procedures include amniocentesis and cytological examination of fetal cells for Down's syndrome, and alphaftoprotein estimation in blood and amniotic fluid for spina bifida. The rubella immunisation programme aims to protect all mothers against this infectious disease before they become pregnant and thereby to diminish the risk of the rubella syndrome. Genetic counselling helps decrease the incidence of certain inherited handicapping disorders.

Improvements in intrapartum care and, in particular the recognition of birth asphyxia, will also do much to reduce handicap rates by decreasing the occurrence of brain damage and mental retardation.

After birth, the prompt recognition and effective management of some disorders also prevents the developement of future handicap: thus, the early recognition and treatment of congenital dislocation of the hip will prevent permanent damage of the hip; the recognition and management of squint prevents the development of amblyopia. Acquired disease can also cause permanent handicap, prompt recognition and management will prevent this; effective treatment of otitis media will prevent the development of chronic middle ear disease and deafness.

4. Recognition and care of at risk groups

a. Those at social disadvantage

The term social disadvantage implies that the living circumstances of some children handicap their growth and development. Some children are able to overcome such disadvantage and to develop normally; others fall short of the level of performance that, given ideal living conditions, they might have achieved.

Children at social disadvantage include those from poor, dirty, overcrowded homes with minimal facilities; those who are neglected or ignored by their parents; those who are discriminated against because of their race, colour or religion; and the children of sick or feuding parents. Adverse social environments hinder physical, emotional and intellectual growth, and such children are more likely to suffer from severe physical disease, psychiatric illness, behaviour disorders and educational failure. As they grow

Table 5.3 Registrar general's classification of social class

I	Professional occupations (such as doctors and lawyers)
II	Intermediate occupations (such as teachers and managers)
III N	Non-manual skilled occupations (such as clerks and shop-assistants)
III M	Manual skilled occupations (such as brick-layers and coal-miners)
IV	Partly skilled occupations (such as bus drivers, conductors and postmen)
V	Unskilled occupations (such as porters and labourers)
Other	Includes those who are unemployed

Table 5.4 Perinatal mortality rate for England and Wales related to social class for the years 1950 & 1977

Social class	1950	1977
All classes combined	33.4	16.2
I	25.4	11.6
II	30.4	13.0
III N	33.6	14.1
III M	33.6	17.1
IV	36.9	18.8
V	40.4	22.0
Other		

older, these children are more likely to progress to unemployment and possibly even to delinquency. Conditions such as dental disease, respiratory infections and diarrhoea are more frequent and often more severe in children from disadvantaged groups; accidents are also more common in these families. Perinatal and infant mortality rates are greater in social class V compared with other groups, and this has been the case for many years.

Table 5.3 shows the Register General's classification for social class. Table 5.4 shows the use of this table in comparing perinatal mortality rates for England and Wales in the years 1950 and 1977.

Table 5.5 Infant mortality rate in England and Wales related to social class 1977

Social class	Infant mortality rate
All classes	12.8
I	9.0
II	10.5
III N	10.8
III M	12.5
IV	15.2
V	19.6
Other	24.3

The perinatal mortality rate for class V patients in 1977 was equivalent to that for social class I patients in the early 1950s. Table 5.5 shows that the infant mortality rate for class V patients in 1977 was more than twice that for those in class I.

Provision for these children requires greater attention from national government and local authorities. Doctors must continue to inform these agencies of the effects of social disadvantage on children's health. This was recognised by the report of the Committee on Child Health Services (Court Report) who reported to the Secretary of State for Social Services in 1976 as follows: 'Children's growth and their experience of illness and health are profoundly influenced by the social circumstances in which they live. Economic prosperity, a sufficient family income, adequate food, satisfactory housing, a widening education and a safe environment are still the foundation of good health in childhood and of services designed to maintain it.' There can be little doubt that general improvement in the standard of living for those who are presently at social disadvantage will do much to improve the health and development of their children. Satisfactory incomes, more adequate food and dry, warm, less crowded housing, will contribute as much to this, if not more, than the efforts of those who provide medical services.

At a personal level, the general practitioner must identify those children on his list who are at risk because of social disadvantage because it is to them that he and the health visitor must direct most of their preventive work. Those in the poorer groups make least use of the preventive medical services that are offered. Table 5.6 shows the percentage of married women in each occupational class in Scotland who 'booked at the antenatal clinic after 20 weeks' gestation. The percentage booking late in

Table 5.6 Percentage of married women in each class making an antenatal booking after more than 20 weeks gestation, Scotland (1973)

Social class	Percentage
I	27.0
II	29.8
III	30.6
IV	35.3
V	40.5

social class V is considerably higher than in social class I. Children from the poorer groups are less likely to be brought to developmental assessment clinics or to have been immunised, and should be followed carefully on this account. Their mothers should be given as much help and educational support as possible in infant feeding and child care and they must be actively encouraged to take their sick children to the doctor.

b. Stressed Families

(i) *Child Abuse. (See also Chapter 6)* Child abuse is the deliberate infliction of harm onto a child which results in physical or emotional injury; such harm may be caused by deliberate wilful act or by neglect and deprivation.

Non-accidental injury is the physical form of child abuse and is caused by beating, burning or poisoning. The incidence of such violence is unknown, but it has been estimated to be 5000 children a year in England; a general practitioner could see one such child every 5–8 years. Almost 10 per cent of battered children die, and a further 10 per cent are left with residual brain damage.

Severely ill-treated children are rare, but general practitioners must remain aware of those who have been less severely ill-used for these children are indicators of stressed families who need help from social and medical services. Most parents become angry with their babies at some time and those additionally stressed by other factors such as poverty, marital disharmony, poor housing or illness are more likely to react in a physically violent way.

Parents who ill-use their children are likely to be unhappy, aggressive, young and socially isolated; they are more likely to have been injured by their parents in their own childhood. They fail to cooperate with helping agencies, including doctors, and miss appointments with the antenatal clinic, well-baby clinic and immunisation sessions. Paradoxically, they may frequently attend surgery sessions, often at awkward times, and may make seemingly unreasonable demands on out-of-hours services. For this reason, they are sometimes regarded as nuisances, and their frequent attendances ,which are probably cries for help, are at risk of passing unheeded. In one-third of cases, the

biological father does not live at home, and in many, the mothers are living with another man.

The clinical features that should arouse a suspicion of child abuse are discussed in Chapter 6.

The general practitioner's role is to prevent child abuse where possible, by recognising the families at stress and by providing emotional support and practical help to diminish this. He will work closely with health visitors and social workers in doing this. Such help may involve rehousing, the provision of social security supplementary benefits and finding places in day nurseries. In some circumstances, it may be necessary to take the child into the care of the local authority, with his parents' consent. Once serious abuse is suspected, then the chid must be taken to a place of safety as soon as possible. At the time of an acute episode, this is most likely to be to the children's ward of the local hospital, thereafter a case conference will be called involving the general practitioner, health visitor and social worker and sometimes a paediatrician and the police. The local authority social worker may arrange for the child to be taken into care and may seek a compulsory order to do this from the local Juvenile Magistrate's Court.

Dealing with child abuse can be very distressing and arouses passionate feelings in those caring for the family. The general practitioner must, whenever possible, maintain contact with the child's parents, help them understand their own feelings and how the child's injury has occurred. His attitude must be non-condemnatory and his efforts must be directed towards helping the parents plan for the future.

(ii) *Cot Deaths.* There are few conditions encountered in general practice that are as stressful to the doctor as sudden death in infancy; for besides helping the bereaved parents, the doctor invariably has to cope with his own emotional reactions to this event. This can be especially difficult if he saw the baby a few days before death and if he feels that appropriate action by him could have saved the child. For then he will have to deal with his own feelings of guilt as well as the anger and blame, real or imagined, of the bereaved parents. He will do well if he can recognise these feelings in himself and understand their origin, for this may then allow him to offer the practical and emotional help that parents sometimes fail to receive.

Cot deaths can occur within a few days of birth and at any time up to the age of 2 years; however, most are between the age of 2 and 4 months. In early childhood, they are the largest single cause of death. The chance of a normal baby being a cot death in the UK is about one in 500. About 2000 babies die in the UK every year for no apparent cause. This means that each general practitioner will encounter this problem about once every 15 years, 2 or 3 times in his professional lifetime.

Whilst some of these babies have been well when put to bed, recent work has shown that many had a variety of symptoms before death. In some, the significance of these was not appreciated by the parents. Obvious symptoms such as skin rashes, vomiting and diarrhoea, coughing and shortness of breath, often lead parents to seek medical advice. Many are unlikely to recognise the significance of their child becoming quiet and drowsy, and this may have serious consequences.

Postmortem findings usually fall into three groups: there is a group of children in whom postmortem examination reveals serious disease such as pneumonia or gastroenteritis leading to hypernatraemia. There is a second group in which there are signs of a disorder such as tracheobronchitis which is not usually a cause of death, and a third group in which there is minimal evidence of disease. In 10 per cent of cot deaths postmortem findings are entirely negative.

Various hypotheses have been proposed as causes of sudden infant death and it seems likely that there is no single cause for this event. Such hypotheses include silent anaphylactic reactions and mininal brain damage disturbing the control of breathing and the action of the heart, leading to prolonged periods of apnoea. Avoidable factors leading to sudden infant death are present in about one-quarter of cases. Over two-thirds of those have been attributed to parental failure and in one-fifth, avoidable factors could be attributed to the general practitioner.

Some babies are at increased risk of cot death. These include the second twin where the first was previously a cot death and babies born into a family in which there has already been a sudden infant death. Preterm babies, particularly if they are drowsy in the first few months of life, also seem to be at increased risk.

Parents' initial reactions to finding their baby unrousable in the cot are usually those of disbelief. There can be no more chilling telephone call than the one from parents who are 'unable to wake the baby up', and no more sickening feeling than the doctor's as he drives to their house. His is the unenviable task of telling parents that their child is dead, for until then, they are likely to deny that this is possible. Their initial reactions will be of shock, anger (which may be physically expressed) and overwhelming grief. Later feelings include guilt and blame, for themselves, each other, and often the doctor and other medical agencies. They will blame themselves for not recognising that their baby might have been ill and may feel that others see them as unworthy parents. The medical profession's inability to provide a concrete cause of death often exacerbates the feelings of bewilderment they may have.

The general practitioner must make himself available to such bereaved parents and to the other members of the family; perhaps the greatest mistake he can make is to assume that they wish to be alone in their grief. He must be able to answer their many questions, as well as anticipate those that they dare not ask. He must prepare them for the trauma they will encounter in dealing with the coroner, possibly the police, a postmortem examination and an inquest. They will require advice on the procedure for registering the death and for the preparations that will be necessary for the burial. The general practitioner has an important role in listening, understanding and helping the family come to terms with all that has erupted around them. Although not invariably required, medication with tranquillisers or hypnotics may be necessary and sometimes lactation may need to be suppressed.

In the months that follow, the doctor must help the family grieve for their lost child; a process that will stretch his emotions and test his skills to the limit. Nevertheless, he must be able to anticipate the difficulties they will encounter. He must warn them of the dreams they may have about their dead baby and how often they may imagine that they hear their child crying. Their feelings of guilt and blame may persist for a long time, and whilst sharing the grief may bring some families closer together, the recrimination caused by their baby's death may drive some couples apart. Whilst mothers may often be able to talk openly about their feelings, fathers may suppress them; they may need as much help and their needs are more likely to pass unrecognised. Help can be obtained from parents who have experienced similar tragedies, such couples can be contacted through the Foundation for the Study of Infant Deaths.

Many parents fear that future children may die under similar circumstances and need to discuss these fears with their doctor. These parents undoubtedly require extra care during future pregnancies, especially as unresolved guilt feelings may reappear at this time.

c. Immigrant Families

Between 3 and 4 percent of the population of the UK are of New Commonwealth origin, (the Carribean, India, Pakistan or Africa). Not all are immigrants in the strict sense; 40 per cent have been born in this country. In some inner urban areas almost 40 per cent of the population is of New Commonwealth origin. These people do not form a homogeneous group; they are from different countries and cultures with differing moral values and religious beliefs. However, they share similar difficulties and stresses in living in Great Britain.

(i) Social factors. On their arrival in the UK, many immigrants settled in the socially and economically depressed areas of our large cities; areas in which infant mortality rates were already high as were the incidences of alcoholism, malnutrition, unemployment and crime. There has since been limited movement away from these areas of original settlement. The gregariousness typical of immigrant communities has led to a concentration of New Commonwealth people that has persisted.

The problems which immigrant people encounter include difficulties with language and communication, antagonism from intolerant sections of the indigenous population, difficulties in finding reasonably priced living accommodation of a moderate standard, and appropriate employment.

Overcrowded housing is a feature of immigrant groups. The 1971 census showed that in 34 per cent of West Indian and in 41 per cent of Asian households there were two or more persons to a bedroom; 11 per cent of the indigenous population lived under such circumstances.

People of immigrant origin experience more difficulty in obtaining employment than the indigenous population. Often immigrants have to take undesirable and unpopular jobs at the bottom of the pay scale with little hope of future promotion. Poor pay often means that a second wage earner is needed in the family and this is particularly so if, as sometimes happens, money is being sent back to the country of origin. Employment amongst mothers is common and in some families, husbands take two jobs, one during the day and the other at night.

Living in crowded conditions with unemployed or overworked parents can adversely affect a child's health, and physical and emotional development. It has been postulated that the lack of a stimulating mother figure inhibits the emotional and intellectual development of West Indian children in the pre-school period. They are then at a disadvantage when they go to school where they may perform badly and often leave with few qualifications. This in turn leads to difficulty in obtaining employment, to disillusionment, depression and possibly even to delinquency. In 1971, the rate of unemployment in West Indian boys aged 16–20 was 16 per cent, twice that for the total population in this age group. More recent figures are likely to be worse.

The West Indian child and adolescent therefore faces difficulties at school and in obtaining subsequent employment. Asian children perform better at school but often experience difficulty in obtaining employment appropriate to their academic achievement. They may have to accept work below their capability. Asian adolescents may also face difficulties within their own families and some come into conflict with their parents as they seek the same freedom that their indigenous school-fellows or work-mates enjoy. Modern British moral values conflict with those of many Asian families; most Asian adolescents eventually conform to their parents' standards and wishes, but a few may break away completely and leave home. These pressures are greater for Asian girls who are often more protected than boys in the Asian family.

Immigrants of New Commonwealth origin face considerable hardships as they settle in our often prejudiced society; these include inadequate, overcrowded housing, educational disadvantage and unemployment. The social and emotional stresses under which they live can lead to the development of symptoms. These may be physical in nature, but such presentation should not blind the general practitioner to their true origin.

(ii) Medical conditions. Exotic tropical diseases do occur in patients of immigrant origin but their occurrence is rare. The commonest is perhaps malaria; the incidence of malaria in the UK has increased rapidly in recent years, and one of the largest groups contributing to this is immigrants living in this country returning from visits to relatives in India. The commonest infecting organism is *Plasmodium vivax*. Rarer infectious diseases that may occur include leprosy, filariasis and trachoma infection of the eye, but these are more likely in patients who have recently arrived in this county.

There has been a substantial decrease in the notification rate of tuberculosis in British born patients in recent years. However, the notification rate for African and Asian immigrants has increased dramatically. Although these groups represent less than 4 per cent of the population, they were responsible for almost one-third of tuberculosis notifications in 1971. The disease has its greatest incidence in immigrants who have recently arrived and especially those from Pakistan. Even in those who have been here for 15 years, there is a greater incidence than in the indigenous population. Tuberculosis in an immigrant patient is associated with a higher incidence of disseminated and non-pulmonary disease (especially meningitis, osteomyelitis and peritonitis) and the incidence of primary drug resistant organisms is high. The spread of tuberculosis is enhanced by the overcrowded living accommodation which is a feature of immigrant communities. BCG immunisation should be offered to newborn babies living in a house in which there is a patient receiving treatment for tuberculosis, or one who has recently arrived from overseas. In some areas such immunisation is recommended for all babies whose mothers are of New Commonwealth origin.

The worm infestation rate of immigrant children is higher than that for indigenous children. The commonest worms are whipworm (Trichuris), roundworm (Ascaris) and threadworm; hookworm may also be found and may be a cause of anaemia. Most children are asymptomatic but should be treated in order to eliminate possible reservoirs of infestation. Giardiasis may also be found in immigrant children arriving in the UK; large numbers of these organisms may cause a malabsorption syndrome similar to coeliac diseases.

The haemoglobinopathies, such as sickle cell disease and thalassaemia, are more common in immigrant patients. The incidence of sickle cell trait in West Indian patients is about 10 per cent and sickle cell disease less than 1 per cent. In the UK, there are about 3000 people with sickle cell disease. Thalassaemia major has been seen increasingly in England in the last 20 years in the children of immigrants from Cyprus, the Far East and the Indian subcontinent. In 1977 there were 300 children in the UK with this disorder. The prevention of severe haemoglobinopathy is possible by antenatal diagnosis using fetal blood samples obtained early in a pregnancy when there is an affected fetus, the pregnancy may be terminated.

The important nutritional disorders that can occur in immigrant patients include iron-deficiency anaemia, osteomalacia and rickets.

Iron-deficiency anaemia is more common in women and children of immigrant origin than in the indigenous population. The cause is usually a dietary deficiency and in infancy this is often related to prolonged breast feeding. The Asian child may be weaned onto a diet of mainly rice and potatoes, low in eggs, meat and fish. Feeding with unmodified cow's milk which, unlike commercial baby milks, is not fortified with iron, may also lead to iron-deficiency anaemia. Prolonged milk feeding, to the age of 2 or 3 years, may also result in an iron-deficiency anaemia and this problem is sometimes seen in Asian children. Hookworm infestation in older children may also cause anaemia.

Studies in Glasgow have shown the increased incidence of rickets in immigrant children, in particular, those of Asian origin. In 1976 a survey of 500 Glasgow children for clinical, biochemical and radiological rickets showed that of 200 Asian children, 10 had florid rickets and 15 subclinical rickets; of 300 African, Chinese and Scottish children, none had florid rickets and 10 had subclinical rickets. A London survey showed that 6 per cent of Asian children aged 6 months had clinical rickets as did 20 per cent of those aged 18 months.

Rickets is most likely to develop at the ages of greatest growth and metabolic activity, that is in infancy and puberty. Rickets occurs in indigenous children only in toddlers, but in Asian children, it is also found in schoolchildren and at puberty. Osteomalacia may also develop in Asian women during pregnancy.

The cause of rickets in toddlers is a dietary deficiency of vitamin D from prolonged breast feeding or the use of unmodified cow's milk. It is especially common in those children who have not been seen by health visitors and those whose mothers work and consequently use baby-minders. Rickets can be prevented by ensuring that these children receive adequate supplements of vitamin D, and this should be recommended by the health visitors and doctors who see these patients.

Rickets in older children and osteomalacia in Asian women is also caused by a dietary deficiency of vitamin D. The cause of this is uncertain, and a combination of factors is probably responsible. This includes a low level of vitamin D in the diet, low exposure to sunlight and the malabsorbtion of vitamin D and calcium from the diet. Chapati flour is said to contain substances that interfere with vitamin D and calcium absorption and the use of vitamin D fortified chapati flour has been shown to reduce the incidence of vitamin D deficiency in Asian patients.

The commonest nutritional disorder in West Indian children is obesity. It is possibly related to a cultural belief that fatness is a measure of wealth and health.

The birth rate amongst New Commonwealth immigrants is higher than that of the indigenous population; in 1975 almost 7 per cent of live births was to mothers of New Commonwealth origin. This higher rate is related to the greater proportion of the immigrant population being of child-bearing age. In previous years there was a tendency for West Indian and Asian families to have more children that indigenous families; recent evidence suggests that family size in both these groups of immigrants is falling and is approaching that of the indigenous population.

A greater proportion of Asian babies is in the low birth-weight category. However, many of these babies do not have the characteristics of the low birth-weight baby and such disproportion in statistics has arisen from the application of British norms to a different population. Normal Asian babies tend to be lighter than normal indigenous babies. Nevertheless, the perinatal and neonatal mortality rates are greater for Asian babies. Although nutritional and obstetric factors must contribute to this, socioeconomic factors must be of much greater importance.

The incidence of asthma and eczema in children of Asian and West Indian origin is higher than that in indigenous children. The incidence is also higher than that of children living in India and the West Indies.

The incidence of burns is higher in West Indian children and is perhaps linked with overcrowded housing and the use of cheap, unguarded oil heaters. Of English children at the age of 3 years, 35 per cent had a history of a previous burn, compared with 60 per cent of West Indian children. Paraffin poisoning is also more common in this group of patients.

The doctor who looks after immigrant patients will occasionally meet the rare and unfamiliar; more usually however, he will see medical conditions that occur in the indigenous population, although the incidences of disorders such as tuberculosis, iron-deficiency anaemia and rickets are higher in the immigrant group. Environmental, cultural and emotional difficulties may lead to the presentation of patients with psychosomatically-induced physical symptoms. These are much more common and their true cause is no less important because it is not physical disease; it should not pass unrecognised.

PRIMARY HEALTH CARE FOR CHILDREN

SEEING THE DOCTOR

Seeing the doctor

As the person of first contact for health care, the general practitioner must be readily accessible; his terms of service dictate that either he or his deputy must be constantly available.

During normal working hours, most children will be seen in the doctor's surgery. He must ensure that those children who require his attention urgently are seen by him as soon as possible. Thus, even if he has organised an appointments system, it must be flexible enough to provide opportunities for sick children to be seen with the minimum of delay. Arranged in such a way, appointments systems need not become a barrier between patients and their doctor, and parents should feel that their doctor is accessible to their child whenever necessary.

Consultation at home

When children are older they are less easy to transport to the doctor's surgery when they are ill, and a consultation at home is then necessary. The number of house calls has fallen markedly in recent years; in the early 1960s between 40 and 60 per cent of a general practitioner's time was used in making home visits. Now, home visiting rates vary between 10 and 20 per cent and seem to be greater in more rural areas and in northern parts of the country. Home visiting remains an indispensable part of the primary care of children, for a home visit gives the doctor great insight into the way in which a child and his family live together. The information gleaned in the home adds much to the doctor's understanding of a family's problems.

The quality of a home environment has a considerable effect on a person's state of health; the state of the home is a reflection of a family's behaviour and attitudes. Overcrowded housing is associated with an increased incidence of respiratory disorders and emotional conditions. On a home visit the doctor is able to note such things as the state of repair of the accommodation — is it well kept or neglected? How much space is there — is it enough for the family? Have they a bathroom? Where are the family's priorities — with warm clothes, food or toys, or with cigarettes, colour television sets and expensive stereo equipment? Is the house clean — is it too clean? Are the rooms lived in or are they just to be looked at and admired? Are there signs of children in the house-

hold? Have they their own room; are their toys in evidence or their pets? Does the house feel lonely or cold or cheerless — is the doctor made to feel at home? Who else lives with the family — is there a father or a grandparent at home? How do they all react to the child's illness? Where do the children play? What hazards seem to be in evidence in the home and would advice on accident prevention be appropriate?

The information that can be acquired from one home visit is enormous. This, together with the patient's ability to express his feelings more freely on his own territory makes the house call a most valuable exercise. Much of the information the doctor acquires helps him in his present consultation with the sick child, but some of the information can be of use in future consultations with other members of the family in the years ahead.

Consultation during special sessions

Much of the child health work undertaken by general practitioners takes place at times set aside for preventive care, and usually in association with a health visitor. Developmental surveillance sessions and immunisation clinics are often arranged in this way. These contacts, free from the parental anxiety that may accompany a surgery consultation with a sick child, also provide opportunities for parents to ask the simpler questions about their child's progress, questions that otherwise would remain unasked. These sessions also provide opportunities for health education and advice on parentcraft and breast feeding.

Many practices have developed age/sex registers which provide the names of children born in specific age ranges. These are especially valuable in the identification of non-attenders to screening and immunisation sessions, and aid their follow-up by the health visitor.

Consultation out-of-hours

To provide primary care services to all his patients for 24 hours every day and to provide time for himself and his family the general practitioner must sometimes employ a reliable deputy. This is often done by organising a rota for out-of-hours work with partners or neighbouring general practitioners. Some doctors make use of the services of commercial deputising agencies.

Almost 10 000 general practitioners in England and Wales use a commercial deputising agency in some way. Most use is made of such services as a long-stop at times of illness, or after 11 pm at night.

Between 15 and 20 per cent of out-of-hours calls are to children under the age of 16 and most of these are needed to allay parental anxiety. Between 10 and 15 per cent are for medical emergencies for conditions such as asthma or convulsions.

Whatever system is used, it is important that parents are clear as to how they can contact their doctor or his deputy in an emergency out-of-hours. Parents should not be discouraged from seeking out-of-hours advice if they are worried about their children. A child's initial symptoms can rapidly develop into serious or life-threatening illness. Education about the significance of symptoms and indications for seeking further advice can lessen parental anxiety and some practices provide pamphlets in an attempt to do this. The presence of a member of the extended family or supportive neighbours also lessens parental anxiety.

The number of out-of-hours calls a practice has is sometimes an indication of its performance during the day. Thus, parents who have been seen earlier that day and who have not been reassured by that consultation may call out-of-hours because they are anxious about their child's progress. The number of such out-of-hours calls can be lessened by giving parents careful explanation of their child's illness when he is first seen. Explanation that temperatures often rise in the evening may prevent a panic call later in the day; failure to give an analgesic as well as an antibiotic to a child with otitis media may result in a late call, and perhaps deservedly so!

An increase in the number of a practice's out-of-hours calls may mean that patients have difficulty in being seen at short notice during the day. Such an increase is an indication to review the practice's arrangements for dealing with the acutely ill earlier in the day and perhaps for determining whether or not the practice's appointments system is being too rigidly applied. If parents know good care is readily and easily available during the day, they will make fewer calls out-of-hours.

Record keeping

Ideally, a patient's general practitioner record should follow him throughout his life. The general practitioner's records belong to the Secretary of State and the Family Practitioner Committee arranges for them to be transferred to the new doctor when a patient changes general practitioner. The information contained in the GP records can, therefore, be very extensive and valuable. Unfortunately, such information is often recorded in such a way that it is extremely difficult to use. The ideal system of record keeping must ensure that the retrieval of information is easy; there are a number of ways of doing this. Some practices use summary cards to list patient's important social, emotional and medical features. Other devices include boxing — in major diagnoses or using a problem-solving list to which active and inactive problems can be designated. An efficient record-keeping system is essential for the provision of good clinical care. It can also be developed to provide a basis for teaching and research in general practice.

Recent studies have suggested that much of the information included in practice records can be stored in computers. This will never be possible unless practice records have been kept manually in such a way that the information contained within them is easily retrievable.

Many practices have developed age/sex registers in which the names of patients are filed according to their date of birth. These enable the doctor to identify those patients within certain age groups and are especially useful in identifying children due for developmental assessment and immunisation. Disease indexes and at-risk registers can also be constructed. The latter is especially useful in identifying those who are likely to fail to take advantage of the services the practice offers and who must be actively sought out and special attempts made to provide the help they need.

Organisation of the practice

General practitioners work in a variety of ways. Many are single-handed, although this proportion of doctors has diminished markedly in recent years (see Table 5.2). Most general practitioners now work together in groups of three or more. This means that they can share premises and equipment as well as develop areas of clinical interest amongst themselves. ·

The general practitioner is responsible for providing his own premises. Some doctors own their own buildings; others rent premises from landlords; some rent health centres from the local health authority. General practitioner premises may have been purpose-built as doctors' surgeries or may have been adapted from private dwellings or shops. The general practitioner is responsible for providing himself with any equipment he may need. He is also responsible for employing the secretarial and receptionist help that his practice may require. District nurses and health visitors are usually employed by the local health authority and sometimes are attached to work with the members of a group practice.

The primary care team

The Receptionist

The practice receptionist is usually employed by the doctors with whom she works, although in health centres she may be an employee of the local health authority. She is the point of first contact with the practice and her duty is to facilitate patients' access to the doctor or one of the other members of the primary care team. She is responsible for the efficient running of the appointments system, for taking requests for home visits, taking telephone messages, filing the patients' records, maintaining the practice age/sex register and for communications with the Family Practitioner Committee. The initial impression she gives patients is most important; her demeanor must in no way inhibit patients from seeking help and yet at the same time she must organise the many requests so that they can be coped with efficiently. The ideal receptionist must be kindly, capable, understanding, discreet, cheerful and have boundless stamina. The work is difficult and the doctors for whom they work are responsible for their training and supervision.

The health visitor

In 1977 there were about 7500 health visitors in England. The health visitor is a state registered nurse or registered general nurse who has had some obstetric experience and who holds the certificate of health visiting. When they have completed their nursing and obstetric experience they undertake a one-year post-registration course in order to obtain this certificate. More recently, integrated courses have been developed during which education for nursing and health visiting are combined and qualification as a nurse and health visitor is obtained.

The health visitor is not actively involved in technical nursing procedures. Her role is to prevent ill health in the community. She has been trained to identify most health and social problems, to recognise needs and to mobilise the appropriate resources where necessary. Much of her work is with families with pre-school children, but it is not confined to these groups. Health visitors have important roles in antenatal health education and in monitoring the elderly and the chronic sick.

A health visitor is required to visit every new baby at about the age of 10 days. Thereafter, she is available to mothers for advice on parencraft, infant feeding, immunisation and the physical and psychological aspects of growth and development.

Many health visitors work closely with general practitioners in attachment. Usually they are based in the doctor's premises and their clients are mainly those registered on the doctor's list. This enables the health visitor and doctor to work together during fixed sessions such as developmental surveillance clinics and communication between them about their patients is informal and easy. However, in some areas, particularly in inner cities, not all people have a general practitioner and in these districts there is often a need for a geographically-designated health visitor.

The geographically-designated health visitor is responsible for the people living in a fixed area. This means that she can visit and be consulted by all people who live within her patch. A disadvantage of this system is that very often she will be working with a number of different general practitioners so that communication may be difficult and, indeed, may lapse altogether.

The district midwife

The work of the district midwife has changed in

recent years with the decline in number of home deliveries. Some are still able to deliver their patients in general practitioner obstetric units, but much of their work for general practitioners is in the provision of antenatal and postnatal care. Many doctors organise separate sessions for antenatal clinics and are joined in them by their district midwife. The increasing popularity of 48-hour discharge after delivery has maintained the volume of domiciliary postnatal care. Most mothers are attended by a district midwife for up to 14 days after delivery; after this, her care is usually undertaken by the health visitor.

The district midwife and health visitor are both employed by the local health authority.

The district nurse

In 1977 there were over 12 500 district nurses in England. The district nurse is also employed by the local health authority. Her work entails the application of practical nursing procedures and she treats most of her patients in their own homes. She is rarely involved in the care of children and most of her patients are elderly. However, she may be called upon to dress wounds, administer injections or to contribute to the education of a new diabetic.

The Court Report proposed that in future there should be a special type of nurse, the child health visitor, whose work with children would be both preventive and include practical nursing. The principal aim would be to treat children at home in order to avoid their admission to hospital. This proposal was not generally accepted; to date there has been no move to implement this suggestion.

The practice nurse

The practice nurse's duties are similar to those of the district nurse, but she is based in the doctor's surgery and does not attend patients in their own homes. Unlike district nurses, most practice nurses are employed by the doctors with whom they work.

The social worker

For many years the relationship between general practitioners and social workers has been an uneasy one. Recent trends, however, have improved the communication between these two groups. Social work liaison is such a trend, this involves the identification of one social worker who works closely with a group of doctors. She attends practice premises at fixed times in the week to see patients that have been referred to her by the general practitioners. She is then able to advise these clients herself or to refer them to her colleagues at the local social services office. She is also able to keep general practitioners informed of the progress of those patients that she may be seeing. Social workers are employed by the local authority.

These are the members of the primary care team who are seen most commonly in general practice. Other members, more rarely encountered include geriatric visitors, counsellors from the Marriage Guidance Council, dieticians, physiotherapists or psychologists. The more members there are in a team, the greater the problems of communication. Communication is usually informal and easy but, nevertheless, many practices organise formal team meetings at which difficult problems can be considered. In this way, all members of the team are kept informed of future plans.

Hospital services

Direct access to laboratories and X-ray departments means that general practitioners can investigate their patients fully and arrange their treatment and follow-up without referral to specialist clinics. In one year, a general practitioner with 2500 patients will refer just over 400 to the hospital outpatient department; 10 of these referrals will be for children. Each doctor has about 12 children admitted as an inpatient each year; the total number of all his patients admitted is about 280 per year.

Patients have direct access to primary care in hospitals in accident and emergency departments. There has been a marked increase in the use of these services in the last 20 years and this has been especially so in urban areas. The reasons for such self-referral are complex and include family tradition, inability or unwillingness to consult their own general practitioner or dissatisfaction with him and the desire for a second opinion.

The NHS provides for domiciliary consultations between a general practitioner and a consultant. This makes it possible for a specialist opinion to be obtained in a patient's home and can sometimes avoid unnecessary admission to hospital. It is also a useful way of general practitioners and consultants meeting and exchanging views. The total number of domiciliary consultations in England and Wales each year is about 333 000, there is one domiciliary consultation for every 15 admissions to hospital and to every 25 new outpatients' attendances. Such an arrangement which might avoid admission to hospital would be particularly suitable for paediatric practice. However, domiciliary consultations are rarely used for children, about 2 per cent of domiciliary consultations are for a paediatric opinion. This contrasts with general medicine and psychiatry, each of which contributed to 20 per cent of domiciliary consultations, and to geriatrics, which contributed to 12 per cent. The cynic might be forgiven for thinking that the domiciliary consultation has become a way of short-circuiting long waiting lists, fortunately, such a manoeuvre is rarely necessary in paediatric practice.

Some general practitioners have access to their own beds in community hospitals; there are over 350 general-practitioner hospitals in England and Wales. Most of the patients admitted to these hospitals have acute medical conditions which cannot be cared for at home but which do not require specialist treatment. The proportion of children admitted to GP hospitals is small.

Community health services

The community health services, including the school health service, are responsible for developmental surveillance and the immunisation of children against infectious diseases. Many general practitioners do this work themselves during sessions in their own premises. Clinical medical officers undertake this service for the patients of doctors who do not provide it. They work closely with health visitors in child health clinics organised by the local health authority.

The work of clinical and school medical officers is in the prevention of illness and in the promotion of health. They are not in a position to treat the illnesses they discover and must refer the child to his own general practitioner for this. At times, this has produced conflict, and it is unfortunate that school and clinical medical officers and general practitioners do not always work closely together in a way that ensures easy and informal communication.

The parents

Much childhood illness does not need medical advice. An important task for the doctor and health visitor is to advise parents how to recognise and cope with self-limiting illness in their children and to distinguish those conditions that need prompt medical help. Many sick and disabled children who do require medical care can also be looked after at home by their parents. The doctor must teach and encourage this, for such an arrangement may avoid a child's admission to hospital and the emotional upset that this may cause.

Of the many resources with whom the general practitioner works, perhaps the most valuable and the most neglected is a child's parents. The doctor relies upon them most in monitoring their child's progress and in administering medication. Ideally, they should be given as much responsibility as is reasonable to care for their child and, rather than take the initiative for care from them, the doctor must support them in their efforts. They must be involved in future planning and their views must not pass unheeded when decisions are being made.

The doctor's relationship with the children on his list will always be important, for besides promoting their health and treating disease, he must also educate them in how to use the health care system appropriately in the future as adolescents, young adults and, in their turn, as parents. His relationship with them is also a way to the rest of the family, for they, too, are his patients. Symptoms in a child as a presentation of illness elsewhere in the family is now well recognised; in general practice it is impossible to care for a child without making some assessment of those with whom he lives.

FURTHER READING

Fry J 1983 Present State and future needs in general practice, 6th edition. RCGP London.

Lobo E de H 1978 Children of immigrants to Britain — their health and social problems. Hodder & Stoughton, London, Sydney, Auckland & Toronto

Royal College of General Practitioners 1979 Trends in general practice — a collection of essays by members of the Royal College of General Practitioners. British Medical Journal, London

6

Accidents, non-accidental injury and child abuse

ACCIDENTS

The child's need for movement, his urge to explore, his inexperience, together with his immaturity in discretion and judgement, make him peculiarly liable to accidents. In addition, lack of safe playing spaces and inadequate supervision and control increase vulnerability for certain groups of children and make accidents a major health hazard. Unfortunately, the environment of children seems seldom designed with their needs in mind; architects and town planners should be better informed on these matters. Parents also urgently need more education on safety in the home as well as outside and on the need for close supervision and control of young children. This should be more thoroughly addressed in child health clinics and in the media, as well as by doctors individually after each accident, however minor. Doctors should also be more diligent at reporting to the authorities facets of the unsafe environment which have already led to accidents or which seem hazardous.

Tables 6.1 to 6.3 show that, in children, deaths from accidents far exceed the other leading causes

Table 6.1 Major causes of death in England and Wales (1979)

| | Age (years) | | | |
| | Under 1 | | 1–15 | |
	Number	%	Number	%
Accidents	201	2.5	925	29.6
Congenital abnormalities	2083	25.5	456	14.6
Respiratory disease	930	11.4	332	10.6
Malignant disease	35	0.4	553	17.7

Table 6.2 Some causes of accidental death in childhood (England and Wales 1979)

| | Age (years) | | | |
	0–4	5–9	10–14	Total
Total accidental deaths	459	331	336	1126
All road deaths	114	205	197	516
Involving pedestrians	80	168	99	347
Involving cyclists	1	16	75	92
All falls	20	13	15	48
Falls from buildings	6	4	7	17
All burns	51	20	20	91
Conflagrations	36	14	15	65

Table 6.3 Some causes of accidental death in childhood (England and Wales 1979)

| | Age (years) | | | |
	0–4	5–9	10–14	Total
Drowning	42	47	16	105
Inhalation and ingestion	129	5	8	142
Homocide and purposefully inflicted	56	14	14	84
Suffocation	43	10	20	73
Poisoning	9	3	10	22
Electrocution	4	2	4	10

of death after the first birthday, and thousands of children are admitted to hospital in pain and distress (Table 6.4). Psychological consequences of hospitalisation such as bedwetting, negative behaviour and fears, are then added to the misery for many children and their parents. Some children are treated in clinics, surgeries or at home and do not appear in accident statistics although they too, suffer considerable pain and distress (Sibert 1981).

Home accidents are a particular hazard for the pre-school child, and, after the toddler years, road accidents including those involving bicycles, cars

Table 6.4 Hospital admissions following accidents (England and Wales 1977)

	Age (years)			
	0–4	5–14	0–14	Adults
All admissions	377 840	429 560	807 400	3 579 660
Admissions following accidents	49 960	83 970	133 930	399 290
Percentage following accidents	13.2	19.5	16.6	11.2

and especially the child as a pedestrian is a major hazard. There has been little research on home accidents although they should be the easiest to prevent (Sibert 1980). Child-resistant containers, now coming into use, should go some way to prevent the enormous toll of admissions and frightening treatment from the ingestion of pills and medicines (Craft & Sibert 1977).

The importance of personal and environmental stress in the cause of accidents has also received scant attention (Bakwin & Bakwin 1948, Burton 1968, Silbert 1970, Margolis 1971, Sibert 1975, Brown & Davidson, 1978, Doege 1978). Sweden has gone further than most countries in research and control of childhood accidents and it is their Joint Committee for Childhood Accident Prevention (Berfenstam 1977) which has led the way for the Childhood Accident Prevention Trust in Britain. Jackson & Wilkinson (1976), Court (1976), Sibert (1977) and Jackson & Gaffin (1983) provide useful further reading.

Management of accidents

Certain principles are vitally important in the management of accidents, especially the ability to recognise a dangerous situation among the many minor accidents seen. When in doubt, the child should be seen again within a few hours and the latent period in poisoning and head injuries should be remembered. Non-accidental injury is common and should be considered in the differential diagnosis. It may be important to know which drugs are present in the child's environment and this includes all other houses visited. It is crucial to keep detailed notes of the history and timing of incidents, together with instructions given to parents. Seeking advice from senior or specialist colleagues is often necessary.

Patience, tolerance, tact and courtesy are indispensible attributes in medical staff and anxious parents may be panicky, aggressive or apparently fussing over trivialities. Careful explanations help, along with the recognition that good parents *should* be anxious until their child is safe and the symptoms and treatment are understood. Parents' worries should always be carefully noted as they usually help in accurate diagnosis.

Frightened children may be difficult to handle. They are best kept close to parents with gentle, patient medical staff who will spend time talking, explaining and reassuring.

It is important to transfer an injured or very ill child immediately to an accident and emergency department where expertise in the diagnostic skills and resuscitation of children is instantly available. Suspected poisoning or head injury, stridor, choking, fits or collapse are some of the common conditions which may need emergency treatment.

Injured children sometimes have other serious illness as the main cause of their symptoms. Meningococcal septicaemia, meningitis, dehydration, intussusception, or acute appendicitis in a pre-school child may present diagnostic problems which require urgent admission and treatment. Illingworth (1978) in her valuable small book addresses many of these issues.

The parents of a child who is seriously ill, dead or dying, after an accident or sudden emergency such as cot death, need careful explanation and support. They need an opportunity, immediately and later, to ask questions and receive reassurance, when appropriate, that they could not have prevented the catastrophe. The need for police investigation and autopsy should be explained.

Parents who may have killed their children equally need medical concern and care in their double anguish over the dead child and their fear of the consequences. This is one of the most delicate situations to handle in the whole of medical practice.

NON-ACCIDENTAL INJURY AND CHILD ABUSE

Child abuse results in a variety of clinical syndromes (Table 6.5) of which non-accidental injury is but a small part (Hall 1974, 1981, Cooper 1977, 1978a). The long-term psychological damage is equally or more severe than the injuries and affects the child's whole personality and development, his learning capacity, his conscience, his social skills and his capacity as a parent later (Martyn 1976, Lynch & Roberts 1982). Abused children usually have parents who were themselves abused whose low self-esteem and inability to trust make them so taxing to understand and to treat (Steele 1980).

Doctors and other health workers need to develop skills in understanding and recognising the injuries as the signal of the abusive environment with its indifference and coldness and its lack of concern for the child's basic needs. Good parenting is characterised by warmth, affection, patience, understanding, encouragement and security, all of which promote the child's optimum development. A hostile environment some or all of the time, with parents who use verbal aggression, ridicule, sarcasm and who belittle the child with fearful threats or cruel punishments is no less damaging than the physical injuries and the two often co-exist. Heated arguments and violence

Table 6.5 Clinical syndromes in child abuse and neglect

1. Physical injuries:
   Bruises, lacerations, grazes, bitemarks, scars (NB mouth, ears and genitals)
   Burns and scalds including cigarette burns and their scars
   Bone and joint injuries
   Brain, eye and ear injuries
   Internal injuries

2. Other disorders or accidents: Poisoning (NB drowsiness, ataxia, coma, fits)
   Drowning
   Suffocation (mimicking cot death or apnoeic attacks)

3. Failure to thrive, psychosocial dwarfism and developmental problems (especially speech and language disorders)

4. Psychosomatic complaints

5. Behaviour problems:
   Repeated problems with crying and feeding
   Overactive demanding and disobedient behaviour
   Withdrawal and apathy with frozen watchfulness
   Persistent rocking, head-banging etc
   Accident proneness
   Hysterical outbursts ⎫
   Running Away ⎬ in older children
   Suicide Attempts ⎪
   Drink and drug problems ⎭

6. Sexual abuse within or outside the family

7. Abuse while in care:
   1. From care-givers due to provocative behaviour
   or 2. From repeated moves and yo-yoing in and out of care or hospital

NB Several forms of abuse commonly exist together.

Table 6.6 Sources of parental problems

1. Psychological vulnerability from:
   (a) lack of affection, attention and encouragement during childhood and/or
   (b) family violence, hostility, neglect or denigration of a growing child's efforts

2. Bonding failure due to:
   (a) mother's unexpected illness or difficulties in pregnancy, labour and subsequent months or
   (b) newborn's illness, feeding problems or excessive crying

3. Family problems:
   Lack of support from/or discord with spouse
   Trouble with relatives
   Another child difficult or handicapped

4. Ill health:
   Depression in either spouse or, rarely, mental illness

   Mother may have several minor ailments, e.g.:
   Anaemia   Toothache
   Backache   Earache
   Bladder problems Migraine
   Gynaecological problems Eczema

5. A loss (unmourned):
   Of a child (miscarriage, death, adoption, removed)
   Of another relative or friend

Social problems:
   Isolation   Violence
   Poor Housing   Alcohol or drug problems
   Overcrowding   Gambling
   Poverty   Poor budgeting
   Mental handicap Discord with neighbours
   Criminality   Etc.

Commonly, mounting stress occurs when several or all of the other problems are added to psychological vulnerability.

between the parents often occur as well, producing fear and insecurity in the child. Drunkenness and criminality produce further stress.

Abusing parents may also show love and concern for the child at times, but their own unmet needs and insecurity make the ordinary frustrations of parenthood intolerable. Unless these signs are recognised, the opportunity to protect the child and assist the parents with their problems is missed. A bruise or other minor injury may be the first opportunity for a health worker to recognise that abuse exists, and to set in train the psychosocial study of the family in order to uncover the problems and to plan appropriate help. A multi-disciplinary team is usually needed for this taxing diagnostic exercise, and it should only be undertaken by senior and experienced practitioners.

Compassion and understanding towards abusing parents must go hand in hand with diagnosis. Seldom are the injuries deliberate, wilful or intentional but they are the result of impulsive outbursts by frustrated parents. The child has usually sparked off feelings of impotence and inadequacy, often by lighting up memories of fear and pain which overwhelmed the parent long ago (Fraiberg 1975, 1980). The devastating damage to the child cannot be overstressed.

Physical abuse — non-accidental injury

The first task of doctors involved with parents and children is to remember that *child abuse is common*; perhaps 1 per cent of children are physically abused and 10 per cent or more are exposed to psychological abuse. Second, unless a detailed history is taken of how the injuries were caused, who was present, what environmental circumstances existed, and what action was taken and by whom, *the discrepant history* will be missed. Even genuine accidents are due to family stress of some kind (Burton 1968) and the details should be gently and thoroughly explored with worried parents. Even when not due to abuse, exploration and advice can assist future prevention.

Third, the parents' attitudes to the injuries often give a clue, and the excessive detail and self-blame of worried parents who genuinely feel they have been careless in failing to prevent an accident can be contrasted with the vagueness, lack of concern and sometimes hostility of abusing parents. Their story may be confused or contradictory, although allowance must be made for semantic problems of inarticulate individuals. Denial of any cause, even for multiple injuries and delay in seeking attention are other significant findings.

Fourth, associated features may be observed in the parents' attitude to the child. They may see him as demanding and difficult or as slow and unrewarding. They may have unrealistic ideas about his personality and expect his skills and understanding to be far in advance of his age and developmental level, showing disappointment or anger at his lack of achievement. They may expect affection and concern from the baby or young child to compensate for their own deprivation.

Fifth, there may be associated features in the family and social background such as youthfulness and social isolation of the parents; absence of the biological father; difficulties surrounding the conception, pregnancy or birth of this particular child causing bonding failure (Ounsted et al 1974, Lynch 1975, Lynch & Roberts 1977); subnormality; mental illness; abuse of alcohol or drugs; criminality; or problems such as poverty, overcrowding and unemployment. Other children in the family may have had injuries, died, been removed through the court or be living with a relative. No single feature is diagnostic but the gradual build-up of psychological and social stresses leads to various forms of severe parental inadequacy and abuse.

The injuries

A detailed discussion of the injuries and their management is beyond the scope of this chapter and has been described elsewhere (Cooper 1978a). Minor injuries on the skin, often of different ages, should lead to routine X-ray of the skeleton. Finger-tip bruises, black eyes, bites, grasp marks, cheek bruises, torn frenulum, petechiae and cigarette burns need particular attention together with periosteal or metaphysical injuries on X-ray. After fresh injuries, repeat X-rays in 2 weeks may show bony lesions although the first films were negative. The brain, eyes and viscera may also be injured

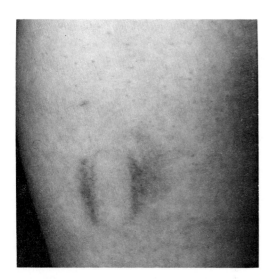

Fig. 6.1 Human bite

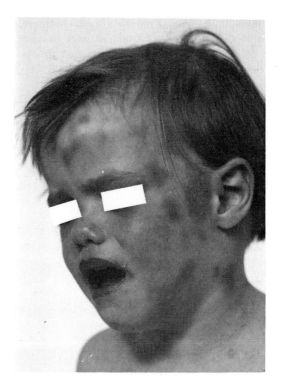

Fig. 6.3 Multiple bruises

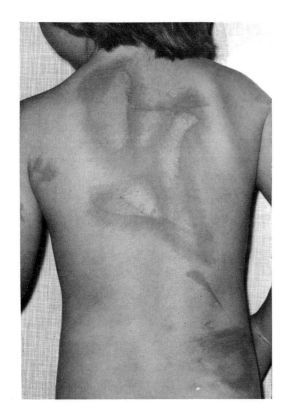

Fig. 6.2 Wheals from a lashing

and internal haemorrhage or brain injury are the commonest causes of death.

Slowly developing subdural haemorrhages after shaking may present puzzling signs at first, with vomiting, irritability and fever. Fundoscopy may reveal the tell-tale retinal haemorrhages before the tense fontanelle and enlarging head suggest the true diagnosis.

Unless there is a high index of suspicion the significance of minor injuries will be missed.

Other disorders

Abuse by *poisoning* may be overt or concealed (Rogers et al 1976, Meadow 1977) with recurrent drowsiness, fits or coma presenting as diagnostic problems.

Drowning may be due to infants being left alone in the bath by frustrated parents, or when a child has actually been pushed into a canal or pond, rather than the reported falling in. Recurrent *apnoeic attacks* are being increasingly recognised as due to partial suffocation. Other *bizarre accidents* such as 'choking on the dummy' should be viewed with concern and carefully assessed.

Disturbed and desperate parents are often frightened after they have hurt a child; they may lie, fabricate and mislead to avoid discovery.

Admission to hospital for tests is the best way of initiating the diagnostic study as well as keeping the child safe. Encouraging the mother to stay in or visit frequently will prevent separation anxiety and provide opportunities for study of the parent-child relationship and the parental problems. Accusing the parents is seldom fruitful, although after a few days a frank discussion of the discrepant findings in the context of the family problems, if carried out with authority and compassion, may elicit the history of abuse.

Failure to thrive

Children do not thrive well in an abusive environment and charting the growth and development is essential for early diagnosis. Neglect and indifference to the child's basic needs for affection and attention, for adequate food and for patience and understanding in feeding and play is the commonest cause of poor growth (MacCarthy 1981). These signs are often present when the minor injuries begin but are missed because weight, length and head circumference are not routinely charted in such cases. Early diagnosis of the mother's uneasiness with her baby can lead to appropriate help and treatment (Fraiberg 1975, 1981). Brain growth and subsequent intelligence are affected (Cooper 1977, 1978a) and many children in special schools for moderately subnormal pupils have suffered these problems. Polansky (1981) has described in detail the apathy–futility syndrome of very damaged and neglectful parents.

Later signs

Doctors in family practice and child health clinics or schools frequently see children with the difficulties listed in Table 6.5 (4 and 5). Too often, sedatives and tranquillisers, which in themselves can release aggression, are prescribed instead of spending time uncovering and helping the basic problems of the child and parents (Lynch et al 1975).

Sexual abuse

Sexual abuse, especially molestation in the family, is increasingly recognised (Foreward & Buck 1981). It is a serious cause of problems and vague symptoms in childhood such as late onset bedwetting, vague pains, sleep disturbance and falling behind at school. Hysterical outbursts and running away are other manifestations in older children and, later on, promiscuity, prostitution and abuse of alcohol and drugs. Boys are affected more often than has been realised, and a high proportion of rapists have suffered sexual abuse when young. Humane forms of investigation and treatment are leading to increasing diagnosis and effective treatment. Kempe & Kempe (1978) provide a useful summary in Chapter 4. An authoritative account of diagnosis and management is Mrazek & Kempe (1981). Other useful references are increasing fast — Burgess et al 1978, Finklehor 1979, Foreward & Buck 1981, Giaretto 1976, Goodwin 1982, Kroth 1979, Meisleman 1979.

ADOPTION & CHILDREN IN CARE

When a child cannot be brought up by his own family, for whatever reason, a permanent family placement offers the best chance of the security and committed parents in the future. The younger the child the more important this is, and adoption offers the best security of all.

Parental agreement is needed before an adoption order can be made but under certain circumstances the court has the power to dispense with these agreements especially if the parents have neglected or ill-treated the child.

Untold damage to the child's development and personality is caused by repeated moves from one care-giver to another. Children who are handicapped or who are older and have been disturbed by their adverse environment and their divided loyalties may need a period of assessment and preparation before family placement. Skills are developing in providing this and in selecting, preparing and supporting a suitable family for each child.

New laws and regulations concerning adoption and children in care have come into force recently and every paediatrician, whether working in the hospital or the community, should be aware of their implications (British Agencies for Adoption & Fostering (BAAF) 1984a).

The Medical Aspects of Adoption

Placement for adoption can now only be arranged by an agency, except for a child placed with a member of the family. The agency may be a private one (which has to be registered with the DHSS) or the statutory social services. Each agency must have one or more medical advisers who will arrange for the medical examinations and reports required on children being considered for adoption. A medical as well as a psycho-social assessment is also required for prospective adopters.

The child's reports will include medical details of the biological parents and their family history. Before the examination and assessment of the child's present status a history of his birth, subsequent care, health, development, behaviour and school progress is needed. The future prognosis can then be given to enable the right family to be chosen for the child and for any necessary treatment, surveillance, special education or other facilities to be planned. The services of a psychologist or child psychiatrist will be needed to complement the paediatric and social assessment of some of the children. The agency's medical advisers should have access to these and to other specialists which will include a geneticist in some cases.

Suitable forms for use in completing the reports are available from BAAF (1984b).

At least one of the agency's medical advisers must sit on the adoption panel which considers the children needing placement and prospective adopters. The panel recommends to the social services adoption committe which children and prospective adopters should be accepted and which family they have chosen for each child.

Legal advice is often necessary in some of the complicated cases now being dealt with and it is helpful if the agency doctors become familiar with main laws and regulations. The welfare principle that first consideration must be given to the long-term needs of the child governs decisions in the agency and in the court.

Medical Aspects of Children in Care

The medical arrangements for children in care are often very sketchy and piecemeal and major medical, sensory, psychological, educational and behavioural problems sometimes go unrecognised and untreated. Normally parents monitor their children's progress and seek advice if they are worried. This close concern and scrutiny is rarely available to children in care unless they are in a long-term family placement when the foster-parents as well as the social worker should oversee the child's progress. When children are in and out of care, or move to different placements, they may not be registered with a family doctor or their medical records do not keep up with them or are lost.

Good practice dictates that every child coming into care should have a preliminary medical form completed with the immediate medical history and details of any treatment he is receiving. Height, weight and skull circumference should be recorded *and charted* and any signs of neglect, ill-treatment or poor development noted.

If the child remains in care more than a week or two a full medical history (including the family medical history) and medical report should be completed to form the basis of the child's medical records which should be updated annually.

Arrangements for the consent to medical examinations and treatment should be formally made each time a child moves to new care-givers. (BAAF 1984c).

REFERENCES

BAAF 1984a A–Z of Changes in the Law. Practice Note No. 6. BAAF, 11 Southwark Street, London SE1

BAAF 1984b BAAF Medical Forms for Children or for Adopting or Fostering Parents

BAAF 1984c Consent to Medical Treatment for Children in Care or Placed for Adoption. Practice Note No. 3

Bakwin R M, Bakwin H 1948 Accident Proneness. *Jr. Paediatrics* Ch 32, pp 749–752

Berfenstam R 1977 The Work of the Swedish Joint Committee for Childhood Accident Prevention in Children. In: Jackson R H (ed) The Environment and Accidents. Pitman, Tunbridge Wells, England

Brown G W, Davidson S 1928 Social Class, Psychiatric Disorder of Mother, and Accidents to Children. Lancet i: 378–380

Burgess A W, Groth A N, Holmstrom L L, Sgrol S M 1978 Sexual Assault of Children and Adolescents. Lexington Books, Lexington, Massachusetts

Burton L 1968 Vulnerable Children. Part 1: Road Accident Involvement in Children (especially Ch VIII). Routledge &Kegan Paul, London

Cooper C E 1977 Child abuse and child neglect. In: Drillien C M,Drummond M B (eds) Neuro-developmental Problems in Early Childhood Ch 20. Blackwell, Oxford

Cooper C E 1978a Child Abuse and Neglect: Medical Aspects. In: Smith S M (ed) The Maltreatment of Children, Ch 2. MTP Press Ltd, Lancaster, England

Cooper C E 1978b Preparing the paediatrician's evidence in care proceedings. In: Franklin A W (ed) Child Abuse: Prediction, Prevention and Follow-up. Churchill Livingstone, Edinburge

Cooper C E 1979 Babies at risk. British Medical Journal 2: 792

Craft A W, Sibert J R 1977 Accidental poisoning in children. British Journal of Hospital Medicine 23: 469–478

Doege T C 1978 An injury is no accident. New England Journal Medicine 298: 509–510

Ebling N B, Hill D A 1983 Child Abuse and Neglect: A guide with Case Studies for Treating the Child and His Family. John Wright, Bristol

Finkelhor D 1979 Sexually Victimised Children. Free Press, New York

Forward S, Buck C 1981 Betrayal of Innocence: Incest and Its Devastation. Penguin Books, Harmondsworth, England

Fraiberg S 1975 Ghosts in the Nursery: A Psycho-analytical Approach to the Problems of impaired Infant-Mother Relationships. Journal of the American Academy of Child Psychiatry 14: 387–422

Fraiberg S 1980 Clinical Studies in Infant Mental Health: The First Year of Life. Tavistock Publications, London

Frude N 1980 Psychological Approaches to Child Abuse. Batsford Academic & Educational Ltd, London

Giarretto H 1976 Humanistic Treatment of Father/Daughter Incest. In: Helfer R E, Kempe C H (eds) Child Abuse & Neglect: The Family and the Community, Ch 8. Ballinger Publishing Co. Cambridge, Massachusetts

Goodwin J 1982 Sexual Abuse: Incest Victims and Their Families. John Wright, Bristol

Hall F, Pawlby S J, Wolkind S 1979 Early Life Experiences and Later Mothering Behaviour: a study of mothers and their twenty week old babies. In: Shaffer D, Dunn J (ed) The First Year of Life. John Wiley, Chichester, England

Hall M H 1974, 1981 The Diagnosis and Early Management of Non-Accidental Injuries in Children. The Police Surgeon No. 6 & No. 19 (Now combined in An Atlas of Non-Accidental Injuries in Children, Police Surgeon Supplement Vol. 12 1982)

Hutchings J 1980 The Behavioural Approach to Child Abuse. In: Frude H (ed) Psychological Approaches to Child Abuse. Batsford Academic & Educational Ltd, London

Illingworth C M 1978 The Diagnosis and Primary Care of Accidents and Emergencies in Children. Scientific Publications, Blackwell, Oxford

Jackson A H, Wilkinson A W 1976 Why Don't We Prevent Childhood Accidents? British Medical Journal i: 1258–126

Jackson R H 1977 Children, The Environment and Accidents. Pitman, Tunbridge Wells, England

Jackson R H, Gaffin J 1983 The Work of the Child Accident Prevention Trust. Archives of Disease in Childhood 58:

Kempe C H, Kempe R S 1978 Child Abuse. Fontana Open Books, Shepton Mallett, England

Kroth J A 1979 Child Sexual Abuse: Analysis of a Family Therapy Approach. Charles C Thomas. Springfield, Illinois

Lynch M A 1975 Ill Health and Child Abuse. Lancet ii: 317

Lynch M, Lindsay J, Ounsted C 1975 Tranquilisers Causing Aggression. British Medical Journal 1: 266

Lynch M A, Roberts J 1977 Predicting Child Abuse: Signs of Bonding Failure in the Maternity Hospital. British Medical Journal 1: 624

Lynch M A, Roberts J 1982 Consequences of Child Abuse. Academic Press, London

MacCarthy D 1974 Effects of Emotional Disturbance and Deprivation (maternal rejection) on Somatic Growth. In: Davis J A, Dobbing J (eds) Scientific Foundations of Paediatrics. Heinemann, London

Margolis J A 1971 Psycho-social Study of Childhood Poisoning: A 5 year Follow-up. Paediatrics 74:439–444

Martin H L 1970 Antecedents of Burns and Scalds in Children. British Journal of Medical Psychology 43: 39–47

Martin H P 1976 The Abused Child. Ballinger Publishing Co. Cambridge, Massachusetts

Meadow R 1977 Munchausen Syndrome by proxy: the hinterland of child abuse. Lancet ii: 343–345

Meiselman K C 1979 Incest: A Psychological Study of Causes and Effects with Treatment Recommendations. Jossey-Bass, Washington

Mrazek P B, Kempe C H 1981 Sexually Abused Children and Their Families. Pergamon Press, Oxford

Ounsted C, Oppenheimer R, Lindsay J 1974 Aspects of Bonding Failure: The Psycho-pathology and Psycho-therapeutic Treatment of Families of Battered Children. Developmental Medicine and Child Neurology 16: 447

Ounsted C, Gordon M, Roberts J, Milligan B 1982 The Fourth Goal of Perinatal Medicine. British Medical Journal 1: 879–882

Polanksky N A, Chalmers M A, Buttenwieser E, Williams D P 1981 Damaged Parents: An Anatomy of Neglect. University of Chicago Press, Chicago

Rogers D, Fupp T, Bentovim A, Robinson A, Berry D, Goulding R 1976 Non-accidental Poisoning: An Extended Syndrome of Child Abuse. British Medical Journal 1: 793

Sibert J R 1975 Stress in Families of Children Who Have Ingested Poison. British Medical Journal iii: 87–89

Sibert J R 1980 Accidents: the child and the home. Journal of Maternal and Child Health 5: 444–452

Sibert J R 1981 Childhood Accidents — An endemic of epidemic proportions. Archives of Disease in Childhood. 56: 225–234

Steele B 1980 Psychodynamic Factors in Child Abuse. In: Kempe C H, Helfer R E (eds) The Battered Child, 3rd edn, Ch 4. University of Chicago Press, Chicago

Wolkind S, Kruk S, Hall F 1983 The Family Research Unit's Study of Women from Broken Homes. In: Franklin A W (ed) Family Matters. Pergamon Press, Oxford

7

The newborn baby

The state of health of a fetus and newborn baby is influenced by the quality of the intrauterine environment and by the mechanics of delivery. Maternal mortality is very low in Western countries, but the mother's physical health, nutrition and social habits are important to fetal welfare (Table 7.1); maternal mobidity may influence fetal

Table 7.1 Maternal factors associated with impaired fetal growth and increased perinatal mortality

Severe undernutrition
Adverse social state
Smoking
Severe and prolonged hypertension in pregnancy
Chronic renal disease
Opiate drug dependence
Alcoholism
High altitude
Cyanotic heart disease

outcome. Maternal diabetes must be well controlled in pregnancy, or preterm delivery of a large fetus with subsequent respiratory distress syndrome and hypoglycaemia may result. Thyroid disorders, anaemia, urinary tract infection and cardiac disease also require careful treatment in pregnancy.

ASSESSMENT OF FETAL WELLBEING

Regular palpation of a growing uterus and maternal perception of vigorous fetal movements are reassuring in the antenatal clinic. If there is concern about the fetus, measurements of the biparietal diameter of the head or abdominal circumference can be carried out using ultrasound. Serial movements can reveal the rate of growth of the fetus. Real-time ultrasound can also show

abnormal positions of the placenta, anomalies of the spine or head and absence of kidneys or bladder. Measurement of oestriol or oestrogen excretion is used as one test of placental function after 28 weeks gestation.

The term *fetal distress* is used to describe a fetus suffering from hypoxia. The causes are listed in Table 7.2. This occurs most commonly during

Table 7.2 Causes of fetal hypoxia

Obliterative vascular lesions in the placental bed
Long-standing placental insufficiency
Placental separation and haemorrhage
Acute compression of the umbilical cord
Fetal anaemia or haemorrhage
Maternal shock or hypoxia
Uterine spasm

labour but may occur before. Fetal distress may be suggested by the passage of meconium *in utero*, or by the presence of fetal heart decelerations, measured by scalp electrode or externally, persisting after a uterine contraction has relaxed (late dips or type-II dips), by a persistent tachycardia over 160 per minute with little variation, or by fetal scalp blood pH below 7.2.

RESUSCITATION OF THE NEWBORN

The need for resuscitation of an asphyxiated newborn can arise at any time and quite unexpectedly. Many hypoxic infants can, however, be predicted (Table 7.3).

The Apgar score is the most common way of recording the degree of hypoxia at birth (Table 7.4)

The Apgar score at one minute is useful in

Table 7.3 A trained member of staff and resuscitation equipment should be present in the following circumstances

Fetal distress
Caesarean section
Breech presentation
Multiple pregnancy
Gestation below 37 weeks
Intrauterine growth retardation
Maternal diabetes mellitus
Rhesus iso-immunisation
Use of large doses of sedatives or analgesic drugs

Table 7.4 Apgar score

Sign	Score		
	0	1	2
Heart rate	Absent	< 100	> 100
Respiration	Absent	Weak Gasping Irregular	Good Crying Regular
Muscle tone	Completely flaccid	Some flexion of extremities	Well flexed
Reflex irrita bility, (response to nasal catheter)	No response	Grimace	Cough Sneeze Gasp
Colour of trunk	White	Blue	Pink

indicating the need for resuscitation and the 5 minute score is a good indication of long-term prognosis. Those infants with a score of 4 or below are more likely to have neurological handicaps later. The most important items are heart rate and respiratory effort. If an infant remains blue after delivery and does not cry, the pharynx should be aspirated with a mucus extractor or power suction catheter. If the infant does not breathe within 10 seconds, place the infant supine on a flat surface preferably under a radiant heater. Apply an infant face-mask and ventilate the baby using 100 per cent oxygen and a Penlon or Ambu bag at 40–50 breaths per minute. Make sure the mask fits tightly over the nose and mouth and that the chest is expanding. Face-mask ventilation produces adequate lung expansion and gas exchange in many babies that are mildly asphyxiated or sedated. However, more severe cases with stiff lungs may not respond.

Endotracheal intubation or face-mask ventilation are required if the heart rate is less than 100 per minute and the baby remains apnoeic, cyanosed and motionless. If the heart rate remains below 40 per minute external cardiac massage with two fingers on the mid-sternum at 120 per minute should be started. Well conducted face-mask ventilation is more effective than a prolonged attempt at intubation. If the mother has received pethidine or morphine within 4 hours of delivery, it is always worthwhile giving maloxone — an opiate antagonist with no sedative properties of its own 0.01 mg/kg can be given intramuscularly by a nurse while the doctor ventilates the baby.

Most babies requiring ventilation by face-mask or endotracheal tube are pink, active and breathing within 5 minutes. The endotracheal tube can be removed after suctioning and the baby observed. If he remains active and well, after a quick general examination he can be wrapped up and given to his mother or father to hold. If the baby develops grunting, cyanosis, indrawing or appears floppy or inactive, he needs to be transferred to a special care baby unit.

ROUTINE EXAMINATION OF THE NEWBORN

Each baby should be examined soon after birth as the parents will want to know if he is normal. The examiner should search for serious congenital abnormalities, adverse effects of intrauterine life or delivery, and should make an estimate of gestational age to see if the baby's growth is appropriate. A final examination before discharge home is necessary to look for congenital abnormalities that might have been hidden at birth, acquired disease, such as jaundice or infection, and to discuss problems such as sleeping, feeding and growth with the mother. It is best to examine the baby with the parents. Gentleness and thoroughness are required: before you handle the baby, observe posture, breathing and colour; is the respiratory rate raised above 60 per minute?; does the baby appear excessively pale, blue, red or yellow? Cyanosis of the extremities is very common in newborns, but the lips and tongue should be pink.

Parents are naturally very concerned about skin blemishes and you may do a great service by explaining these. Milia are small cysts in the epidermis; they are white or pale yellow papules usually less than 1 mm in diameter around the nose and resolve during the first month. Stork bites (macular haemangioma) are flat salmon-pink or red blotches most commonly over the bridge of the nose, the eyelids and the nape of the neck. They are extremely common, but the marks on the face usually disappear within a few months. The marks on the nape of the neck may persis longer, but are covered by hair. A strawberry naevus is usually not visible at birth, but appears and grows rapidly in the first few weeks after birth. The lesions are raised, red and bumpy. They may grow rapidly in the first 6–9 months and may produce an alarming appearance if they are near the eyes. These lesions are capillary cavernous haemangiomas and are extremely vascular. They nearly always begin to regress by the end of the first year, the earliest sign is the development of pale patches in the centre, and spontaneous resolution is very likely before the child is 5 years old. Plastic surgery is extremely difficult because of the vascular nature of these lesions and should not be recommended because of the good prognosis. A port-wine stain is flat and is due to persistent dilatation of capillaries. The lesion may be extensive and, unfortunately, is usually permanent. Neonatal urticaria (erythema toxicum) affects many babies within the first 2–4 days. It usually starts on the trunk as erythematous patches with a white papule in the centre. The rash may be extensive and shows a tendency to vary from hour to hour. The cause is not known but you can confidently reassure the mother that it will disappear without any treatment. Spetic spots may occur in small groups particularly in the axillae, the groins and around the neck. The lesions are pustules and may or may not have surrounding erythema. Petechiae are small purple spots which do not blanch when pressed. They may be a normal finding around the head because of trauma during delivery. However, they are not a normal finding on the rest of the body after vertex deliveries and their presence suggests a bleeding disorder particularly thrombocytopenia.

The occipito-frontal head circumference should be measured carefully and compared with the range for the baby's gestational age. A cephalhae-matoma is a swelling produced by bleeding under the periosteum of one of the cranial bones. This is most common on the parietal bones. The swelling is limited by the suture lines and the lesion usually increases during the first few days after birth. The haematoma leads to jaundice and the swelling may persist for months. A caput succedaneum is oedema of the part of the head presenting through the cervix, there is no limitation to particular bones of the skull and the swelling disappears in a few days.

The face should be examined. A cleft lip is obvious but the palate should also be inspected and felt to exclude a cleft. Note any purulent discharge from the eyes and try to open them so that you can exclude cataracts or corneal opacities. Subconjunctival haemorrhages are harmless and disappear in one to 2 weeks. Down's syndrome is suggested not only by slanting eyes and epicanthic folds but also obvious hypotonia, single transverse palmar creases, short incurved little fingers, a flat occiput, small head circumference, simple ears and abnormal dermal ridge patterns.

If the baby's breathing and colour are normal do not waste time listening to the lungs. Auscultate the heart, and if you hear an ejection systolic murmur in an otherwise well baby re-examine the heart in a few days time. The murmur may disappear during these few days. Significant cardiac signs include the presence of a pansystolic mumur loud in intensity, a gallop rhythm, absent femoral pulses, central cyanosis not relieved by oxygen and congestive cardiac failure with rapid respiration, rapid heart rate and a large liver. The abdomen should be observed for distension. Gently feel each side of the abdomen for enlargement of the liver, spleen, kidneys or any other mass. Feel for a hernia in the groin, scrotum or labia. Note whether both the testes are in the scrotum. Small hydroceles usually resolve without treatment. Note the position of the urethra and make sure that there is a normal anal opening. In a girl make sure that the urethra and vagina are normally situated. Enlargement of the clitoris or fusion of the labia may be due to masculinisation by adrenal hyperplasia. Turn the baby over and examine the whole length of the spine for openings. Examine all four limbs and make sure that the normal number of digits is present. You will not impress the mother with your competence if you have omitted to notice that the baby has an extra finger.

It is best to leave the examination of the hips until last because this is the one part of the examination where it is legitimate to produce some temporary discomfort in the baby. This must be explained to the mother before you test for congenital dislocation of the hips. Hold the baby's legs as shown in Figure 7.1; test one hip at a time.

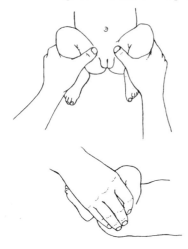

Fig. 7.1 The position for testing the stability of a baby's hips (from Brown & Valman 1979, by kind permission of the authors and publishers)

Adduct the hip pressing downwards along the line of the femur; a dislocatable hip will slip over the posterior edge of the acetabulum with this manoeuvre. Then abduct the femur pressing medial with the middle finger on the greater trochanter. If the head of the femur re-enters the acetabulum a clunk is also felt.

LOW BIRTH-WEIGHT INFANTS

Babies born at less than 37 completed weeks from the last menstrual period are termed preterm and babies with birth weights below the 10th centile for gestational age are small-for-dates. If the mother is certain of the date of her last menstrual period and was not on the contraceptive pill, her estimated date of delivery is likely to be accurate. However, this is not the case with many mothers and the expected date of delivery may have been

estimated by palpation of the uterus or ultrasound measurements of the fetus early in pregnancy. The most widely used method of assessing gestational age in the newborn is that compiled by Dubowitz et al (1970). This uses external physical characteristics and neurological characteristics, particularly tone. In babies that are ill at the time of examination, tone may be reduced and this will depress the neurological part of the score.

Preterm infants

Cervical incompetence, pre-eclamptic toxaemia, placental abruption and placenta praevia are causes of preterm delivery but, in many, the aetiology is unknown. Preterm babies may develop a number of serious complications after birth due to their immaturity.

1. Hyaline membrane disease

(Respiratory distress syndrome)

2. Feeding difficulties

Babies of less than 35 weeks gestation are usually unable to suck adequately their own nutritional requirements. Nasogastric feeding of milk may be required in small volumes at frequent intervals. The capacity of the stomach may be very small and regurgitation and aspiration are possible hazards.

3. Hypothermia

The preterm baby has little insulating subcutaneous fat, has an increased surface to weight ratio compared with term babies and reduced energy stores. Because of his other medical problems he is likely to be more exposed when being handled and treated. Cold stress has been shown to increase oxygen requirements, calorie requirements and mortality. Low birth-weight babies require a thermoneutral environment. For most babies under 2000 g a closed incubator is the best way of achieving this. The ranges of temperature for thermoneutrality have been determined for different birth weights and at different ages after birth (Hey, 1972).

4. Apnoea

Infants of less than 32 weeks gestation are prone to periods of stopping breathing with bradycardia. These may be short lived and self limiting but in some cases obvious hypoxia occurs. Although apnoea may be a symptom of almost any underlying disease in preterm infants, it may occur purely as a result of immaturity. Infants of less than 34 weeks gestation need to be on a respiration or heart rate monitor so that apnoea or bradycardia can be automatically detected and stimulation or resuscitation given as required.

5. Sepsis

6. Hyperbilirubinaemia

7. Maternal deprivation

Because of the factors listed above, babies who are significantly preterm tend to spend a number of weeks, if not months, in special care nurseries before they are able to be looked after at home. It may be difficult for a young mother, particularly with her first baby, to feel emotionally close to her tiny infant in a perspex incubator. Besides the physical separation and the difficulties of travelling from home to the special care nursery, the mother may have a feeling of inadequacy because she cannot provide all the care that the baby needs. Emotional difficulties between mother and child, and child abuse have been reported as being more common in infants who have been in special care nurseries.

8. Intracranial bleeding

Ultrasound and CT scanning has shown that intracranial bleeding from the sub-ependymal germinal matrix occurs in approximately 40 per cent weighing less than 1500 g at birth. Bleeding frequently extends into the cerebral ventricles (intraventricular haemorrhage). Neurological signs include hypotonia, tight popiteal angles and roving eye movements. Large haemorrhages into the cerebral substance (parenchyma) and post-haemorrhagic ventricular are associated with a high rate of cerebral palsy.

SMALL-FOR-GESTATIONAL-AGE INFANTS

Table 7.1 shows a list of factors which may produce fetal growth retardation with delivery of a small-for-gestational-age infant. In severe pre-eclamptic toxaemia, intrauterine growth may come to a halt and there may be shrinking of the abdominal circumference on ultrasound. Such a fetus is in a state of starvation and is in danger of total asphyxiation with intrauterine death before or during labour. The obstetrician may well decide to deliver the baby by Caesarian section, arguing that the environment in the uterus is more hostile than the environment outside. Such a baby often requires resuscitation at birth but, if this is successfully managed, most of these babies do well with modern techniques. They are prone to hypoglycaemia having very small energy stores of glycogen and fat. They are also likely to develop hypothermia. Less commonly, small-for-gestational-age babies have polycythaemia; this is thought to result from chronic intrauterine hypoxia. If the venous haematocrit is above 70 per cent the viscosity of the blood may be excessive and tissue perfusion may be impaired. A successfully delivered small-for-gestational-age baby of 1000 g with a gestational age of 35 weeks is likely to have a much smoother postnatal course than a 1000 g infant of 27 weeks gestation. The prognosis for small-for-gestational-age babies depends very much on the underlying reasons for their small size. If a baby has suffered from intrauterine rubella or has a multiple congenital malformation syndrome the outlook is poor. On the other hand, a successfully managed pre-eclampsia or multiple pregnancy with careful monitoring postnatally of blood glucose and body temperature should result in a health infant. Babies who have had a brief period of intrauterine growth retardation have the capacity to catch up in their somatic growth if they are well nourished. However, babies who have had a prolonged period of intrauterine growth retardation (10–20 weeks) may not catch up fully in their growth later in childhood (Fancourt et al 1976).

NUTRITION

Babies require adequate calories for basal metabolism, temperature regulation, muscular activity and growth; amino acids for protein synthesis; electrolytes, minerals and vitamins. The feed should be palatable, easily digested, non-allergenic and free from infection. Breast feeding meets all the needs of full-term babies. Untreated cow's milk is very far from being suitable for newborn babies. Pasturisation may remove most bacteria, but cow's milk provides no added protection against infection and is capable of stimulating an allergic response. The main protein in cow's milk is casein. This tends to form a bulky curd in the baby's stomach and the proportions of amino acids in casein are not optimal for human babies. The fat in cow's milk is more saturated than that in human milk and fat absorption is reduced. The phosphate content of cow's milk is very much higher than in human milk and this may result in hyperphosphataemia with hypocalcaemic tetany. The sodium content of cow's milk is considerably higher than human milk; under most conditions a healthy baby will be able to handle this increased sodium load but if the baby develops fever and diarrhoea, the water loss involved may result in hypernatraemia.

Recently, cow's milk has been highly modified in order to reduce the above disadvantages. Initially, the milk was diluted to lower the protein content and the calorie content was maintained by the addition of sucrose. It was prepared as a powder which could then be diluted with boiled water. This feed was used for many years as National Dried Milk in the UK. However, the milk was unsatisfactory and further modifications have now been made to cow's milk. The casein content has been greatly reduced and most modern milk are based on demineralised whey. The sodium content of the modern baby milk is approximately the same as in human milk. Polyunsaturated fats have replaced much of the butter fat resulting in improved fat absorption. The phosphate content has been substantially reduced. Vitamins A, B group, C, D, E, iron, copper and zinc have been added.

Although modern baby milk are a great improvement on their predecessors, breast milk still has a number of advantages. The physical closeness involved in breast feeding helps the emotional attachment between mother and baby. Human breast milk contains its own lipase and thus helps its own digestion at a time when the baby's own pancreatic lipase secretion may be inefficient. Human breast milk contains 5 mg per 100 ml of taurine but cows milk and artificial formula feeds contain less than 0.3 mg per 100 ml; newborn kittens have developed retinal degeneration and taurine deficient diets but no deficiency syndrome has yet been defined in humans. Vitamin D sulphate is water soluble and its concentration in the breast milk of well-nourished Caucasian women is 30–40 units per 100 ml, 80 times that of the fat soluble form. Thus, a breast-fed infant would have almost full requirements from breast feeding without any supplements. Breast milk also has a number of protective factors including IgA, lactoferrin, lysozyme, an anti viral substance, white blood cells and produces a low stool pH which favours the growth of *Lactobacillus acidophilus* rather than *Escherichia coli*. Matthew et al (1977) reported that infants of allergic parents had significantly less eczema in the first 6 months of life if they were purely breast fed or received only soya bean milk when compared with babies fed with a cow's milk formula and supplemented with cereal and animal solid foods after 3 months.

NEONATAL JAUNDICE

Neonatal jaundice may need investigation and treatment because of the possibility of bilirubin encephalopathy (kernicterus) and because the jaundice may be due to an underlying disease which is dangerous in its own right. Approximately one-third of all newborn infants become clinically jaundiced during the first week. In what is often called physiological jaundice no kernicterus occurs and the jaundice fades by 10 days of age. This jaundice is due to the normal breakdown of red cells and is exacerbated by a transient deficiency of glucuronyl transferase and by reabsorption of bilirubin from the gut. Unconjugated bilirubin has a high lipid-solubility and at high concentrations may saturate the bilirubin-binding capacity of plasma albumin thus allowing free unconjugated bilirubin to circulate in the plasma and enter nervous tissue. Bilirubin glucuronide (conjugated bilirubin) is poorly soluble in lipid and being water-soluble can be excreted in bile and urine. Kernicterus affects the brain stem nuclei and basal ganglia particularly. Nerve deafness and choreoathetoid cerebral palsy are the commonest long-term effects but, if the condition is very severe, mental retardation and death may occur. There is a risk of kernicterus if the unconjugated plasma bilirubin rises above 400 μmol/l (24 mg/100 ml) in a full-term baby.

Preterm infants and hypoxic or acidotic infants may have a lower bilirubin-binding capacity and thus kernicterus may occur at unconjugated bilirubin levels lower than 340 μmol/l (20 mg/100 ml). Neonatal jaundice should be considered abnormal if jaundice appears before 24 hours; the plasma

Table 7.5 Causes of neonatal jaundice before 24 hours

Haemolytic disease	Rhesus incompatibility ABO incompatibility Red cell defects
Haematoma	Cephalhaematoma Bruising to breech
Polycythaemia	Small-for-gestational-age Twin-twin transfusion

Table 7.6 Causes of unconjugated hyperbilirubinaemia after 24 hours

Haemolytic disease
Haematoma
Polycythaemia
Prematurity
Sepsis
Dehydration
Slow intestinal transit

Table 7.7 Causes of prolonged unconjugated jaundice

Haemolytic disease
Breast milk jaundice, a diagnosis of exclusion in a well, breast-fed baby
Hypothyroidism
Sepsis , e.g. urinary tract infection

Table 7.8 Causes of prolonged conjugated jaundice (cholestasis)

Severe haemolytic disease
Urinary tract infection
Neonatal hepatitis
Biliary atresia
Galactosaemia
Cystic fibrosis
Tyrosinaemia

unconjugated bilirubin is greater than 255 μmol/l (15 mg/100 ml); the jaundice persists beyond 10 days; or the conjugated bilirubin is greater than 34 μmol/l (2 mg/100 ml) (Tables 7.5, 7.6, 7.7 and 7.8).

Treatment

If no underlying cause demands treatment, the main objective is to prevent kernicterus. If the plasma bilirubin is rising rapidly and may approach toxic levels, the baby should be treated with phototherapy. Light at a wavelength of 450 nm degrades unconjugated bilirubin in the skin to water-soluble substances which can be excreted in the bile. If, despite phototherapy, the plasma bilirubin approaches toxic levels, exchange transfusion provides a reliable way of lowering the bilirubin level. In many neonatal units, the exchange level for term infants is 340 μmol/l unconjugated bilirubin.

NEONATAL RESPIRATORY DISTRESS

The clinical signs of respiratory distress are tachypnoea (rate over 60/min), expiratory grunting, nasal flaring, cyanosis in air, and sternal, subcostal, intercostal or supraclavicular recession on inspiration. There are numerous possible causes (Table 7.9).

Hyaline membrane disease

In hyaline membrane disease (HMD) there is a deficiency of surfactant, a complex phospholipid which reduces surface tension and thus prevents collapse of small airways. HMD is associated with preterm delivery and asphyxia. In affected babies, progressive collapse of small airways occurs and

Table 7.9 Differential diagnosis of neonatal respiratory distress

---

Pulmonary causes
   hyaline membrane disease (respiratory distress syndrome)
   retained lung fluid (transient tachypnoea)
   meconium aspiration
   pneumonia
   pneumothorax
   diaphragmatic hernia
   hypoplastic lungs
   tracheo-oesophageal fistula
   congenital lobar emphysema
   lung cyst
Cardiac failure
Upper airway obstruction
Overheating
Anaemia or blood loss
Neurological damage (in the brain stem respiratory control
   centre)
Polycythaemia
Metabolic acidosis

---

the lungs are very stiff requiring increased work for breathing. Ventilation-perfusion mismatching and decreased alveolar ventilation results in progressive hypoxaemia and hypercapnoea. Chest X-ray shows a diffuse granularity throughout the lungs and an air bronchogram. Management consists of maintaining arterial PO_2 6.7–12.0 kPa (50–90 mmHg) and nutritional support until the lungs recover after about one week. Some babies can maintain an adequate arterial PO_2 by breathing a humidified air-oxygen mixture in a head box. In more severe cases, continuous positive airway pressure (CPAP) is required to keep small airways open. This can be delivered by face-mask, twin nasal cannulae, nasopharyngeal tube or endotracheal tube. Mechanical ventilation with positive end-expiratory pressure becomes necessary if CPAP fails to maintain adequate blood gases, if respiratory acidosis allows the pH to fall below 7.2 and if the baby becomes opnoeic. Frequent or continuous monitoring of arterial PO_2 or transcutaneous PO_2 is necessary to avoid brain damage from hypoxia or retrolental fibroplasia from hyperoxia.

Retained lung fluid

This can affect term or preterm infants particularly after Caesarean section. The chest X-ray shows fluid streaks radiating out from the hila and fluid in the lung fissures. Although oxygen may be required, the prognosis is good.

Asphyxiation

Asphyxiated fetuses may pass meconium and then gasp, thus inhaling meconium. Meconium is irritating to the lungs and may obstruct airways causing collapse or a ball-valve effect with distal air-trapping and the risk of pneumomediastinum. If a baby is born with meconium in the mouth, the larynx should be inspected and any meconium sucked out with as large a tube as possible. Chest X-ray shows coarse shadowing with overinflation, often with a pneumomediastinum.

Pneumonia

Group B streptococcal pneumonia may present a similar clinical and radiological picture to hyaline membrane disease. Death may occur within 12 hours. Factors favouring pneumonia would be a term infant, prolonged rupture of the membranes, maternal fever, foul smelling liquor or a low neutrophil count (below $1500/\mu l$). If this diagnosis is suspected, blood and a gastric aspirate should be taken for culture and ampicillin and gentamicin should be given.

INFECTION IN A NEONATE

Intrapartum and postnatal infection

Newborn infants are much more vulnerable to infection than are older children because they have very low levels of IgA and IgM, low levels of complement, and reduced bactericidal capacity in polymorphs. Ill and low birth-weight infants tend to be looked after together, 10, 20 or more in one unit, with opportunities for cross-infection between babies and acquired infection from staff. Infection may ascend to the fetus from the vagina if the membranes are ruptured for over 24 hours before delivery. Invasive procedures such as endotracheal intubation and umbilical vessel catherisation may provide a portal of entry for infection.

Because of the limited ability of neonates to localise infection, sepsis in one site is likely to become generalised with septicaemia and meningitis.

If a baby becomes ill with any of the features listed in table 7.10, sepsis should be considered.

Table 7.10 Clinical features of sepsis in neonates

Nurses concern about baby
'Going off feeds'
Fever (> 37.5°C rectal) or hypothermia
Vomiting
Apnoea
Tachypnoea
Jaundice
Lethargy
Convulsions
Purpura
Palpable spleen or kidneys

If the signs persist for 2 or 3 hours or more appear, it is often safest to take blood, urine and CSF for culture and start the baby on antibiotics. Ampicillin 100 mg/kg and gentamicin 2.5 mg/kg by i.m. or i.v. injection every 12 hours (Nelson & McCracken 1977) provide bactericidal blood levels against all likely neonatal bacterial pathogens (Table 7.11). Babies with sepsis may deteriorate rapidly and prompt treatment substantially improves the results.

Table 7.11 Neonatal infections

Intrapartum pathogens	
E. coli	
Group B streptococcus	
Listeria monocytogenes	generalised infection
Herpes simplex	
N. gonorrhoeae	
Chlamydia	conjunctivitis
Postnatal pathogens	
E. coli	
Klebsiella	
Pseudomonas	generalised infection
Group B streptococcus	
Staphylococcus aureus	septic skin lesions, omphalitis or generalised
Candida albicans	skin and mouth lesions

Purulent conjunctivitis

This may be due to *Neisseria gonorrhoeae*. Gram stain of pus can confirm this diagnosis. Treatment is urgent to prevent corneal damage and penicillin eye drops should be given every 15 minutes until the pus clears. Intramuscular penicillin 50 000 units 12 hourly is also necessary.

Urinary tract infection

UTI may be very insidious in neonates producing only poor weight gain or prolonged jaundice. Because of the difficulties in collecting uncontaminated urine, diagnosis of UTI should be made on suprapubic aspiration.

Gastroenteritis

Epidemics of diarrhoea and vomiting are fortunately rare in neonatal units but, Salmonella, Shigella, enteropathogenic *E. coli* and rotavirus can all spread easily from one baby to another. Management should be maintenance of fluid and electrolyte balance and isolation.

HYPOGLYCAEMIA

Hypoglycaemia (blood glucose below 1.1 mmol/l (20 mg/100 ml) is a potent cause of brain damage in infants (Table 7.12). The brain may be able to

Table 7.12 Infants at risk of hypoglycaemia

Small-for-gestational-age infants (particularly if fed only from the breast)
Infants of diabetic mother
Preterm infants not absorbing milk feeds
Infants with severe haemolytic disease
Asphyxiated infants
Hypothermia
Septicaemia

---

compensate temporarily for a low blood glucose if there is plenty of oxygen and alternative substrate, such as lactate or ketone bodies but, eventually, neurological abnormalities such as convulsions are likely. There is a high incidence (up to 50%) of permanent neurological damage in babies with symptomatic hypoglycaemia

All at-risk babies should have regular blood glucose screening with Dextrostix. If the reading is 1.4 mmol/l (25 mg/dl) or below, the blood glucose must be measured in the laboratory. If the baby appears neurologically abnormal, 1 g/kg of glucose should be given intravenously immediately, followed by a continuous intravenous infusion of 10 per cent glucose starting at 100 ml/kg daily. The rate and concentration of the intravenous glucose can then be adjusted in the light of repeated blood glucose estimations. Asymptomatic hypoglycaemia may be treated initially with frequent intragastric milk feeds, but if the blood glucose does not rise above 1.1 mmol/l (20 mg/dl) intravenous glucose should be used.

VOMITING

Nearly all babies regurgitate some milk at some time. Vomiting is abnormal if it is bile-stained, blood-stained or persistent. Bile-stained vomit (i.e. greenish) is likely to be due to intestinal obstruction at any level below the sphincter of Oddi. There may be atresia, stenosis or malrotation with volvulus of the small intestine or aganglionosis of the large gut (Hirschsprung's disease). Erect and supine X-rays of the abdomen may confirm obstruction by showing dilated loops of intestine with fluid levels.

Blood-stained vomit may be due to haemorrhagic disease but this should be preventable by the injection of all newborns with 1 mg vitamin K in the delivery room. An acute gastric erosion may cause a haematemesis. Swallowed maternal blood may be vomited by the baby but the adult haemoglobin can be distinguished because sodium hydroxide denatures maternal but not fetal haemoglobin. Persistent vomiting may be due to sepsis, neurological damage, hiatus hernia and, later in the neonatal period, adrenal hyperplasia and pyloric stenosis.

DIARRHOEA

Breast-fed infants may pass rather loose stools up to four to six times a day. In spite of this the babies look well and thrive. Diarrhoea is only a problem if watery stools are copious, frequent and cause weight loss. Gastroenteritis is the most likely cause. If the diarrhoea is bloody, then necrotising enterocolitis and a bleeding tendency are also possible. Green stools often worry parents but do not signify disease.

NEUROLOGICAL ABNORMALITIES

Spina bifida

Spina bifida may result in an open lesion of the spinal cord with disorganised nervous tissue and meninges forming a swelling in the lumbar area (myelomenigocele) or a closed lesion with a swelling of the meninges containing CSF overlying the spine (meningocele). In the case of myelomeningocele, spinal cord function is often absent at and below the lesion whereas it may be intact at and below a meningocele. A paediatric surgeon can close an open defect and remove a swelling but this does not restore spinal cord function, although further damage from infection and drying is prevented. In a severe lower thoracolumbar myelomeningocele, there may be total paralysis below the umbilicus with resulting dislocation of the hips and talipes equinovarus deformities of the feet. There may be dilatation of the bladder and ureteric reflux. Even with successful surgery, the patient is paralysed below the waist and incontinent of urine and stool. Spina bifida is often associated with a downward displacement of the medulla resulting in defective circulation and reabsorption of CSF. This causes CSF to accumulate inside the cerebral ventricles with resulting hydrocephalus. This can be treated by insertion of a ventricular catheter connected to a one-way valve and leading to the right atrium or peritoneal cavity. Many experienced paediatricians feel that babies with extensive spina bifida and hydrocephalus have no chance of an independent happy life even with multiple surgical procedures. For a review of these issues see Lorber (1972).

Focal paralysis

The commonest lesion is Erb's palsy caused by traction on the upper nerve trunk in the brachial plexus (C5,6). The deltoid, biceps and supinator muscles are weak and the arm lies pronated by the side of the trunk. The grasp is normal. Muscle strength usually returns over 1–3 weeks unless the nerve trunks have been avulsed.

Convulsions

(See Chapter 22) The causes of convulsions in the newborn are given in Table 7.13. EEG studies

Table 7.13 Causes of convulsions in the newborn

Birth asphyxia
Intracranial haemorrhage
Hypoglycaemia
Hypocalcaemia + hypomagnesaemia
Hyponatraemia
Meningitis
Maternal opiate withdrawal
Pyridoxine dependence
Cerebral malformations
Hyperammonaemia

have shown that subtle changes in eye movements and apnoea may be manifestations of seizure activity. However, a clinical diagnosis of convulsions in practical terms, means repetitive clonic movements with or without altered consciousness, respiratory changes or extensor rigidity.

The immediate management of convulsions is to clear the airway and give oxygen if required. Exclude hypoglycaemia as a possible cause and investigate the other possibilities as indicated. Phenobarbitone 15 mg/kg i.v. or paraldehyde 0.1 ml/kg with 200 units hyaluronidase i.m. (from a glass syringe) gives rapid anticonvulsant cover.

Hypotonia

A full-term infant has a considerable degree of flexor tone, will resist extension of all limbs and will not let the head flop backwards more than about 45 dg when lifed forwards from supine. Excessive head lag and limbs without flexor recoil indicate hypotonia. If the baby is hypotonic but alert with open eyes there is likely to be a muscle or anterior horn cell disease but if the baby is not alert, the possibilities include maternal sedative or analgesic drugs, sepsis, severe intracranial damage, or Down's syndrome.

Hypertonia

The neonatal brain reacts to various types of insult by producing extensor hypertonus. The neck extensors override neck flexion producing head retraction.

The limbs tend to be extended and adducted with feet crossed. The extensor tendon reflexes, such as the knee and ankle jerks, may be exaggerated and with sustained clonus. There may also be pathological irritability. Extensor hypertonus may occur with birth asphyxia , subarachnoid harmorrhage, hypoglycaemia, hypocalcaemia and raised intracranial pressure.

THE OBJECTIVES OF GOOD PERINATAL MEDICINE

Modern obstetrics and neonatal paediatrics has been strikingly successful in improving survival of babies and each year's mortality rate is usually lower than the last. There is now much emphasis on the prevention of handicap. The majority of children with cerebral palsy have had a perinatal mishap, most commonly preterm delivery, apnoea or birth asphyxia. Some children with mental retardation, epilepsy, deafness or blindness have perinatal causes for their handicap, such as hypoxia, hypoglycaemia, intraventricular haemorrhage, meningitis, kernicterus, gonococcal ophthalmia and retrolental fibroplasia. Good perinatal care can reduce these handicaps. Newborn infants in the UK are screened at one week for elevated blood levels of phenylalanine (phenylketonuria), tyrosine (tyrosinaemia) and, in some cities, thyroid stimulating hormone (hypothyroidism). Further handicap is prevented by the early treatment of these serious biochemical disorders.

The final objective of perinatal medicine is a happy and healthy family. Modern medicine need not drive a wedge between mother and baby. In the past, measures to prevent infection caused much separation of mothers and newborn infants and, in a few cases, made bonding difficult. Sensitive staff can promote the natural physical and emotional closeness of mother and baby even if the baby requires observation, investigation and treatment.

FURTHER READING

Brown R J K & Valman H B 1979 Practical neonatal paediatrics, 4th edn. Blackwell, Oxford, pp 14, 29

Dubowitz L M S, Dubowitz V & Goldberg C 1970 Clinical assessment of gestational age in the newborn infant. Pediatrics 77: 1–10

Fancourt R, Campbell S, Harvey D & Norman A P 1976 Follow-up study of small-for-dates babies. British Medical Journal 1 1435–1437

Hey E 1971 The care of babies in incubators. In: Hull D, Gairdner D (eds) Recent advances in paediatrics. Churchill Livingston, London, p 171

Lorber J 1972 Spina bifida cystica. Archives of Disease in Childhood 47 854–873

Matthew D J, Norman A P, Taylor B, Turner M W & Soothill J F 1977 Preventiion of eczema. Lancet 1: 321–324

McCracken G H & Nelson J D 1978 Antimicrobial therapy for newborns. Grune & Stratton, New York

8

Infant feeding and nutrition

A sound nutritional intake forms the basis of normal health, growth and development in childhood. As understanding of infant nutrition has increased, the technology required to manufacture sophisticated artificial milks has progressed rapidly. The range of formulations currently available reflects both the demand and the industry's continuing aim to match the elusive subtleties of human breast milk.

NUTRITIONAL REQUIREMENTS

The nutritional demands of the infant are unique. They are related to the requirements for growth,

Table 8.1 Approximate daily requirements of younger infants (0–5 months) for calories, protein and water

Water	125–150 ml/kg
Protein	1.9 g/100 kcal
Calories	100–110 kcal/kg (430–470 kJ)

Energy values of nutrients as kcal/g = protein 4, carbohydrate 4, fat 7 (1 kcal 4.2 kJ, 1 MJ 240 kcal).

Table 8.2 Advisable vitamin and mineral intakes daily in infants (per kg body wt)

Vitamins		Minerals	
A (retinol)	150 μg	Sodium	2–6 mmol
D	10 μg	Potassium	2–6 mmol
C	20 mg	Iron	5–10 mg
Thiamine	0.2 mg	Calcium	500 mg
Riboflavin	0.4 mg	Magnesium	20–25 mg
Niacin	5.0 mg	Phosphorous	150 mg
E	4.0 iu	Iodine	35–45 μg
K	15 μg	Copper	60 μg
Folic acid	50 μg		

homeostasis, and the maintenance of a high metabolic rate. A balanced diet is essential and must include water, protein, fats and carbohydrates with their associated energy, vitamins and minerals. The requirements necessary in infancy are given in Tables 8.1 and 8.2. They should be regarded as guidelines, since individuals vary in their efficiency of food utilisation, and the values given were calculated theoretically on the basis of the intake found necessary to avoid deficiencies and promote normal growth in healthy children.

Fats

Most fat is ingested in the form of triglycerides (triacylglycerols), that is glycerol molecules in which three hydroxyl groups have each been esterified with fatty acids. These fatty acids may be long, medium or short chain according to the number of carbon atoms contained in each molecule. One-half of the fatty acids in human milk are long chain (more than 12 carbon atoms); medium chain fatty acids (8–12 carbon atoms) are of interest since they are absorbed from the gut more readily. Fatty acids are also classified according to the number of unsaturated or double-bond linkages between the carbon atoms. Some of the polyunsaturated acids are not synthesised by the body and are essential in the diet, notably for prostaglandin production. These fatty acids include linoleic (18:2) arachidonic (20:4) and linolenic acids (18:3), vegetable fats are particularly rich sources. Other important constituents of fat are cholesterol and phospholipids. Cholesterol is the precursor of steroid hormones and bile acids, phospholipids are essential components of cell membranes and various other cellular components, and they play a part in the absorption and transfer of fatty acids.

Fat absorption is a multi-step process. In the intraluminal phase, lipolysis and emulsification of triglycerides occurs in the duodenum secondary to the action of pancreatic lipase which requires colipase and bile salts for optimum activity. Monoglycerides, free fatty acids, and glycerol are released and interact with bile salts to form micelles. Micelles are water soluble and are able to diffuse to the microvillous membranes of the intestinal epithelial cells to enter the mucosal phase of fat absorption. Fatty acid uptake is facilitated by a binding protein which is concerned with transport to the endoplasmic reticulum of the cells. Triglycerides are resynthesised there and chylomicrons are formed in association with apoproteins. The final phase of absorption is the passage of these chylomicrons into the mesenteric lymphatics and to the portal venous system.

Carbohydrates

Carbohydrates provide the major source and bulk of calories in the diet. The disaccharide, lactose, containing the monosaccharides glucose and galactose forms the major carbohydrate in milk. Cereals contain sucrose (glucose and fructose) and the starches, which are complex carbohydrates consisting of glucose units linked into dextrins and amylopectin. Carbohydrates also constitute an energy store in the form of glycogen, another polysaccharide of glucose. It should be noted that the major sites of glycogen storage are the liver and muscle which, in the infant, represent only a fraction of the adult reserves.

The intraluminal phase of carbohydrate digestion commences in the mouth with the action of salivary amylase on starch. Amylase is also secreted by the pancreas. Enterocyte brush border disaccharidases are then responsible for the mucosal digestion of lactose, maltose and sucrose. Glucose and galactose are absorbed by active transport systems, some of which are sodium dependent; fructose does not share the same mechanisms.

Proteins

Proteins provide nitrogen as well as calories. They contain amino acids linked by CO-NH bonds into long peptide chains. Eleven amino acids, at least, cannot be synthesised by the newborn and are essential in the diet. These include histidine, tyrosine and cystine, in addition to those necessary to avoid a negative nitrogen balance in adults, which are isoleucine, leucine, lysine, methionine, phenylalanine, threonine, tryptophane and valine. The structural proteins of the body can only be formed when the correct balance of amino acids is available. A high quality protein is one which supplies all the essential amino acids in sufficient amounts to fulfil the requirements for body maintenance and growth. Such proteins are said to have a high biological value. The balance between grams of amino acid nitrogen in the diet and non-protein calories is also critical, since the energy supply available forms a limiting factor to their efficient metabolism.

Protein digestion is initiated in the stomach by a group of proteases which are activated from precursor pepsinogens. The polypeptides released stimulate cholecystokinin and secretin which promote pancreatic enzyme secretion, and also enterokinase activity from the intestinal brush border membrane. The enzymes released include trypsin, chymotrypsin, elastase, the carboxypeptidases and aminopeptidases. There are several different transport mechanisms for the products of intestinal hydrolysis. Uptake of dipeptides and tripeptides occurs and is quite distinct from amino acid transport systems.

Water, minerals and vitamins

Water is second only to oxygen as a necessity for life and is even more important to babies than to older children. It represents 70 to 75 per cent of their body weight; the intake volumes required are high and are also related to caloric consumption and the kidney's limited ability to conserve water in infancy.

The major minerals necessary include sodium, potassium, calcium, iron, phosphorus and magnesium. Many trace elements are also recognised to be essential, these include iodine, copper, manganese, zinc, cobalt, molybdenum, selenium, chromium, tin, vanadium, fluorine, silicon and nickel. Vitamins A, D and C are of particular importance since supplementation is required. The vitamin B complex, vitamin E and folic acid must also be available.

GASTROINTESTINAL FUNCTION DURING INFANCY

Many aspects of gastrointestinal function are less well developed in the newborn than in the older infant and child. Gastric acid and pepsin activity are reduced in preterm neonates. Tryptic activity in duodenal juice and pancreatic lipase levels are low and increase rapidly after birth. Bile acid concentrations in the duodenum are often below the level required for micelle formation; this may be an important factor in the newborn's lesser ability to absorb fats. The activities of brush border sucrase and maltase increase during gestation and reach maximal activity by the eighth month, whereas lactase concentration increases close to term.

MILK FEEDING

Human Milk

Most of the normal nutritional requirements for the young infant are provided in breast milk. The advantages of human milk over cows milk mean that whenever possible mothers should be encouraged to breast feed. Even a period as brief as 2 weeks has been shown to be valuable, although ideally breast feeding should be continued for the first 4–6 months of life.

The advantages of breast milk include:

1. Its chemical composition. This differs from cow's milk, see Table 8.3 and below.
2. It is sterile, cheap and attractively packaged.
3. It does not contain proteins which will provoke allergic reactions.
4. It encourages a bowel flora favouring lactobacilli and discouraging *Escherichia coli*.
5. It contains antibodies and immunocompetent cells which are important in the development of the infant's immune system.
6. The intimacy of breast feeding promotes bonding with the infant.
7. Metabolic disorders in the newborn such as hypocalcaemia and hypernatraemia are less common.
8. Certain conditions such as gastroenteritis, eczema and cot death occur less frequently.

There are few contra-indications to breast feeding; these are essentially confined to serious health problems in the mother. Acute or chronic maternal illess may impair the supply of milk, in which case supplementary feeds will be required to achieve satisfactory growth. A breast abscess may infect the milk with staphylococci or other organisms and is an indication for at least temporary artificial feeding. Active open tuberculosis is a contra-indication until the infant is immunised; this is often done with isoniazid-resistant BCG and the baby is also given a protective course of isoniazid. Nearly all drugs ingested by the mother can be assumed to be excreted into the milk to some extent. Most antibiotics, salicylates, antihistamines and barbiturates are clinically insignificant to the infant in the concentrations commonly found. Breast feeding should be discouraged if the mother needs to take phenindione, lithium, antithyroid or antimitotic drugs. Specific information should be sought about new or unusual drugs.

In the baby, immaturity, illness or anatomical abnormalities such as cleft palate may impair sucking, necessitating the administration of expressed breast milk. Infants with certain metabolic disorders, such as phenylketonuria or galactosaemia will deteriorate if dietary modifications are not carried out. Neonatal jaundice associated with an icterogenic factor in breast milk has been described, its existence is, however, controversial and breast milk jaundice must be regarded as rare. Even when it is suspected, only a temporary period of artificial feeding will be required.

Artificial Milks

The differences in chemical composition which exist between human and cow's milk are shown in

Table 8.3 Composition of human, cow's milk and a demineralised whey formula (per litre)

		Human	Cow	Demineralised whey
Calories	(MJ)	2.9	2.7	2.8
Protein	(g)	11	35	15
Fat	(g)	38	37	36
Lactose	(g)	68	49	72
Sodium	(mmol)	7	22	6
Calcium	(mg)	340	1170	420
Phosphorus	(mg)	140	920	330
Iron	(mg)	1.5	1.0	12.7
Vitamin A	(μg)	570	400	790
Vitamin C	(mg)	43	11	43
Vitamin D	(μg)	0.1–2.5	0.1–1.0	1.1

Table 8.3. Cow's milk contains more curd protein and the mineral content is higher, while the levels of polyunsaturated fatty acids and the lactose concentration are lower. Ordinary pasteurised cow's milk (doorstep milk) is thus unsuitable for feeding newborn infants. Evaporated milk has the advantage that if unopened it will keep for months in liquid form without refrigeration. During processing the fat globules have been homogenised and this contributes to a reduction in casein curd formation. The sugar content is unchanged and dilution must be carried out before use. This preparation is however little used in this country. Condensed milk has a high concentration of sucrose added to it and is generally unsuitable for infants.

Early approaches to modifying cow's milk included reducing the protein content by simple dilution with water, increasing the carbohydrate concentration by adding sucrose, or removing the fat as in skimmed milk, a by-product of butter manufacture. Iron and vitamins were then added.

There are currently three major modifications which are made to cow's milk to bring its composition closer to that of breast milk. These are the added carbohydrate, substituted fat and demineral-ised whey formulae (Table 8.4). Any one of these milks is suitable for infant feeding.

The addition of carbohydrate dilutes the protein content and reduces the concentration of phosphate, sodium and other minerals, which would otherwise represent a high solute load and predispose the infant to hypocalcaemia or hyperosmolar states. The carbohydrate added may be maltidextrin, which reduces the increased osmolar load on the gut caused by supplementary lactose or sucrose or, alternatively, fat and lactose may be added.

The substituted fat or filled milks substitute a mixture of vegetable and animal fats for cow's milk fat and aim to mimic the polyunsaturated fatty acid composition of human milk. The theoretical advantages of this approach have yet to be confirmed in infants and their use necessitates various other manipulations to the formulations, such as the addition of vitamin E, during manufacture.

Demineralised whey formulae contain much lower concentrations of the less well digested curd protein, casein. Whey is demineralised by electrodialysis and then minerals, vegetable oils, lactose and a small amount of skimmed milk are added. It is, therefore, a highly modified preparation.

The choice of an artificial formula for a normal baby can be any of the milks discussed above. The final decision will depend on availability and price as much as on nutritional factors.

Special Milk Formulae

Most infants thrive well on breast milk or the commercially available artificial milks. Despite this, there are many parents who become dissatisfied with some aspect of their baby's behaviour, such as his mood, stool character or sleeping pattern, and then attribute the problem to the milk given. There is a temptation to change the formula used quite empirically. This practice should be

Table 8.4 Modified cow's milk formulae

Added carbohdyrate	Substituted fat	Demineralised whey
Cow & Gate Baby Milk Plus	Cow & Gate V Formula	Cow & Gate Premium
Ostermilk Complete Formula	SMA	Gold Cap SMA
	Milumil	Osterfeed

Table 8.5 Artificial feeds for infants: Comparison of infant formulae with breast milk and cow's milk (Breast feeding should normally be encouraged; if formula feeding is necessary infants should be given a modified artificial milk which is nutritionally similar to human milk. These milks are sometimes known as 'low solute' or 'humanised' milks. It may be beneficial to continue with a modified formula up to one year rather than change to cow's milk)

Composition per 100 ml*	Kcal	Protein (g)	Fat (g)	CHO (g)	K+ (mmol)	Na+ (mmol)	Ca+ (mg)	P (mg)	Fe (mg)
Cow's milk	65	3.3	3.8	4.1	3.83	2.17	120	95	0.05
Human milk — transitional	67	2.0	3.7	6.9	1.74	2.1	25	16	0.07
— mature	69	1.3	4.1	7.2	1.49	0.6	34	14	0.07
Modified artificial milks									
Gold Cap (Wyeth)	65	1.5	3.6	7.2	1.44	0.65	45	33	0.67
SMA/S₂₆ Nan (Nestlé)	66	1.6	3.4	7.3	1.46	0.83	50	34	0.8
Osterfeed (Farley Health)	68	1.45	3.82	6.97	1.5	1.0	46	31	0.65
Premium (Cow & Gate) — ready to feed	65	1.8	3.45	6.9	1.54	0.78	48	31	0.65
— reconstituted from powder	68	1.5	3.8	7.2	1.49	0.69	40	27	0.65
Similac PM 60/40 (Ross)	68	1.57	3.54	7.57	1.54	0.87	40	20	0.26
Nenatal — premature formula (Rousell)	76	1.8	4.5	7.2	2.4	2.6	100	50	0.8
Prematalac — premature formula (Cow & Gate)	79	2.4	5.0	6.6	2.03	1.3	67	53	0.65
Improved Formula (Farley Health)	62	1.8	2.4	8.3	2.21	1.17	65	53	0.65
Ostermilk — 2	68	1.9	3.1	8.4	1.79	1.3	71	55	0.7
Milumil (Milupa)	65	1.7	2.6	8.6	2.28	1.22	61	49	0.65
Ostermilk Complete (Farley Health)	65	1.9	3.5	6.9	1.9	1.1	66	53	0.65
Plus (Cow & Gate)	65	1.5	3.6	7.			56	44.5	0.67
SMA (Wyeth)	68	1.55	3.61	7.23			51	39	1.2
Similac with Iron (Ross)	68	1.55	3.61	7.23			51	39	39
Similac (Ross)									Trace

Notes (right-hand column):

For the humanised group (Gold Cap, SMA/S₂₆ Nan, Osterfeed, Premium, Similac PM 60/40): These milks have a correlated casein-whey ratio such that the amino acid composition is nearer to human milk. The milks contain mainly blends of butter, fat and vegetable oils with lactose as the source of CHO. The milks are fortified with vitamins and minerals, except Similac PM 60/40 which requires Fe supplement

For the modified whole-milk group: Modified milks based on whole milk with added vitamins and minerals. CHO may be lactose or lactose + maltose/amylose. Based on whole milk protein — needs Fe supplement

*Figures from *The Composition of Foods* 4th ed. Paul & Southgate

Table 8.6 Specialised infant formulae and products used in paediatrics (These products should only be used as directed by specialist medical and dietetic advisors)

Name	Manufacturer	Source of nutrients	Supplements needed especially when used as only source of nutrition	Indications for use and further consideration
Lactose-free formulae				
A1 110	Nestlé	Purified casein, cream, corn oil, glucose, vitamins and minerals	Complete formula	Lactose intolerance/galactosaemia. As unmodified formulae special dilution/additives advisable for infants under 6 months to meet individual requirements
Galactomin 17 and Galactomin 18 (reduced fat)	Cow & Gate	Partially demineralised casein, coconut and maise oils, glucose, same vitamin and minerals	Cow & Gate vitamin & mineral tablets (contain trace of sucrose) + source of vitamins A & D	
Galactomin 19 (fructose formula)	Cow & Gate	Partially demineralised casein, coconut and maise oils, fructose, some vitamins and minerals	Sucrose free complete vitamin & trace element supplement	Glucose-galactine intolerance. Unmodified formula for feeding special dilution/additives for infants under 6 months to meet individual requirements
Isomil	Ross	Soya protein isolate, methionine, coconut and soy oil, corn syrup, sucrose vitamins and minerals	Iron	Cows milk protein for lactose intolerance galactosaemia
Formula S	Cow & Gate	Soya protein isolate & methionine, glucose syrup, vegetable oil, vitamins and minerals	Complete formula	As above. Also sucrose free
Prosobee powder	Mead Johnson	Soya protein isolate & methionine, corn syrup solids, coconut and corn oils, vitamins and minerals	Complete formula	Cow's milk protein intolerance +/or lactose intolerance. Galactosaemia, sucrose free
Prosobee liquid	Mead Johnson	Soya protein isolate & methionine, corn syrup solids, soya and coconut oils, vitamins and minerals	Complete formula	As above
Wysoy	Wyeth		Complete formula	As above
Velactin	Wander	Soya flour & methionine, glucose syrup, dextrose soya & arachis oil, vitamins and minerals	Complete formula	Cow's milk protein +/or lactose intolerance. Presence of galactosides contra-indicative of use for treatment of galactosaemia in infancy. Soya flour contains sucrose
Pregestimil*	Mead Johnson	Enzymatically hydrolysed casein, + tyrosine, cystine & tryptophan, corn syrup solids, modified tapioca starch, corn oil, MCT oil, soya lecithin, vitamins and minerals	Complete formula unless severe steatorrhoea or other malabsorption exists	'Elemental' formula used in malabsorption problems including intractable diarrhoea, steatorrhoea intestinal resection, sensitivity to instant protein, lactose +/or sucrose intolerance. Pancreatic insufficiency (CF)

Table 8.6 (continued)

Name	Manufacturer	Source of nutrients	Supplements needed especially when used as only source of nutrition	Indications for use and further consideration
Nutramigen*	Mead Johnson	Enzymatically hydrolysed casein (low in cystine), sucrose, modified tapioca starch, corn oil, vitamins and minerals	As above	Unmodified formula for use in malabsorption problems (particularly for abnormalities) including biliary obstruction, pancreatic insufficiency, intestinal resection, lactose intolerance
MCT (1)*	Cow & Gate	Partially washed casein, glucose syrup, MCT oil, some vitamins and minerals	Cow & Gate vitamin, vitamin & mineral tablets (contain trace sucrose) + source of vitamins A & D	Unmodified formula, very low in cystine and devoid of essential fatty acids and may require sodium supplement. More suited for older infants with fat abnormalities and can be used in treatment of intestinal lymphangiectasis and chylothorax
MBF (meat base formula)*	Gerber	Beef hearts, cane sugar, sesame oil, modified tapioca starch, vitamins & minerals	Complete formula unless severe malabsorption exists	Hypo-allergenic liquid formula used in treatment of cow's milk intolerance, milk-induced steatorrhoea
Comminuted chicken meat*	Cow & Gate	A dispersion in water of finely ground chicken meat	Requires added CHO and fat of choice with complete vitamin & mineral supplements	A modified infant fromula can be prepared by appropriate dilution and additives for use in malabsorption states including intractable diarrhoea, cow's milk protein intolerance, CHO intolerances according to CHO added, steatorrhoea, intestinal resection
Albumaid hydrolysate complete	Scientific Hospital Supplies	Hydrolysed beef serum with some added vitamins and minerals	Requires source of CHO, fat, vitamins & minerals according to individual requirements	Adaptable for use in malabsorption syndromes particularly where there is failure to absorb whole protein

* These formulas can, theoretically, be used for infants with lactose intolerance, but it would be more appropriate to use a modified lactose-free formula based on cow's milk protein or soya-based formula as these are less expensive

Table 8.7 Products used in mineral abnormalities

Edosol — minimal sodium formula	Cow & Gate	Partially demineralised casein, lactose, coconut & maize oils, some vitamins	Cow & Gate vitamin and mineral tablets & source of vitamins A & D	Development of low solute artificial feeds has mainly replaced occasion to use such a low sodium feed. As unmodified milk special dilution/additives advisable for young infant and used with extreme care with constant biochemical follow up of infant sodium levels.
Locasol — low calcium formula	Cow & Gate	Partially demineralised casein, lactose, coconut and maize oils, some vitamins and minerals	Cow & Gate vitamin and mineral tablets and source of vitamin A. Vitamin D is frequently required	Unmodified formula used in treatment of hypercalcaemia

Table 8.8 Products used in disorders of amino acid metabolism

Disorder	Product	Manufacturer	Amino acid(s) lowered in product
Phenylketonuria	Minafen	Cow & Gate	Phenylalanine
	Albumaid XP	Scientific Hospital Supplies (SHS)	
	Lofenalae	Mead Johnson	
	Aminogram	Allen & Hanbury	
	Cymogram	Allen & Hanbury	
	PKU Aid	SHS	
	Maxamaid XP	SHS	
Maple syrup urine disease	MSUD Aid	SHS	Branched chain amino acids
Homocystinuria	Albumaid (methionine low)	SHS	Methionine
Cystinosis	Albumaid (cystine low)	SHS	Cystine
Histidinaemia	Albumaid (histidine low)	SHS	Histidine
	Formula HF (2)	Cow & Gate	
Tyrosinosis	Maxamaid XP	SHS	Phenylalanine, tyrosine

All products require supplements of natural protein or L-amino acids and most require suitable source of energy with vitamin and mineral supplements. Specification of all products and nutritional guidelines vary from county to county

discouraged and replaced by appropriate counselling of the parents. Specialised milk feeds should only be used to treat specific conditions. The use of elimination diets may lead to an inadequate general nutrition if care is not taken. Cow's milk protein allergy is unusual although often suspected; lactose intolerance is more common but is usually short-lived and it is seen if brush border damage to the small bowel mucosa has occured such as after gastroenteritis. These conditions and the use of special formulae are discussed in Chapter 14. The formulations available are shown in Table 8.5–8.8. The changes involve the replacement of lactose with other carbohydrates, the replacement of cow's milk protein with casein hydrolysates or soya protein to render the milk hypo-allergenic, and the modification of the fat content to include medium-chain triglycerides. The latter milks are readily absorbed in the absence of pancreatic enzymes and bile salts. Some of these milks, require the addition of mineral and vitamin mixtures. It is important to note that the use of these formulae may, in fact, mean several changes in the diet, for instance, many of the cow's milk protein-free products are also lactose free. If goat's milk is given, folic acid supplements are required.

FEEDING PRACTICES

Breast Feeding

The success of lactation depends on both physical and emotional preparation, generally begun in pregnancy. Cracked or inverted nipples reduce the chances of success, while the physiology of lactation can be affected by the mother's emotions. An actively sucking infant enhances both the secretion and ejection of milk; the hormone prolactin promotes secretion of milk and oxytocin the ejection of milk by the let-down reflex.

Breast feeding should begin at birth or shortly after. The breast should subsequently be offered on demand and at least every 3–4 hours with suckling at both breasts for as long as the mother wishes. Advice which suggests restricting the time or frequency of suckling reduces the chances of successful breast feeding. A newborn baby at about 6 days may often feed 12–14 times a day. A normal newborn baby does not need routine supplements of water or artificial milk.

Attention must be paid to maternal hygiene and nutrition, and the advice and encouragement given regarding details of technique and expected newborn behaviour.

Bottle feeding and Introduction of Solids

Milk powders must be reconstituted in a sterile fashion according to the manufacturer's instructions. The total volume of milk offered per day is calculated from the infant's expected weight. An average amount is 150 ml/kg divided into five or six feeds, giving an energy intake of 462 kJ/kg. As the infant gets older the calorie requirement falls to 420 kJ/kg. After the age of 4 months the nutritional requirements for optimal growth cannot be supplied by milk alone; as the infant becomes heavier the volume of milk that would be required

become less manageable. The first solid food to be introduced is usually a cereal, which in Europe is usually wheat or rice-based with added iron and vitamin D. By the age of 6 months or so most children are developmentally ready to chew solids as distinct from taking thickened feeds. They begin to start drinking from a cup and various diluted fruit juices may be introduced. The variety of solids soon needs to be increased to provide the essential components of the diet. Most babies take to a new food readily if it is given in teaspoon amounts initially.

New food additions should be made gradually. Many manufacturers produce strained foods for the younger infant and less finely divided foods for the older child. When mixed feeding is well established doorstep milk may replace powdered milk. At around one year a liquidised mixed adult diet is usually adequate; this is given three to four times a day with up to 600 ml of milk daily. Providing the child is thriving, accurate dietary assessments are usually not necessary. By 18 months most children are anxious to feed themselves and puréed meals have given way to cut-up and minced foods. Most parents start introducing finely chopped foods from about 9 months.

Vitamin and Mineral Supplements

Vitamins supplements are recommended for breast-fed infants. The British DHSS vitamin drops contain vitamins A, C and D (0.2 ml or 7 drops, contain 300 µg of vitamin A, 30 mg of vitamin C and 10 µg of vitamin D). Supplementation is not usually essential for babies given formula feeds since these are fortified, but become necessary when doorstep milk is given. Additional folic acid may be required in some preterm infants. Deficiency of the B complex vitamins is rarely encountered in Europe and specific supplementation is not given. Vitamin E and K deficiencies are occasionally seen in neonates.

It is uncommon for mineral deficiencies other than iron to develop spontaneously. Calcium, phosphorus and magnesium are well provided for in most milks. The normal child does not require trace element supplements, although their importance has been emphasised following the use of synthetic diets for the treatment of inborn errors of metabolism, the development of intravenous nutrition, and the recognition of the hazards of environmental pollution.

FEEDING PROBLEMS

Refusal to suck, slow weight gain, continual crying, vomiting and colic are all common problems in infants and often cause great anxiety to their parents. In the vast majority of cases there is no underlying infection, metabolic, cardiac or respiratory abnormality, although these should always be considered. The first observation must be to watch the mother feeding her baby. Simple mechanical problems such as a small or blocked teat, or engorged breasts may be corrected, while errors of technique such as allowing the baby to swallow excessive amounts of air may become obvious. Under-feeding and over-feeding must be recognised, the former being more common in breast-fed, and the latter in bottle-fed babies. Test feeding the breast-fed baby and then weighing him before and after may not give an answer, since individual feeds are so variable in quantity. Monitoring for a 24-hour period may be necessary. The effect of a mother's anxiety or depression on her baby's behaviour should not be underestimated. Sympathetic discussion and follow-up is often fruitful.

Food refusal is a normal phase in many toddlers. Ignoring it is the treatment of choice lest it becomes an attention-seeking device thereby provoking anger, bribery or even violence in the parents. The paediatrician should demonstrate that, despite the most alarming history, the child is pursuing a relentless course along the appropriate height and weight centile lines.

The older pre-school child who has a small appetite may also cause concern. It should be appreciated that the rapid growth rate of infancy declines in the 3–5-year-old with a proportionate decrease in calorie requirements and hence appetite. If the parents have an unrealistic demand for food intake and their child takes the offensive, meal times may be transformed into a battleground of opposing wills. Parents should be aware that the pre-school child's appetite will reduce, and the child should be encouraged into an active life-style

avoiding an excessive intake of milk, carbohydrates, and between-meal snack foods.

WEIGHT GAIN

The Underweight Child

Weight gain normally averages 20 g per day for the first 5 months of life, and approximately 15 g per day for the remainder of the first year. The full-term infant will thus usually have doubled the birth weight by 5 months and tripled it by one year of age. The small or thin child is not necessarily failing to grow. Birth weight and genetic factors must be taken into account. Weight loss or failure to gain weight consistently, should be taken seriously and investigated thoroughly if the cause is not immediately obvious. The commoner causes are discussed in detail elsewhere but will broadly fall into those listed in Table 8.9.

Table 8.9 General causes of failure to thrive in infancy

Deficiency energy intake	Increased catabolism
inadequate feeds	infections
feeding difficulties	urinary
faulty preparation,	respiratory
poverty,	malignancy
poor parent-child	
relationship	
local, oral or	
upper respiratory	
abnormalities,	
mental retardation	
Excess energy loss	**Miscellaneous**
vomiting	metabolic disorders
hiatus hernia	congenital abnormalities
malabsorption	emotional deprivation
coeliac disease	

The Overweight Child

Obesity is the commonest nutritional disorder of children in wealthy countries. It is a matter of concern because of the high proportion of overweight children who become obese adults, and the high morbidity of the condition in later life. The definitions used are arbitrary, but clearly, any infant whose rate of weight gain greatly exceeds height velocity is at risk, particularly if the parents are also overweight.

The pathogenesis is multifactorial, involving both genetic, environmental and psychological factors. Endocrine disturbances are unusual. The evidence that early nutritional experiences in man effect cellularity and hence body weight is still debated. Recently, it has been found that obese people show an unusually small increase in metabolic rate in response to many stimuli such as food, cold and thyroxine. It is suggested that they store ingested fat as triglyceride in their expanding fat stores, rather than dissipating it as heat. The tissue responsible for the thermogenesis induced by dietary fat is thought to be brown adipose tissue, which is found not only in babies, but also in the para-aortic, renal and perirenal fat depots of adults.

There is no doubt that the fat infant is at a disadvantage. He suffers more respiratory infections and is less mobile than his normal weight contemporary. Feeding practices should limit bland carbohydrates and desserts and other high calorie infant foods. It may be necessary to ask the whole family to change its eating habits and become involved in energy-expending activities if the recalcitrant 5 year old is to successfully lose weight.

NUTRITIONAL DEFICIENCIES

Vitamin D Deficiency (Rickets)

Nutritional rickets is a disorder of adequate mineralisation of bones during rapid growth. It may be prevented by ensuring an appropriate intake of vitamin D (10 µg or 400 iu per day) and of calcium. Pathogenesis depends on altered or decreased endocrine action of 1,25 dihydroxycholecalciferol $(1,25(OH)_2D)$ on the gut, bone and kidneys. The long recognised association of lack of sunlight with rickets is explained by the poor synthesis of cholecalciferol (vitamin D_3) in the skin together with decreased ingested ergocalciferol (vitamin D_2). Vitamin D_2 and D_3 undergo 25-hydroxylation $(25(OH)D)$ in the liver, and a further hydroxylation in the kidney to give the active form $1,25(OH)_2D$. Studies or nutritional rickets of

pigmented ethnic groups, who have a higher incidence of nutritional rickets in the UK than do the indigenous population, have suggested that the skin is probably a more important source of 25 $(OH)D$ than the diet.

Clinical Features

Rickets is characterised clinically by abnormalities in those bones which are undergoing active growth. In the infant, the skull vault bones become thin and softened (craniotabes), and later thickened (bossed), while the long bones and rib ends become broadened; the wrists are swollen and the costochondral junctions show a rickety rosary. As the child sits up the spine and pelvis become deformed and as he starts to walk the tibiae begin to bow and short stature becomes apparent. Motor development may be delayed as a result of generalised muscle hypotonia.

Investigation and Management

Radiological changes include demineralisation of the long shafts and cupping and fraying of the ends of long bones with widening of the epiphyseal plate. The biochemical changes depend on the extent of vitamin deficiency and the degree of secondary hyperparathyroidism. There is, in general, a rise in plasma alkaline phosphatase and a fall in phosphorus with normal or low serum calcium concentrations.

Neither human or cow's milk contain sufficient vitamin D_2, so most artificial milks are fortified. Breast-fed and older infants established on doorstep mild should begin oral vitamin supplements.

Rickets may be treated with 250 µg of vitamin D_2 daily. If healing is not initiated within one month, further investigation of renal and gastrointestinal function is required. An excessive intake of vitamin D_2 produces toxic effects such as vomiting, anorexia and failure to thrive with associated hypercalcaemia. This was a particular problem before the levels of vitamin D fortification of cow's milk were reduced; some patients, however, appear to be unduly sensitive to the vitamin.

Scurvy

The fact that scurvy is extremely rare in the UK should not obscure the importance of an adequate dietary intake of vitamin C (ascorbic acid) of 10 mg per day. Breast milk usually contains sufficient for the newborn unless the mother is on an inadequate diet. Cow's milk contains much less and a large proportion is destroyed on heating. The artificial milks now have adequate supplements. In the past daily fresh fruit juice was advised as a main source. In scurvy there is defective formation of mesenchymal intercellular ground substance. Fibroblasts, osteoblasts and odontoblasts are all affected.

Clinical features

Petechiae are seen, while bruising occurs readily, and pseudoparalysis results from subperiosteal haemorrhage and fractures. Symptoms appear between 6 and 12 months of age; the infants are pale, fretful, anorexic and feverish. The gum changes are similar to those seen in adults but are confined to areas where teeth have erupted. A hypochromic anaemia frequently develops.

Investigation and Management

The radiological features are characteristic, and include decalcification and atrophy of the bony trabeculae while leaving the denser cortical bone unaffected. The corners of the long bone ends pull away, epiphyseal displacement occurs and subperiosteal haematomas calcify. Measurement of plasma levels of ascorbic acid is often unhelpful, since there is a considerable normal variation. Daily treatment with oral vitamin C, 200 mg, gives rapid improvement.

Vitamin A Deficiency

The major sources of vitamin A (retinol) are animal tissues (e.g. liver) and milk. Precursors of the vitamin occur in carrots, dark green leaves, red palm oil, and wheat, but not rice. Its absorption is promoted by fats so that in situations where animal fat is rarely consumed deficiency is common. This is particularly seen in those rice-eating areas of the world which are nutritionally deprived. The main function of retinol is for the synthesis of visual purple (rhodopsin) in the retina. It is also essential for the integrity of epithelial tissues.

Clinical Features and Management

The earliest sign of vitamin A deficiency is night blindness, but this is rarely clinically evident in young children. More severe deficiency causes xerosis of the conjunctiva and Bitot's spots. These consist of grey, raised plaques of desquamated epithelial cells on the temporal conjunctiva. Xerosis causes haziness, thickness and drying of the eyes and leads to corneal scarring. It is the major preventable cause of blindness in the world. Keratomalacia requires urgent treatment with intramuscular water-miscible vitamin A (3000 ug/kg body weight) followed by an equivalent oral dose for 5 days, and then 1500 g daily until the eyes are normal. Associated protein energy malnutrition is common in such children.

Vitamin B Complex deficiency

Thiamine (B₁)

Thiamine is a coenzyme involved in the hexose-monophosphate shunt and in the decarboxylation of alpha-ketoacids. Deficiency particularly occurs in communities who eat parboiled rice. Its presentation is protean, beri-beri in infants can cause cardiac failure, pseudomeningitis or hoarseness due to laryngeal oedema or laryngeal nerve paralysis. Emergency treatment involves parenteral thiamine 50–100 mg, followed by maintenance 5–10 mg daily.

Nicotinic Acid (Niacin)

Nicotinic acid in the form of phosphorylated nicotinamide adenosine dinucleotide (NADP) is an essential coenzyme in many oxidation-reduction reactions. Deficiency is seen in maize-eating communities where it causes pellagra. This dermatosis is symmetrical and appears on exposed parts of the body. Mucocutaneous junctions are often fissured and sore while the tongue becomes red, swollen and painful. Diarrhoea and neurological changes may also be seen. Treatment with

20 mg/day oral niacin should be accompanied by a diet containing adequate tryptophan from milk, meat and eggs.

Riboflavin (B₂)

Riboflavin (B₂)

Riboflavin also forms part of coenzymes involved in oxidation-reduction reactions. It rarely causes an isolated deficiency but its absence is characterised by angular stomatitis, cheilosis and the appearance of a magenta colouration of the tongue. The usual dose used in treatment is 20 mg orally.

Iron deficiency

Neither breast milk nor cow's milk contains sufficient iron to meet nutritional needs after the age of 4–6 months. In the fetus, the greatest accummulation of iron occurs at the end of intrauterine life. During the first 2 months after birth there is a minimal requirement for iron due to the physiological decreases in the circulating red cell mass. From the second to sixth month, active haemoglobin synthesis begins. Preterm and low birthweight infants are, therefore, liable to develop iron deficiency later in infancy. Many milk formulae and infant cereals contain added iron and other important dietary sources include meat and green leaf vegetables such as spinach. It should be noted that the iron content of food does not correlate well with the iron available for absorption. Inorganic iron is absorbed better than food iron and ferrous salts more efficiently than ferric. Dietary phosphate and phytate reduce iron absorption.

The clinical features of iron deficiency are those of anaemia and are discussed in Chapter 19. Pallor is the most common sign and splenomegaly may occur. Cardiac failure complicates extreme cases. Haematological features include hypochromic microcytic red cells and a low ferritin concentration. Investigation must also exclude the possibility of blood loss, particularly from the gut. Treatment should be given using oral ferrous salts in a daily dose of 6 mg of elemental iron/kg.

MALNUTRITION

A prolonged period of inadequate nutritional intake, interacting with infection may precipitate protein energy malnutrition (PEM). The clinical presentation varies with the degree and duration of deprivation, the age of the individual concerned, and the effects of associated vitamin and mineral deficiencies. The spectrum of growth failure extends from marasmus to kwashiorkor, with mixed features of both extremes in some children. The onset is most common after weaning, between the ages of 9 months and 2 years. Recognition of current and past malnutrition is based on measurements of weight, height, mid-arm circumference, head circumference and skin fold thickness. Classification is related to the weight for age, weight for height and height for age. The clinical features of marasmus and kwashiorkor are discussed in Chapter 25.

Children with protein-energy malnutrition experience profound changes in both body composition and organ function. The total body water is increased with a proportionate rise in extracellular fluid. Protein catabolism is regulated independently of anabolism, the total body proten and especially muscle mass is reduced. Lipid accumulation in the liver, probably as a result of decreased synthesis of transport proteins, and the release of fatty acids from adipose tissue occurs. The total body fat is reduced unless the carbohydrate content of the diet has been high. Potassium is depleted more than other minerals with a disproportionate loss occurring in those patients with diarrhoea. Secondary changes in cellular metabolism are thus widespread. Gastrointestinal function is impaired as a result of reduced exocrine secretions, functional and morphological mucosal changes, and infection. Many of the endocrine glands are atrophic; concentrations of cortisol, growth hormone and thyroid stimulating hormone, however, are usually maintained or increased, although plasma insulin responses to glucose are low. Immune function, particularly cell-mediated immunity, is usually compromised. Gram-negative bacteria and viral infections are common but may exhibit few typical clinical signs on presentation.

Management

The management requires more than just nutritional rehabilitation. Electrolyte disturbances, dehydration, hypoglycaemia, infections, anaemia and hypothermia must all be corrected. Dehydration may be difficult to assess because of muscle wasting or oedema. Fluid overload may lead to cardiac failure in the presence of a low reserve in myocardial function, anemia, hypokalaemia, and a diminished glomerular filtration rate. In the absence of renal failure additional potassium is required as well as calcium and magnesium. Hypoglycaemia and hypothermia are easily overlooked and are often associated with a septicaemia which should be suspected and treated. Dietary treatment is complicated by the presence of diarrhoea and vomiting. Long-term intravenous therapy is rarely practical, oral/water and electrolyte solutions should be given and within 2 or 3 days increasing concentrations of milk administered. If carbohydrate intolerance is confirmed by finding that the stool water has a pH less than 6 and contains glucose, a lactose-free feed may be necessary. Vitamins A and D must be given and a mixed diet appropriate to the locality gradually introduced. Vitamin K should be given parenterally. Early iron supplementation has been shown to be associated with an increased incidence of infection and is is, therefore, usually commenced only when the general condition of the patient has started to improve.

In severe PEM normal vigour and growth may not be regained for many months. The long-term effects on growth and brain development are debated since the interaction between malnutrition and other environmental factors is complex. The unfavourable social circumstances which frequently accompany an inability to provide an adequate diet contribute materially to morbidity. On the other hand, there is no doubt that a foundation of good nutrition in the pre-school years enables a child to make the most of his environment and fulfil his potential for both physical and intellectual growth.

FURTHER READING

Arneil G C & Stroud C E 1978 Infant feeding. In: Forfar J O & Arneil G C (eds) Textbook of paediatrician, 2nd edn. Churchill Livingstone, Edinburgh, Ch 6, p 231

Fomon S J 1974 Infant nutrition, 2nd edn. Saunders, Philadelphia & London

McLaren D S & Burman D (eds) 1976 Textbook of paediatric nutrition. Churchill Livingstone, Edinburgh

Report on Health & Social Subjects No 9 1974 Present-day practice in infant feeding. HMSO, London

9

The handicapped child

A handicap is any impairment of function which prevents a person leading a full life. An impairment does not, however, necessarily consititute a handicap. Moderately poor vision, for example, may not hinder an academically-inclined child. The relationship between the impairment of function and the handicap it causes depends upon many factors including the impaired person's intelligence, his environment and the attitudes of others, especially those close to him. When assessing the handicapped it is important to consider separately the defect (e.g. cataracts), the impairment of function (poor vision) and the resulting handicap.

Associated abnormalities

In this chapter handicapping conditions are considered singly but it must be remembered that handicaps are often multiple. The presence of additional handicaps, which should be carefully sought in any one case, complicates management considerably, and even relatively minor additional handicaps can have a significant effect on overall function and developmental progress.

Emotional disturbance

In view of the difficulties faced by the handicapped and their families, the higher incidence of emotional and behaviour disturbance is not surprising. For the physically handicapped, especially those with spina bifida, adolescence is a difficult time. Continuing physical dependence at a time when young people are asserting their abilities and independence is hard to bear. One third or more of adolescents with spina bifida will show emotional disturbance, especially depression.

Emotional disturbance is equally common among the mentally retarded. The spectrum of disorders is not different from that found in the general population except among the severely retarded where autistic symptoms are commoner.

The multidisciplinary team

The range of problems presented by handicapped children is wide, covering many disciplines including paediatrics, orthopaedics, neurology, psychology, psychiatry, speech and physical therapies and social work. The needs of most handicapped children go beyond the limits of any one person's expertise and it has become common practice to adopt a team approach. A team assessment is time consuming, but there is often no other way to adequately assess the needs of a child and to plan a realistic and coordinated programme of management.

Early diagnosis

Neurological maturation, experience and practice operate together to produce rapid developmental progress in the first few years of life. The handicapped child will not be able to benefit from all these experiences. For example, the deaf child's learning of language will be impaired. The earlier these handicaps are recognised, and either corrected or circumvented, the less severe will be the developmental consequences. In addition to the immediate effects of handicapping defect, secondary effects can develop if appropriate help is not given. For example, a child with impaired speech may become withdrawn having repeatedly experienced failure in communication. These secondary effects can profoundly influence the child's behaviour and may become as detrimental as the original handicap.

Special education

The Warnock committee estimated that one in five or six children will require some form of special education provision during their school life. For the majority, this would consist of a period of

Table 9.1 Categories of handicapped children (England and Wales)

1. *Blind pupils:* Pupils who have no sight or whose sight is likely to become so defective that they require education by methods not involving the use of sight
2. *Partially-sighted pupils:* Pupils who by reason of defective vision cannot follow the normal regimen of ordinary schools without detriment to their sight or to their educational development, but can be educated by special methods involving the use of sight
3. *Deaf pupils:* Pupils with impaired hearing who require education by methods suitable for pupils with little or no naturally acquired speech or language
4. *Partially-hearing pupils:* Pupils with impaired hearing whose development of speech and language, even if retarded, is following a normal pattern, and who require for their education special arrangements or facilities though not necessarily all the educational methods used for deaf pupils
5. *Educationally subnormal pupils:* Pupils who, by reason of limited ability or other conditions resulting in educational retardation, require some specialised form of education wholly or partly in substitution for the education normally given in ordinary schools
6. *Epileptic pupils:* Pupils who by reason of epilepsy cannot be educated under the normal regime of ordinary schools without detriment to themselves or other pupils
7. *Maladjusted pupils:* Pupils who show evidence of emotional instability or psychological disturbance and require special educational treatment in order to affect their personal, social or educational readjustment
8. *Physically-handicapped pupils:* Pupils not suffering solely from a defect of sight or hearing who by reason of disease or crippling defect cannot, without detriment to their health or educational development, be satisfactorily educated under the normal regime of ordinary schools
9. *Pupils suffering from speech defect:* Pupils who on account of defect or lack of speech not due to deafness require special educational treatment
10. *Delicate pupils:* Pupils not falling under any other category in this regulation, who by reason of impaired physical condition need a change of environment or cannot, without risk to their health or educational development, be educated under the normal regime of ordinary schools.

From: the Handicapped Pupils and Special Schools Regulations 1959 as ammended

remedial help in one or more areas, usually given in normal schools. There is a much smaller group of children, at present about 1.5 per cent of all school children in England, who are educated in special schools because of the severity and extent of their handicaps. Special schools are classified under 10 headings (Table 9.1), although each school is unique in the spectrum of disabilities for which it caters.

The education act 1981

This Act seeks to improve the use of special educational resources; by legislation it strengthens good practice already in operation in many areas. The main changes in procedure introduced by the act include:

1. Statement of Special Educational Needs. Instead of seeking a school a child might best fit into, a comprehensive assessment leads to a statement of special educational needs. The change of emphasis from what is available to what is required is intended to make provision more sensitive to all of the child's requirements.

2. Assessment. Either the child's parents or the Education Authority can request an assessment which may lead to a statement if the child is found to have special educational needs.

3. Appeal. Legislation gives parents the right to make representations concerning an assessment, and to appeal against the contents of a statement or proposals (such as a school placement) arising from such a statement.

4. Statutary Provision of Special Education from Two Years of Age. From two years of age special education is available (but not compulsory) as of right. Previously provision was often made for children before the age of five years, but on a discretionary basis.

5. Duty to Inform. A Health Authority has a duty to inform the Education Authority of a child whom they believe may have special educational needs.

Talking to parents

The need for full and sympathetic explanation to parents of the implications of a child's handicap is obvious. The issues may be complex, requiring repeated explanations before they are grasped, but because the problem is a continuing one, and because the parents' role in management is so vital they cannot be left out. At many points there will be alternatives to chose and parents will often have a vital influence over these decisions.

Genetic counselling

The possibility of having another handicapped child is a vital issue for most parents. Where the exact cause of the handicap is known an informed recurrence risk can be given. Indeed, this is one of the main values of an exact diagnosis; in contrast with acute medicine where management and prognosis are based more upon the nature of the problem than its underlying cause. When the diagnosis remains imprecise (e.g. cerebral palsy, non-specific mental retardation) after reasonable attempts to discover the aetiology, an empirical recurrence risk can still be given.

Progressive disorders

The majority of handicapped children have suffered some specific insult, damaging the brain or body but, once caused, the damage does not progress. Despite their impairments these children are able to make developmental progress using their residual abilities. There is a smaller group of children who have not had one major insult, but who suffer progressive impairment (e.g. muscular dystrophy, Tay-Sach's disease), usually leading ultimately to death. These children are usually managed by a paediatric neurologist, but it is important for the doctor dealing with the handicapped to recognise such conditions when they present to him. Because of the inevitability of deterioration management goals are often limited with concentration on preservation of function for as long as possible.

VISUAL HANDICAP

The approximate prevalence of visual handicaps is shown in Table 9.2 and the causes of severe visual handicaps in Table 9.3.

In young children minor visual problems, such

Table 9.2 Prevalence of visual handicaps among children (per 1000)

Squint	30
Refractive error	50
Registered blind	0.25
Registered partially-sighted	0.3
Attending school for blind or partially-sighted	0.4

as squints, are usually detected during routine screening examinations; even in older children visual problems are often not recognised by the children themselves. Refractive errors can usually be substantially corrected.

Children with myopia tend to be more academically inclined than their peers. Squints may result

Table 9.3 Causes of severe visual handicap in children

Optic atrophy	secondary to perinatal insult
	inherited
Inherited retinal degenerations	
Ocular malformations	anophthalmia
	microphthalmia
	coloboma
	aniridia
Cataract	genetic
	prenatal rubella
	metabolic
	other
Postnatally acquired	infection ⎫ to either eye
	trauma ⎬ or brain
	other ⎭
Cortical blindness	perinatal insult
	prenatal infection
Perinatal insults	oxygen toxicity
	other
Retinoblastoma	
Glaucoma	
Severe refractive error	
Other	

in suppression of the image from the squinting eye (amblyopia), and it is important to prevent this by patching the good eye or surgery. By about 7 years of age the vision in the suppressed eye is unlikely to improve. Squints do not impair vision greatly, at least not in the better eye, but true binoccular vision is unlikely to develop, and subtle perceptual problems have been noted.

Definitions of blindness and partial sight

The usually quoted figures for blindness (an acuity of 6/60 or less in the better eye) and partial sight (an acuity of 6/24 or less in the better eye) are arbitrary and not entirely suitable when dealing with children. Even with an acuity of 6/60 a child may have useful residual vision, but the use of this residual vision depends as much upon the visual fields, eye movements and cortical processing of the visual input, as upon measured acuity. The developmental effects of visual impairment depend more on the near vision than that at 6 m. The definitions used for educational purposes are better in that, although imprecise, they are concerned with visual function rather than one aspect (acuity) of it.

Registration of blindness and partial sightedness (form BD8, normally completed by an ophthalmologist) is optional, but helps in obtaining certain benefits and services.

Developmental effects of severe visual handicap

The presence of severely impaired vision in a young child may be suspected on the grounds of an obvious ocular abnormality, the lack of visual fixation, abnormal eye movements, such as roving, coarse nystagmus, and the absence of optokinetic nystagmus.

Many severely visually handicapped children have developmental delays due to associated handicaps (Table 9.4), but among those who are otherwise normal their visual handicap has a profound effect upon developmental. Vision is one of the most important channels through which the child is informed about his environment, and it is vital in coordinating experiences. Thus, early development is delayed in all areas in children with severe visual impairment.

Table 9.4 Severe visual inpairment — associated handicaps

Severely subnormal	30%
Epilepsy	15%
Behavioural/emotional problem	13%
Deafness	10%
Cerebral palsy	6%

Management

Correction of refractive errors is important.

Residual vision

Where a child has some residual vision the value of this can be improved by training, increasing his awareness and understanding of what he does see.

Non-visual awareness

The severely visually handicapped child's use of other senses is initially poor because vision plays an important part in the development of these senses. Touch, sound and smell give only an incomplete picture of the world, unless the information is coordinated by vision. The use of the other senses can, nevertheless, be encouraged and will improve the child's ability to learn from his surroundings.

Specific developmental items

Blindness inhibits the development of some important skills and concepts such as manual exploration, sound localisation and object premanence. The lack of these can retard development, and specific training is often needed to overcome these delays.

Other

Feeding problems are common in blind children. Associated handicaps (Table 9.4) may also add a variety of difficulties.

Education

Many children with visual handicaps cope in normal schools, often with the assistance of low vision aids. Placement in a school catering specifically for children with visual handicaps will depend upon a variety of factors including intelligence, and the presence of other handicaps in addition to visual function. Very severe visual impairment renders reading of print impossible, or at least very inefficient and a tactile code (Braille) is used.

PRENATAL RUBELLA AND DEAF-BLINDNESS

The probability of congenital abnormalities following infection with rubella during pregnancy is high, at least 25 per cent if infection occurs within the first month of pregnancy. Multiple anomalies are common, and prenatal rubella is the commonest cause of severe combined deafness and visual handicap in children (Table 9.5), although deafness or pigmentary retinopathy may occur singly.

Table 9.5 Causes of severe deafness and visual handicap

Prenatal rubella
Other prenatal infections
  cytomegalovirus
  syphylis
Insults affecting optic and acoustic nerves (or organ of Corti)
  prematurity
  meningitis
  trauma
Inherited conditions affecting both senses
  Usher syndrome (deafness with retinitis pigmentosa)
  other

Features of prenatal rubella

Deafness

This is sensorineural although there may be an additional conductive component. Deafness may appear or progress after birth.

Heart defects

Persistent patent ductus arteriosus and pulmonary artery stenoses are commonest.

Eye

The salt and pepper pigmentary retinopathy does not impair vision. Cataracts are common and do cause visual impairment. Glaucoma occurs sometimes.

Mental retardation

The reported frequency of retardation varies according to the population studied. A further complication is that retardation may be difficult to exclude in a child with severe sensory handicaps. Severe retardation is associated in about 10 per cent of cases.

Other

Low birth-weight, neonatal hepatitis and thrombocytopenia.

Management of the deaf-blind child

Impairment of both vision and hearing is an uncommon but devastating handicap. With impairment of the two main routes of learning, development will ineveitably be interfered with, even without the mental handicap which is often present. If the child's awareness of the world is sufficiently impaired he is unlikely to establish meaningful contact with his parents or surroundings and he is likely to withdraw into a self-centred state reminiscent of autism.

Maximising residual vision and hearing with appropriate aids is important, as is training of the residual vision and hearing. It is often difficult to assess the degree of residual function and a period of training is usually worthwhile even if it appears initially that no useful function is present.

Developmental training attempts to establish an awareness of self as an individual within the world, to enlarge experience of the world and to promote communication through touch and movement, using residual vision and hearing where appropriate.

DEAFNESS

The approximate prevalence of hearing impairments is shown in Table 9.6 and the causes of severe hearing impairment in Table 9.7.

Testing hearing in the early months of life is difficult because of the lack of clearcut responses to sound. The diagnosis of deafness may be rejected on the grounds that the child responds to sounds such as traffic, but these sounds may be of very high intensity and their preception does not exclude even severe deafness. Children with early

Table 9.6 Prevalence of hearing impairment in children (per 1000)

Mild	35–50 dB	13
Moderate	50–70 dB	2
Severe	more than 70 dB	1

The normal average threshold at each frequency is desingated zero decibels (dB). Other sound levels are related to this:

$$\text{decibel no} = 10 \times \log 10 \frac{\text{sound pressure level}}{\text{threshold sound pressure level}}$$

thus 20 dB represents a sound pressure level 100 times greater than the threshold. For a given individual thresholds up to 20 dB are within the normal range.

Table 9.7 Causes of severe deafness

Inherited
  recessive
    Pendred's syndrome (deafness with goitre)
    Usher's syndrome (deafness with retinitis pigmentosa)
    and many others
  dominant
    Waadenburg syndrome (deafness with white forelock)
    other
  X-linked
Inner ear malformations
Malformations of the face and ears involving the middle ear
  cleft palate
  Treacher Collins' syndrome
  other
Following meningitis
Prenatal infections
  rubella
Perinatal
  asphyxia
  jaundice
  other insults
Other

deafness, due to conditions such as inherited disorders with severe deafness, prenatal rubella, and perinatal insults, are likely to have a severe loss rather than the mild losses common after 6 months but, despite this, attempts to detect deafness at birth, by techniques such as auditory evoked response have not been completely successful. An alternative is to identify children at risk of deafness (Table 9.8) and to follow them with regular hearing tests.

Table 9.8 Risk factors for deafness

Family history of hereditary childhood deafness
Rubella or other prenatal non-bacterial infection
Physical malformations around the ear
Low birth weight
Severe neonatal jaundice

About 8 per cent of children will fall within these criteria including 70–80 per cent of those with early deafness

Characteristics of deafness

1. Degree of hearing loss
2. Nature of hearing loss — conductive, typically due to chronic middle ear disease
   — sensorineural
3. Age at onset — generally the earlier the onset of deafness the more severe are the developmental consequences

4. Duration — deafness due to middle ear disease is often intermittent
5. Frequencies involved
   — low, below 1 kilohertz (kHz)
   — middle, 1–4 kHz
   — high, above 4 kHz.

The functional effects of hearing loss will depend upon all the above characteristics. Hearing losses of up to 35 dB generally cause little handicap, but greater losses will cause difficulties. The human ear perceives sound over the range of 30 to 10 000 H_2. Speech covers a rather smaller range. The vowel sounds carry most of the power of speech and fall in the middle and low frequencies, while the consonant sounds which convey the intelligibility of speech fall into the upper frequencies. Thus high-tone deafness tends to impair understanding of speech rather more than low tone deafness.

Vowels — low and middle frequencies, convey most of the power of speech, but not much intelligibility:

__a_ __a_ a _i_ e _a_

Consonants — predominantly high frequencies, convey most of the intelligibility of speech:

M__ry h__d __ L_ttl_ L_mb

Developmental effects of severe hearing loss

Severe deafness during the first year of life prevents a child from hearing speech, and thus his speech development will be delayed. When deafness is profound (90 dB or more) speech development is likely to be prevented altogether. However, the deaf child will learn to communicate using strategies such as gesture, and facial expression.

Deafness beginning after the child has begun to communicate verbally has generally less severe effects.

Management of severe deafness

Amplification

Hearing aids are used to make optimum use of residual hearing.

Understanding

Using residual hearing, vision (lip reading) and touch (feeling the vibration of the larynx) awareness, and later, understanding of speech is encouraged.

Speech training

The speech production of the deaf is either absent or distorted because of their lack of auditory feedback. Sound production and its refinement is encouraged by the teacher monitoring the correctness of the sound for the child.

Alternative methods of communication

Sign language can be used as an alternative or an adjunct to speech. The use of a sign system tends to stimulate rather than inhibit speech development.

Education

The language training of the early years is vital. At school age most children with useful hearing will be integrated into the normal school system, often in units for the hearing-impaired within normal schools. Those without useful residual hearing are more likely to require separate education, and continuing difficulties with understanding and production of speech may contribute to poor educational progress.

Mild hearing impairment

Mild transient hearing loss following ear infections is usual. Failure of resolution of an ear infection resulting in a middle ear full of viscous exudate (chronic secretory otitis media or CSOM) is the commonest cause of mild and moderate hearing loss in childhood, affecting up to 7 per cent of children, and being commonest in the age range from 6 months to 7 years. Typically, the tympanic membrane looks dull and retracted, and the findings of low middle ear pressure with reduced compliance on impedance audiometry are diagnostic. Decongestant medication sometimes clears the condition, but aspiration of the middle ear is often required, sometimes with the insertion of grommets, which are small tubes inserted into the drum, constituting an artificial perforation to ensure middle ear ventilation.

Although the deafness of CSOM is not severe, it may contribute a significant additional handicap for a child who already has a language or other problem. At school age behaviour problems or poor progress are common features.

SPEECH DELAY

Speech makes greater demands on motor coordination and intellect than any other activity of the young child, and it is not surprising that speech delay is common (Table 9.9).

Table 9.9 Prevalence of speech delay (%)

Unintelligible at school entry (poor articulation)	5
Reduced speech content at school entry	1
Severe language difficulty (not due to deafness or mental retardation)	0.1

The causes of speech delay are outlined in Table 9.10. The deaf child does not hear speech, and so his learning to speak is impaired. He does develop the symbolic understanding upon which language is founded and he will communicate in other ways, for example by gesture.

Table 9.10 Causes of speech delay

Constitutional
Mental retardation
Deafness
Abnormalities of the speech apparatus
  neurological
    cerebral palsy
    cranial nerve abnormalities
  physical abnormalities
    cleft palate
  lip and tongue dyspraxia
Specific language disorder
Psychiatric
  autism
  elective mutism

The speech delay of the retarded child is part of the overall picture of developmental delay, although it is not uncommon for speech to be more severely delayed than other areas of development.

Abnormalities of the speech apparatus impair the child's speech production (articulation), but not the sense he is trying to convey (content). The majority of young children with poor articulation do not have any obvious physical or neurological abnormality and their immaturity of speech production will generally resolve in time.

Of the pre-school children with speech delay (content) not due to deafness or retardation, most will have caught up within the first few years. This developmental pattern is known as constitutional speech delay, and there is often a history of delayed speech in other family members. A much smaller number have more severe and persisting problems with speech. This group of children with specific developmental language disorders is not completely distinct from those with constitutional delay, but rather the groups merge into one another.

Later, there is an increased incidence of reading and writing difficulties in children who have or have had speech delay.

Management

Where comprehension of language is normal and the problem is one of expressive language only, the outlook for development is good and little intervention is required unless the speech difficulties are severe. The child may be aware of his difficulties making him reluctant to speak. Gentle encouragement is needed to overcome this. When there is a problem of articulation, speech training may be required, but this often has to wait until the child is old enough to cooperate and is motivated to improve his speech.

When there is impaired comprehension of language the outlook is less good. Developmental help, often provided in units for language-delayed children, for example in nursery classes, is indicated. The child's language development is fostered by gearing the level of language to which he is exposed to his level of understanding.

Alternative methods of communication

Where a child's language abilities are grossly impaired, especially where expression is affected leaving comprehension intact, a sign system may improve communication, possibly stimulating language development at the same time.

MENTAL RETARDATION

The dividing line between normal and subnormal intelligence is taken as IQ 70 (corresponding to an IQ test score of two standard deviations below the mean), and includes about 3 per cent of the population (Table 9.11). For educational purposes retardation is classified as moderate (IQ 70–50) and severe (IQ less than 50).

Table 9.11 Prevalence of mental retardation

Retardation	IQ	Incidence (per 1000)
Moderate	70–50	30
Severe	50–20	
Profound	below20	3

The degree of mental retardation depends upon a variety of factors in addition to the insult primarily responsible for the retardation (Table 9.12). Deprivation and the presence of additional handicaps can increase the deficit, while an optimum environment maximises developmental potential.

Investigations

Where clinical examination does not suggest the diagnosis, the following investigations should be considered: plasma amino acids; urine for amino

Table 9.12 Causes of mental retardation

Prenatal (75%)

Genetic
1. Chromosomal disorders — Down's syndrome commonest
2. Gene mutations
    biochemical disorders: phenylketonuria
    neurocutaneous syndromes: tuberous sclerosis Sturge
    Weber syndrome
Recognisable syndromes and those with dysmorphic features, but not falling into a recognisable syndrome
Prenatal infections

Perinatal (15%)

Birth asphyxia
Trauma
Severe jaundice
Hypoglycaemia

Postnatal (10%)

Trauma
Infections: meningitis
    encephalitis
Severe metabolic disturbance

acids and organic acids; plasma electrolytes; serology for congenital infections, rubella, herpes cytomegalovirus, toxoplasmosis, syphylis; chromosomes; thyroxine, thyroid stimulating hormone.

If clinically indicated, further investigations such as skull X-ray, CT scan and electroencephalogram may be done. The results of these tests are often abnormal but are less often clearly diagnostic. There are few remediable causes of retardation, although hypothyroidism is an important but uncommon exception, and investigations should be kept to a reasonable minimum. Greater thoroughness may, however, be required for genetic counselling.

Management

Many retarded children will be brought by their parents for medical advice and more will be detected on routine developmental screening. Some, especially the less severely retarded, will not be picked up until school entry, but early identification is desirable.

Early management consists of optimising opportunities for development after having attended to remediable problems such as hearing loss. This may be achieved by encouraging parents to provide stimulation, getting the child into a playgroup or, in a more structured way in a nursery for the handicapped or, by an educational adviser working through the parents, nursery, or both. Work on particular problems temporarily blocking development, for example poor attention, may enable learning to procede more efficiently. It is important to work at the appropriate developmental level, otherwise learning efficiency will be very poor.

The school placement of the retarded child is not made on the basis of IQ alone. The child's motivation, behaviour and ability to use his learning potential all influence placement, especially in borderline cases. While schools for moderately retarded children pursue the usual type of education, albeit at a slower pace, schools for the severely subnormal will tend to concentrate on behaviour, communication and social skills.

Prognosis

One can never be confident about the future of a child with delayed development but, in general, the pace of development exhibited so far is likely to continue in the absence of significant external changes, although there may be early levelling off of developmental progress, especially in the more severely retarded. The ability to live independently and to be economically self-supporting, depending as it does upon personality, sociability and learned skills is even harder to predict. The child leaving a school for the moderately subnormal is likely to be placed in employment by the schools' careers service, but their prospects for long-term employment are less good.

DOWN'S SYNDROME

This is the commonest single cause of severe mental retardation with an incidence of approximately one per 1000 births. The common clinical

Table 9.13 Clinical features of Down's syndrome

Present in about three-quarters of Down's children
    upslanting palpebral fissures
    flat facies
    flat occiput
    loose skin on neck
Present in about one-half of Down's children
    broad hands
    short fingers
    incurved 5th fingers (clinodactyly)
    single transverse palmar crease
    malformed auricles
    epicanthic folds
    speckled iris (Brushfield's spots)
    protruding tongue
    hypotonia
    broad space between 1st and 2nd toes

Table 9.14 Down's syndrome — associated abnormalities

Cardiac defects
    atrioventricular canal defect
    verticular septal defect
Intestinal malformation
    duodenal atresia
Strabismus
Convulsions
    although less frequent than among other children with severe retardation, convulsions are more common than among the general population
Deafness
    mainly conductive
Occasional endocrine abnormalities   hypothyroidism
                                    diabetes

features and associated abnormalities are shown in Tables 9.13 and 9.14.

Cytology

The underlying defect is an autosomal trisomy. In 95 per cent of cases there is simple trisomy of chromosome 21. In the remainder the additional chromosomal material is translocated onto chromosome 14 (or occasionally 15).

Maternal age

The chances of non-disjunction, (producing simple trisomy 21) increase with maternal age, it is about 1 per cent when the mother is 40. This age-related effect accounts for around one-half of all babies with Down's syndrome.

Intelligence

Early development is generally delayed, but not grossly so, with average performance being around two-thirds of the chronological age in the first 2 years. In later years progress is slower, the average intelligence is around IQ 50 with most Down's children falling within the range of IQ 20 to 70.

Life expectancy

Life expectancy of Down's children has increased during this century. There is a high early mortality of approximately 25 per cent in the first 2 years, cardiac defects being the commonest cause of death. After the first 2 yeras, infection is the commonest cause of death. The overall life expectancy is about 30 years.

PHYSICAL DISABILITIES

Approximately 25 children in every 10 000 suffer from a significant physical handicap; one-half of them require special education because of their handicap. The commoner causes of physical handicap are shown in Table 9.15.

Cerebral palsy

Cerebral palsy is a non-progressive disorder of movement resulting from a brain insult before or during birth. A similar clinical picture can be

Table 9.15 Conditions causing physical handicap

Cerebral palsy
Congenital and rheumatic heart disease (The handicap is usually relatively mild; and these children are generally educated in normal schools)
Spina bifida
Congenital limb deformities
Muscular dystrophy
Post-poliomyelitis (becoming rarer)
Perthe's disease
Haemophilia
Juvenile rheumatoid arthritis
Arthrogryposis
Other

caused by an insult occuring after birth. The incidence of cerebral palsy is 2–3 per 1000 births. Various patterns of cerbral palsy are seen (Table 9.16). Many cases show features of more than one type. There may be athetoid features in the movement disorder of a predominantly spastic child and vice versa and, limbs apparently spared, for example in hemiplegia, will often show slight abnormalities.

Table 9.16 Patterns of cerebral palsy

Spastic	
quadriplegia	15%
hemiplegia	30%
diplegia	5%
Athetoid	20%
Hypotonic	5%
Ataxic	5%
Mixed	20%

Features of cerebral palsy

Posture There are many typical postures. Adduction and internal rotation of the legs with equinus at he ankles is common, as is adduction and internal rotation at the shoulders with flexion at the wrists and elbows.

Responses Primitive reflexes, Moro, grasp, tonic neck, are late disappearing, and the secondary responses, parachute and propping reactions, are dealyed in development.

Movement The abnormalities of movements have several components including weakness, poor coordination involuntary movements (athetosis) and poor postural control and abnormal responses.

Tone Muscle tone varies with time and posture and is different in different muscle groups. Thus, a predominantly spastic child will have low tone in some muscle groups. The muscles of the spine and neck are often weak and hypotonic.

Tendon reflexes These can vary. They are often increased.

The manifestations of cerebral palsy evolve with time. Most affected children are initially hypotonic, with spasticity or athetosis developing later. There is a tendency for the earlier onset of spasticity or athetosis to indicate a better porgnosis, while the persistence of generalised hypotonia into the second year of life is a poor prognostic sign. In addition, an apparent deterioration in neurological state may occur at adolescence. The growth spurt in height, which puts greater demands upon balance, may contribute to this as may the reluctance to persevere with physiotherapy often seen at this age.

In addition to the movement disorder of cerebral palsy there are often other problems (Table 9.17). Only about one third of children with cerebral palsy will be able to cope in normal schools.

Table 9.17 Cerebral palsy — associated problems

Epilepsy	40%
Squint	30%
Severe visual handicap	10%
Speech delay	
not speaking at 5 years	20%
poor articulation at 5 years	50%
Deafness	15%
Subnormal intelligence (IQ below 70)	50%

Management

The presence of associated problems will complicate management and, in some children with very complex handicaps, integrating the various aspects of management will itself be a major task. The mainstay of the management of the movement problems in cerebral palsy is physiotherapy. Surgery can correct some deformities and may be beneficial, but elongating and, therefore, weakening already weak muscles can cause its own problems, while the period of immobility following surgery may be detrimental to the programme of education and physiotherapy. Thus, the selections and timing of cases for surgery is critical.

There are a variety of non-surgical methods to reduce hypertonia. These include nerve and muscle infiltration with alcohol, and drugs such as baclofen and diazepam.

The aims of physiotherapy are to prevent muscle contractures and deformities which are inhibiting to movement in the less severely affected, and make management difficult in the severely affected. Physiotherapy also aims to improve ability to balance and perform movements, for example walking, dressing, as appropriate to the child's developmental level. A wide variety of therapy techniques have been used to inhibit the abnormal patterns of muscle activity and promote more normal activity.

Spina bifida
(See chapter 23)

The problems associated with spina bifida include infection; spinal cord damage, weakness of the legs (may require braces to control weakness, tendon transfer to avoid deformity), sensory loss, incontinence (bladder managed by regular expression, penile appliance, ureteric diversion, regular catheterisation), constipation (managed by diet, laxatives and manual evacuation); hydrocephalus; kyphosis and scoliosis; renal problems (reflux, chronic infection); squint; emotional and behaviour problems; and intellectual impairment (nonverbal skills often more impaired than verbal, hydrocephalus lowers intelligence still further).

CONDITIONS CAUSING SEVERE OR PROGRESSIVE WEAKNESS
(Muscular dystrophies, spinal muscular atrophy)

The management of these disorders aims at preserving function for as long as possible. The development of contractures is prevented or delayed by physiotherapy; calipers can prolong the period of ambulation. Various splints may improve hand functions. Immobility, for example during intercurrent illness, must be minimised as rapid loss of function can occur during these times.

Although in the later stages of the ambulatory period, the child may be very restricted, not being able to manage steps, slopes or rough ground, persisting with walking is worthwhile because once the child is chairbound, scoliosis, which may become gross, joint contractures, respiratory problems and constipation tend to develop.

10

Genetic disorders

Genetic disease is now relatively more common as infections and perinatal trauma have decreased. Among livebirths, single gene disorders occur in 1 per cent (0.7 per cent autosomal dominant, 0.05 per cent X-linked recessive and 0.25 per cent autosomal recessive), chromosome disorders in 0.4 per cent and polygenic malformations in around 2 per cent. These are population figures and the proportions of diseases that are wholly or partly determined genetically are much greater in medical practice (Table 10.1). Genetic diseases

SINGLE GENE DISORDERS

These conditions are the simplest to understand; they are caused by an abnormal mutation in one or both members of a single pair of genes. The family patterns are logical and consistent.

Autosomal dominant diseases

Autosomal dominant conditions are those which are caused by a single mutant gene present on one

Table 10.1 Genetic contribution to illhealth in childhood (%)

Among	Single gene or chromosome disorders	Malformations that are partly genetic
Stillbirths & neonatal deaths	6—10	30—40
Paediatric inpatients	4—8	20—25
Severely mentally-retarded children	46	10
Deaf schoolchildren	50	1—2
Blind schoolchildren	42	8

often give rise to longer and more frequent admissions to hospital and to more outpatient visits than other problems. In 1959, 26 per cent of institutional beds in Northern Ireland were occupied by patients with genetically-determined illnesses, and in British Columbia in 1964 about three-quarters of children registered as handicapped had a condition that was entirely or partially genetically determined.

It helps families with genetic problems to give them the risks of recurrence and an understanding of basic genetics is required by any doctor caring for children.

of the 22 pairs of autosomes. Since a child inherits half his father's genes and half his mother's genes, he has a one in two chance of inheriting the abnormal gene from whichever parent is affected. Thus he or she, has a half chance of developing the disease if one parent is affected. Some examples of autosomal dominant conditions which can affect children are achondroplasia, tuberous sclerosis, neurofibromatosis, myotonic dystrophy, and lobster-claw syndrome. A pedigree illustrating the inheritance of dominant optic atrophy is shown in Figure 10.1

Autosomal dominant conditions are often very

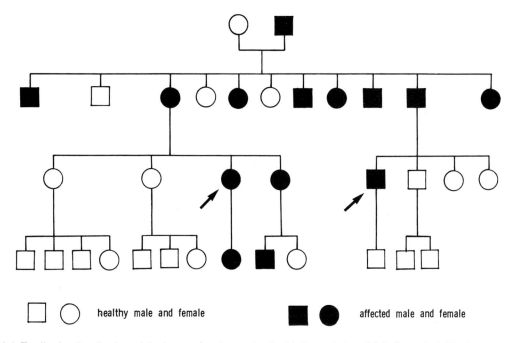

| □ ○ | healthy male and female | ■ ● | affected male and female |

Fig. 10.1 Family showing dominant inheritance of optic atrophy (by kind permission of S B Crews & G Harding)

variable, both in severity and in age of onset. It may be difficult to decide whether a symptomless relative carries the gene (i.e. is a heterozygote). For example, while 60–70 per cent of patients with tuberous sclerosis are mentally retarded and around 90 per cent are epileptic, there remain 10 per cent who are without symptoms and who only have skin or eye lesions. It is these 10 per cent who are likely to become parents, not knowing that they run a 1 in 3 risk of having a mentally handicapped child. Thus, when counselling the parents of a child with severe tuberous sclerosis it is essential to know whether one of them is mildly affected. Each parent must have a careful examination of the skin and optic fundi. The skin and retinal features that are pathognomonic of tuberous sclerosis usually occur together, but each has been described in a parent as the only manifestation of the disorder. These features are: adenoma sebaceum, shagreen patch, subungual fibromas, pale white macules and retinal phakoma. At least one of these features should have appeared by adult life in an individual who is a heterozygote for tuberous sclerosis. If neither parent has one of these lesions, then they may be reassured that their child is affected by a new mutation, and that recurrence in another sibling is most unlikely.

(There is a slight caveat here, for two families have been described in which apparently normal parents have had more than one child with tuberous sclerosis. Such families are clearly extremely rare.)

This leads to the next point about dominant conditions, namely that a proportion of patients are affected by a new mutation. This mutation would have occurred during meiosis (the formation of either ovum or sperm); in this situation, the parents are normal and therefore there is little chance of the disorder occurring again in another child. In dominant disorders, the proportion of patients affected by new mutations is directly related to the overall fertility of patients. For example, in achondroplasia, the average number of children born to patients is about one-fifth of the average number of children born to unaffected individuals. This is partly due to failure to marry as dwarfism is a social handicap, and partly due to the patients' knowledge of the genetic risks. The proportion of achondroplasts who are new mutations and who have healthy parents is four-fifths, in neurofibromatosis the proportion is one-half, and in tuberous sclerosis, about four-fifths.

If two individuals with the same dominant

condition marry, there is a one in 4 chance that a child could be homozygous abnormal, that is, possess two similar dominant genes. This has been observed with achondroplasia, Thomsen's disease or myotonia congenita, and distal myopathy as well as in other disorders. In each case the homozygous child was more severely affected than the parents.

disorders, and these are useful if the condition is common. For example, the carrier state for Tay-Sachs disease (hexosaminidase A deficiency) can be recognised. Since the carrier state for this condition in Ashkenazi Jews lies between 1 in 20 and 1 in 30, it is worthwhile testing Jewish couples on marriage, and certainly worthwhile to test the siblings of patients and their spouses. The

Table 10.2 Frequencies of some commoner autosomal recessive conditions

Disease	Frequency of disease	Frequency of carrier state
Cystic fibrosis in Europeans	1 in 2000	1 in 22
Tay-Sachs disease in Ashkenazi Jews	1 in 2000	1 in 22
Thalassaemia in Cypriots	1 in 150	1 in 6
Sickle-cell disease in West Africans	1 in 900	1 in 15
Phenylketonuria in UK	1 in 12 000	1 in 55
Werdnig-Hoffmann disease in UK	1 in 25 000	1 in 80

Autosomal recessive conditions

These conditions occur when a child possesses two abnormal members of a gene pair, one inherited from the mother and one from the father. The parents are both symptomless carriers (or heterozygotes) and are not usually identified as such until they have had an affected child. Once this has happened, it is clear that there is a 1 in 4 risk of recurrence and the parents should be told this. The risk of recurrence is very small for half-siblings, or for a sibling conceived by donor artifical insemination (AID). Autosomal recessive diseases, in contrast to autosomal dominant ones, are fairly consistent in age of onset and in severity. Some examples are phenylketonuria, Tay-Sachs disease and acute spinal muscular atrophy (Werdnig-Hoffmann disease).

The recessive diseases are thought to be caused by specific enzyme abnormalities, either an enzyme deficiency, or a structural change in an enzyme which impairs its activity. In some cases, a specific enzyme abnormality has been identified and, moreover, may be demonstrable in amniotic cells or fluid, thus making prenatal diagnosis possible. The list of conditions that can be diagnosed prenatally is growing, and an up-to-date authority should be consulted when one comes across a family at risk. In addition, there are tests for the carrier (or heterozygote) in certain recessive

healthy sibling of a child with an autosomal recessive disease has a 2 in 3 chance of being a carrier.

Table 10.2 lists the frequencies of some commoner autosomal recessive diseases. Most, however, are less frequent, and perhaps the average frequency of the carrier state of a particular recessive disease is 1 in 100. This means that if a man or woman is a carrier (and probably everyone is a carrier for at least one recessive gene), then the chance of marrying someone who carries the same gene is about 1 in 100 and, therefore, the chance of having an affected child is about 1 in 400. Of course, the chance of marrying a carrier is increased in marriages between relatives. A carrier who marries a first cousin, for example, has a 1 in 8 chance of marrying another carrier, since cousins have one-eighth of their genes in common. This is why there is an excess of cousin marriages among the parents of children with less common recessive diseases. On the other hand, the empirical risk for married first cousins having a child with a recessive disease is relatively small, about 1 in 30.

In autosomal recessive diseases genetic counselling is easy, for there is, inevitably, a 1 in 4 risk of recurrence for further children of a couple who are carriers for the same disorder. Since recessive conditions are often serious it is important to recognise a condition as being recessive after the first case in the family. Diagnosis must depend upon clinical features, and not upon the presence of an affected relative.

Finally, here is a warning about phenylketonuric women who are leading normal lives as a result of treatment or because they have a mild form of the disease. It is now clear that women with serum phenylalanine levels that are over 15 mg/100 ml during early pregnancy, have a high risk (almost 100 per cent) of having children who are retarded in growth, microcephalic and mentally retarded and, of whom, some also have congenital heart disease or other malformations. It is important that such women are placed on a low phenylalanine diet before pregnancy occurs.

X-linked recessive diseases

X-linked diseases are those produced by a gene on the X chromosome. Although the X chromosome in a woman is paired, that in a man is not, for he has a small Y chromosome in place of the second X. Thus, a recessive gene on one of a woman's X chromosomes will usually show no ill-effects. A recessive gene, however, on the X-chromosome of a male will manifest itself fully since there is no normal homologue.

The family patterns obtained are very characteristic. If a man is affected, all his sons will be normal (for in order to be sons they will have inherited their father's Y chromosome) and all his daughters will be carriers. If a woman is a carrier, half her sons will be affected and half her daughters will be carriers. A family tree showing the inheritance of X-linked retinitis pigmentosa is given in Figure 10.2. The propositus in this family had visual problems from an early age and was registered partially-sighted at the age of 7. His mother had not previously been given genetic advice, but now says that she certainly would have liked it. Examples of other X-linked conditions are Duchenne muscular dystrophy, haemophilia, Lesch-Nyhan disease, Menkes' disease. Becker muscular dystrophy, adrenoleucodystrophy, and certain types of mental retardation.

Some of these diseases are serious and affected males never reproduce. Since the diseases are not disappearing, this means that some new cases arise because of new mutations, in the same way that some patients with severe autosomal dominant conditions are affected by new mutations. The relationship between severity of disease and the proportion of X-linked mutants is not straightforward as with the dominant conditions, since a mutation occurring in a female is not immediately apparent: with lethal conditions such as Duchenne muscular dystrophy, the proportion of boys who

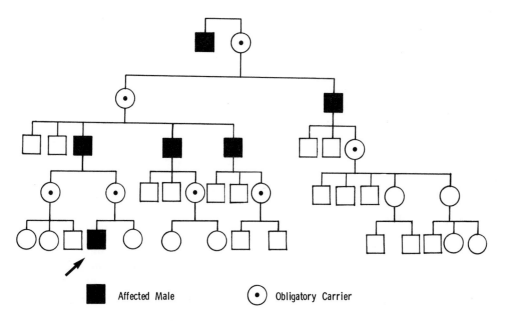

Fig. 10.2 Family with X-linked retinitis pigmentosa

are affected by new mutations and who have mothers who are not carriers, can be calculated as one-third. Looking at it differently, the mother of an isolated male with a lethal X-linked disorder has a two-thirds chance of being a carrier. (These are useful working figures but, in fact, the calculations are only correct if the mutation rate is equal in the two sexes, which is not always so.)

From the point of view of genetic counselling, it is important to know precisely whether a female relative is a carrier. For some diseases, for instance, Menkes' disease and Lesch-Nyhan disease, there are accurate carrier tests, although these are often tedious to carry out. The basis for these tests is the phenomenon described by Dr Mary Lyon in the early 1960s, namely that only one X-chromosome is active in each cell of a female, and that inactivation of the second occurs early in development and at random. This means that a woman is composed of two populations of cells, in one of which the maternal X is active, while in the other it is the paternal X that is active. If cells from skin are cultured *in vitro* and then cloned, so that each clone is derived from a single skin cell, then some of the clones will demonstrate the activity of one X chromosome and some the other. In Lesch-Nyhan disease and Menkes' disease, a specific metabolic abnormality can be demonstrated, not only in patients, but also in clones from carrier females, and in amniotic cells from an affected fetus.

Unfortunately, however, in some other X-linked disorders, a precise biochemical abnormality has not been demonstrated and accurate carrier tests are not available. Genetic counselling is therefore less reliable; it depends upon assessing two sets of data: first, the information from the pedigree and second, information derived from carrier tests that are only partly discriminating, such as the serum creatine kinase level in Duchenne muscular dystrophy. Pedigree analysis consists of halving a woman's chances of being a carrier for each step in the female line that she is from, and reducing her chances further if she has unaffected brothers or sons. A family showing the results of such calculations is shown in Figure 10.3. Carrier testing (in this example, the mean of three serum creatine kinase levels) adds further information, for the laboratory should be able to give the relative odds

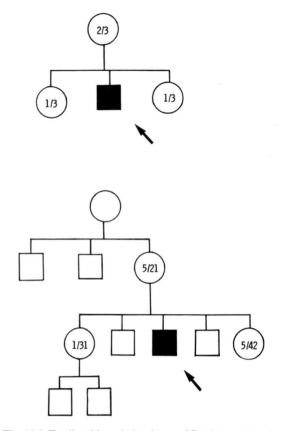

Fig. 10.3 Family with an isolated case of Duchenne muscular dystrophy, showing the risks that his mother and two sisters have of being carriers; (top) when the family information is incomplete; (bottom) when the pedigree is completed

for such a mean level belonging to the normal distribution compared with the carrier distribution. The two sets of odds are then multiplied to give the woman her final probability of being a carrier. The methods of calculation are described by Emery (1976). In Duchenne muscular dystrophy it is not yet possible to detect disease in a fetus. Possible female carriers can only be offered the option of fetal sexing during pregnancy with abortion of all male fetuses.

X-linked dominant inheritance

Examples of conditions showing X-linked dominant inheritance are vitamin-D-resistant rickets and Albright's syndrome of pseudohypoparathyroidism. The characteristics of this type of inheritance are that more females are affected than males; females are usually less severely affected; all the daughters but none of the sons of affected males are affected; and one-half of the offspring of affected females are affected.

There are two disorders thought to be due to X-linked dominant inheritance, with lethality in males. These are incontinentia pigmenti and the Aicardi syndrome. All patients with the Aicardi syndrome have been females; there has been no recurrence in siblings and the sex ratio is equal in unaffected siblings. It has been suggested that all female patients are new mutations, and that the mutations in male fetuses lead to intrauterine death. In incontinentia pigmenti about two-thirds of patients are new mutations, since some females are mildly affected and become mothers. Occasional male cases have been reported.

OLIGOGENIC INHERITANCE

Oligogenic inheritance describes those conditions where a genetic predisposition to disease is produced by a few (oligo) genes. The aetiology of such diseases is not entirely genetic; usually there are environmental causes as well.

HLA complex

The diseases which are associated with specific HLA antigens show oligogenic inheritance. The HLA complex (also called the major histocompatibility complex) comprises a short stretch of chromosome number 6 and is known to include the five or more loci for A, C, B, and D antigens, and three of about 15 loci for the complement components. There are many different A C B D antigens but any one individual will possess only eight; four coded by genes on the maternal chromosome and four coded by genes on the paternal chromosome. Some of these A C B D antigens are much commoner than others, for example A2 and B12 are very common in Europeans, and A1 and B7 are the next commonest. In addition, some antigens are found together more frequently than would be expected by random association; for example, the combination A1, B8 is five times commoner in Europeans than would be expected from the individual frequencies. These non-random associations of antigens (also called linkage

disequilibrium) probably reflect some advantage that they conferred on their possessors many generations ago. Chromosomal crossing-over within the HLA complex is uncommon (occurring once or twice per hundred generations) so these HLA associations must have been present for a long time.

Coeliac disease

The association of coeliac disease with B8 was the most marked disease-HLA association at the time it was observed in 1972. There is a fourfold increase of B8 in patients with coeliac disease compared with healthy controls, and the presence of this antigen gives its possessor a risk of coeliac disease eight times greater than the population risk. The association of coeliac disease with the A1 antigen is due to linkage disequilibrium with B8. It has recently been shown that the strongest association of coeliac disease is with Dw3 (the w refers to a workshop assignment) so that the risk to Dw3 possessors of developing coeliac disease is 64 times the population risk. Among those patients who do not possess the Dw3 antigen, there are many with the Dw7 antigen.

Family studies have shown that the B8 antigen of an affected patient is distributed more or less equally between his affected and unaffected children. This means that the B8 gene is not itself responsible for coeliac disease, and probably there is a 'coeliac-susceptibility' gene in linkage disequilibrium with the B8 gene. Recently, a much stronger association has been shown with Dw3 (and Dw7); it is likely that the susceptibility gene is nearer to the D locus than the B locus, and possibly identical to Dw3.

Family studies looking at the haplotypes of pairs of siblings, both of whom have coeliac disease, show that affected siblings almost always share one HLA haplotype (Table 10.3) and that there is no excess of pairs sharing both haplotypes. This finding indicates that the disease susceptibility gene is likely to be dominant. On the other hand, the risk of coeliac disease in first-degree relatives of 5–10 per cent (according to whether or not a jejeunal biopsy is carried out), is much less that the 50 per cent expected if the disease were entirely caused by an autosomal dominant gene.

Table 10.3 Distribution of HLA haplotypes in pairs of affected siblings

	One haplotype in common	Both haplotypes in common	Neither haplotype in common
Theoretical			
at random	0.50	0.25	0.25
if disease susceptibility is produced by one dominant gene in the HLA complex	0.50	0.50	0
if disease susceptibility is produced by two genes, one from each parent	<0.50	>0.50	0
Observed			
coeliac disease	0.55	0.38	0.07
juvenile-onset diabetes mellitus	0.40	0.60	0

Certainly gluten is one environmental agent involved; perhaps there are others, or a second genetic mechanism.

Juvenile-onset insulin-dependent diabetes mellitus

Clinical indications for heterogeneity in diabetes mellitus have been supported by genetic studies and by finding that juvenile-onset insulin-dependent diabetes is associated with specific HLA antigens, whereas maturity-onset insulin-independent diabetes is not. The association with juvenile-onset diabetes mellitus is most marked with Dw3 and Dw4 and with B8, B18, B15 and B4. The associations suggest that there may be more than one diabetes susceptibility gene and this belief is strengthened by family studies. Affected sibling-pairs are most likely to share both maternal and paternal haplotype (Table 10.3), in contradistinction to coeliac disease, suggesting that genes from both parents confer susceptibility to juvenile-onset diabetes. These genes need not be recessive; it is more likely that they are independent and additive.

Antibody titres to coxsackie-B viruses are unusually common in juvenile-onset diabetics who have B8 and B15 antigens. It is probable that the susceptibility genes influence the immune response to viruses which can cause pancreatic damage. From the practical point of view, the empirical risk of recurrence of juvenile-onset insulin-dependent diabetes in the sibling or child of a patient similarly affected is about 5 per cent.

POLYGENIC INHERITANCE

In this type of inheritance many genes are involved; each are of little individual effect, but they act together to produce an additive predisposition to disease. Usually some factors in the environment act upon this genetic predisposition.

This type of inheritance was first used to explain those characteristics, such as height, which show a continuous variation in the population; it was then applied to human diseases by C O Carter. The distribution of height in the population has a normal or Gaussian shape, which can theoretically be caused by the action of many discrete factors, such as genes. Family studies show that adult height is almost entirely genetically caused, and the patterns in relatives fit the expectations from polygenic inheritance with a few exceptions due to assortative mating and the presence of at least one pair of dominant genes for shortness. Similarly, studies on relatives, twins, and adopted children demonstrate that the genetic component of the normal range of intelligence is also due to polygenic inheritance. With both height and intelligence there are individuals at each extreme who do not conform to the Gaussian distribution, and whose deviance has different causes. These are the dwarves and the giants; the imbeciles and the geniuses.

With diseases it is not possible to measure the underlying genetic predisposition, and this has to be inferred from observations in patients and their relatives. In polygenic inheritance it is assumed that there is an underlying genetic liability to a particular disease, which is normal or Gaussian in shape, and that patients are at one extreme of this distribution. One assumes a threshold beyond which individuals are susceptible to environmental factors. On such a polygenic model, the following family patterns would be expected and are in fact observed.

If the patients represent one extreme of a polygenic predisposition, their relatives must share some of this predisposition to an extent related to the proportion of genes shared with the patient. Thus, relatives must have an increased risk of disease; the incidence of disease in first-degree relatives approximates to the square root of the population incidence and, therefore, is absolutely greater, but proportionately less increased as the population incidence increases.

The incidence in second and third-degree relatives falls off sharply and some illustrative risk figures for neural tube malformations are given in Table 10.4.

Table 10.4 Risks of neural tube malformations*in South-East England

Random population risk	1 in 340
If one sibling is affected**	1 in 22
If two siblings are affected	1 in 10
If a half-sibling is affected	1 in 50
If a parent is affected**	1 in 22
If an aunt, uncle, nephew or niece is affected	1 in 70
If a cousin+ is affected	1 in 148

*Term includes anencephaly, iniencephaly, encephalocele, myelomeningocele and meningocele
** Similar risks are found if the affected relative has spinal dysraphism or multiple vertebral anomalies
+ This risk figure refers to the incidence in mother's sisters' children, where knowledge of abnormalities is likely to be greatest

Furthermore, the polygenic model predicts that those patients who are the greatest deviants from the underlying genetic predisposition will need fewer environmental triggers than the less genetically predisposed patients. If such patients can be identified, their relatives should show a higher incidence of disease than the relative of patients with less genetic predisposition. Sometimes a particularly severe malformation indicates extreme genetic predisposition, and this is seen for example, with bilateral cleft lip and palate,

following which the recurrence risk is 1 in 16, whereas the recurrence risk after unilateral cleft lip ± palate is only 1 in 40. On the other hand, an extensive neural tube defect does not mean that the patient is particularly genetically predisposed; on the contrary, individuals who have multiple vertebral abnormalities but no overt spinal lesion have the same risk of having a child with a neural tube malformation as if they had overt spina bifida.

A second way by which a patient can be identified as being particularly genetically predisposed, is by being the unusual sex for that malformation. For example, it is five times more common to find pyloric stenosis in a boy than in a girl; the risk of recurrence after a boy with pyloric stenosis is 1 in 30 but after a girl it is 1 in 16. Finally, families of increased genetic susceptibility may be recognised when they have had more than one affected individual; in South-East England the recurrence risk after one sibling with a neural tube malformation is 1 in 22, but after two affected siblings the risk increases to 1 in 10. In Northern Ireland the risk of recurrence after one affected sibling is 1 in 12, but after two it rises to 1 in 5. Risks of recurrence after the other polygenically inherited malformations are given in Table 10.5.

The important point about these polygenically inherited malformations is that environmental factors usually play some part in their development and, therefore, there is hope for preventing the condition if the environmental triggers can be recognised and controlled.

It has been known for some time that environmental factors are important in the aetiology of neural tube defects, for there is a seasonal variation consisting of an excess of February, March and April conceptions, and there is a marked and consistent social class effect with a greater incidence in social classes IV and V. These observations, together with the finding of a low red cell folate level and low leucocyte ascorbic acid level in early pregnancy in women who later gave birth to babies with neural tube defects, led to the suggestion that poor nutrition with vitamin deficiencies could be causative factors in some women at risk. In a prospective controlled study of pregnancies at risk because the woman had at least one

Table 10.5 Risks of recurrence in those congenital malformations that are polygenically inherited (after British Medical Bulletin, 1976)

Malformation	Population incidence per 1000 total births	Risks of recurrence	
		after one affected child	after two affected children
Club foot	2.0	1 in 35	?
Persistent dislocation of the hip	1.0	1 in 22	1 in 12
Cleft lip± cleft palate	1.0	1 in 28	1 in 12
Congenital heart defects	6.0	1 in 25*	1 in 10
Pyloric stenosis in males	5.0	1 in 30	1 in 7
in females	1.0	1 in 16	1 in 4
Neural tube defects in South-East England	2.9	1 in 22	1 in 10

* For the same heart malformation as in the index patient

previous baby with a neural tube defect, a lower risk of neural tube defects has been found if the woman had received vitamin and iron supplements for one month prior to conception and for 6 weeks afterwards. This observation gives rise to optimism that neural tube defects may be prevented in some women at risk. In the meantime, tests on amniotic fluid (that is, the levels of α-fetoprotein and acetylcholinesterase) and ultrasound examination can detect all cases of anencephaly and the great majority of babies with spinabifida. Women at higher than usual risk, who should be offered these prenatal tests, can be recognised by a family history of neural tube malformation or by a high level of α-fetoprotein in their serum.

CHROMOSOME DISORDERS

Techniques

The 46 chromosomes can be distinguished from each other by their length, the position of their centromeres (those points where the chromatids meet), the pattern of cross striations, and by the presence or absence of distinctly staining markers near to the centromeres. A chromosome preparation is made from cells (usually white cells, fibroblasts, or amniotic cells) which have been encouraged to divide in culture. The chromosomes have divided into two halves, or chromatids, by the time of fixation, and so show their well known bipartite appearance. Untreated chromosomes in non-dividing cells are single stranded.

Current techniques for staining chromosomes can distinguish each one and demonstrate individual bands and polymorphisms. In brief, the staining methods consist of: (a) the use of fluorescent quinacrine derivatives which stain different bands of a chromosome to different extents, giving rise to a characteristic Q banding pattern; (b) the use of Giemsa stains which similarly produce differential staining of a chromosome; the dark G bands approximate to the bright Q bands. The Giemsa stains also produce very intense areas of fluorescence on the Y chromosome and certain autosomes, which can be seen in fixed cells as well as in dividing cells; (c) a differential staining method called C banding demonstrates those areas near the centromeres which contain highly reiterative DNA; and (d) there is recent technique which reduces the amount of folic acid in the culture medium, thereby demonstrating 'fragile' sites in a few specific conditions, notably one of the X-linked mental retardation syndromes. These techniques not only identify each chromosome but also allow detection of structural abnormalities not easily seen before, such as an inversion or a symmetrical translocation, and can often distinguish the paternally-derived chromosome from the maternally-derived.

Frequency of chromosome abnormalities

The frequency of overt disease due to a recognisable chromosomal abnormality is about 4.1 per 1,000 livebirths. Only around 5 per cent of patients with a chromosome abnormality have inherited it from a parent; the remainder are due

Table 10.6 Incidence of chromosome abnormalities (per cent)

Abnormality	In livebirths	In stillbirths	In abortuses
Autosomal trisomies	0.12	5.0—6.0	20.0—50.0
Unbalanced structural rearrangements	0.05	0.1—0.5	3.0—4.0
Sex chromosome abnormalities	0.24	1.0—1.5	7.0—20.0 (XO only)

to a recent error of meiosis or of postzygotic development. The incidence of chromosome abnormalities in abortuses and in stillbirths is much higher than the incidence in livebirths (Table 10.6), and is greatest in the early abortuses. The incidence of chromosome abnormalities in conceptuses of women over 40 could be as high as one in 2.

Clinical features of chromosome abnormalities

Numerical abnormalities of the autosomes always give rise to clinical disease, and some distinguishing clinical features are listed in Table 10.7. The clinical features that are common in a baby with a chromosome abnormality are low birth-weight, poor feeding and failure to thrive, an abnormality of tone, an odd appearance with or without specific malformations, and developmental delay.

Structural abnormalities of the autosomes (such as a translocation or an inversion) only give rise to clinical signs if they are unbalanced; that is, if a segment of a chromosome is actually lost or triplicated. However, for carriers of balanced translocations there is a risk of producing unbalanced gametes and thereby abnormal offspring. One danger here is that an abnormality which appears to be 'balanced' may in fact be unbalanced and a small deletion may be unnoticed. The empirical risk of clinical abnormality for the possessor of a *de novo* apparently balanced structural abnormality (for example, one found in cultured amniotic cells) is about 1 in 10.

Numerical abnormalities of the sex chromosomes give rise to less morbidity, and often only

Table 10.7 The most distinctive features of some chromosome disorders which are present in a baby

Trisomy 21 (Down's syndrome)
Low to normal birth-weight
Hypotonia
Brachycephaly
Oblique palpebral fissures
Small flat nose, rosebud mouth, darting tongue
Congenital heart malformation
Duodenal atresia

XO (Turner's syndrome)
(This is often not recognisable at birth)
Slightly low birth-weight
Loose folds of skin of neck
Oedema of hands and feet
Hypoplastic, hyperconvex nails

Trisomy 13 (Patau's syndrome)
Low to normal birth-weight
Microphthalmia, coloboma
Deformed ears
Post-axial polydactyly
Cleft palate and lip
Exomphalos
VSD
Hydronephrosis

Trisomy 18 (Edwards' syndrome)
Low birth-weight
Long narrow skull
Prominent occiput, small chin
Low-set faun-like ears
Finger flexion, small nails
VSD
Hips limited in adduction
Rocker-bottom feet, short big toe

4p- (Wolf syndrome)
Microcephaly
Frontal bossing, high forehead
Ocular malformation
Harelip±cleft palate
Vertebral malformations
Hypospadias

5p- (cri-du-chat syndrome)
High-pitched mewing cry
Microcephaly
Anti-monogoloid slant to eyes
Widely set eyes
Moon face

after puberty; the XO condition or Turner's syndrome is the only sex chromosome abnormality which often produces clinical signs at birth.

Down's syndrome

This autosomal disorder is the one that is of greatest significance in older children and in adult life, because most of the other autosomal disorders are associated with a short life span; it accounts for around one-third of all mentally retarded children. The commonest cause of Down's syndrome is trisomy-21, due to non-disjunction occurring in either maternal or paternal meiosis. The 21 chromosome shows several normal variations in its staining pattern, and in around 75 per cent of patients the paternally-derived chromosome-21 can be distinguished from that maternally-derived and, therefore, the source of the non-disjunction can be identified. Usually the non-disjunction is maternal in origin.

Less commonly, Down's syndrome is due to an unbalanced translocation where an additional chromosome 21 is attached to a chromosome-13, -14, -15, -22 or to another -21. This may arise *de novo* or it may have been inherited from a parent whose translocation was balanced. Recurrence risks for the different forms of Down's syndrome are shown in Table 10.8. With the inherited translocations the risk to offspring varies according to whether the mother or the father is the carrier, probably due to selection against the translocation-bearing sperm.

Two factors appear to be concerned with the aetiology of Down's syndrome. One is advanced parental age, particularly the mother's and the other is therapeutic radiation to the mother many years previously. The relationship with radiation is not firmly substatiated as it is based on retrospective studies, but the relationship with increased parental age is very clear (Table 10.9).

Table 10.9 Maternal age and trisomy-21

Maternal age group	Incidence of liveborn mongols	Incidence of trisomy-21 at amniocentesis
under 20	1 in 2000	
20–24	1 in 1600	these age groups
25–29	1 in 1000	are not screened
30–34	1 in 760	by amniocentesis
35–36	1 in 390	1 in 196
37–38	1 in 225	1 in 122
39–40	1 in 120	1 in 72
41–45	1 in 60	1 in 37

There is a smaller but definite association of other trisomies with advanced maternal age. Because of these associations, 'elderly' pregnant women are offered karyotyping of amniotic (fetal) cells. As a result of this practice it has been observed that the incidence of chromosome abnormalities in amniotic cells at 16 weeks' gestation is nearly twice the incidence in livebirths. This is partly explained by the condition in stillbirths not being recognised, but there may also have been a real increase in the incidence of Down's syndrome during the last decade.

Indications for chromosome studies

First, chromosome studies on the blood of a

Table 10.8 Counselling in Down's syndrome

Abnormaltity	Relative frequency (per cent)	Recurrence risk for siblings
Trisomy 21	93	1 in 100
Mosaicism	2	Small
de novo translocation	2	Random risk
Inherited translocation 14/21, 13/21, 15/21, 22/21	2	Mother is a carrier: 1 in 3 to 1 in 5 Father is a carrier: 1 in 12 to 1 in 20
Inherited translocation 21/21	1	100 per cent

patient should be requested if there are definite indications of a known chromosome syndrome, if there are suspicious features of such (for example, low birth-weight, failure to thrive and odd appearance) or if several malformations are present in either a still- or livebirth. Other indications include ambiguous or incongruous genitalia, primary amenorrhoea, secondary amenorrhoea with short stature, infertility in a man, a couple who have had three or more spontaneous abortions, or a mentally-retarded male who is thought to have the Martin-Bell syndrome. In all these instances the chance of finding a chromosome abnormality is at least 5 per cent.

Second, chromosome studies on amniotic (fetal) cells should be offered if the mother is aged 35–38 (depending upon local resources), if the father is aged over 55, if one parent carries a balanced structural abnormality, if there has been a previous trisomic child, or if there is a high risk of an X-linked disorder in a son.

GENETIC COUNSELLING

Genetic counselling is essentially a service to patients or to their families. It is provided for those who ask for advice, and should be offered to those who do not, if there is a high risk of a serious disease or a lower risk for a disease that can be detected prenatally. Genetic counselling should also be available for those women who know of no disease in their family, but who find themselves in a high risk category; such as those with a high serum α-fetoprotein level in the second trimester of pregnancy, or those women who have an increased risk of having a chromosomally abnormal child because they are elderly.

The first aim of genetic counselling is to give accurate risks of recurrence to couples, and to put those risks into perspective. Some indications of the risks in genetic or part genetic disorders have already been given. The counsellor should explain to couples the range of severity likely if another child is affected, and whether treatment of the condition, or prenatal detection of it, is possible now or likely to become so in the future.

The second aim is to alert the obstetrician, paediatrician or general practitioner to the risk of a particular disease developing in a neonate. Some

diseases should be treated promptly to prevent complications, e.g. galactosaemia, to prevent cataract formation, and congenital adrenal hyperplasia (21-hydroxylase deficiency, which may be difficult to recognise in a male) in order to prevent collapse and death during intercurrent illness.

The third aim of genetic counselling is to reduce the birth frequency of severely handicapped children in the population. This is a general aim, for on an individual basis there is no pressure by the genetic counsellor to persuade couples to behave in a certain way. The decision is left to them once they know the accurate risks on which to base it.

It is often not easy to give accurate risks of recurrence for those conditions where the aetiology is mixed or is not clear. Table 10.10 lists the empirical recurrence risks for some clinical disease categories. In an undiagnosed but possibly genetic condition in a male, one should always think 'could this be X-linked?' for the genetic advice given to the mother and sisters in such a case is very different from that given for an autosomal recessive condition.

Malformation syndromes may present a difficult problem in diagnosis. If single gene causes are eliminated (usually by the clinical expertise of the paediatrician or geneticist) and chromosome

Table 10.10 Some empirical risks used in counselling heterogenous conditions

Condition in child	Recurrence risk for siblings
Idiopathic microcephaly without neurological signs	1 in 8
Unexplained cerebral palsy which is symmetrical	1 in 9
Asymmetrical cerebral palsy	<1 in 100
Undiagnosed severe mental retardation	1 in 25
Male with IQ 35–50 and no abnormal neurological signs	1 in 5 for brothers
Hydrocephalus without spinabifida	1 in 100
Hydrocephalus in a male with aqueduct stenosis	1 in 10 for brothers
Idiopathic infantile spasms	1 in 50
Petit mal epilipsy	1 in 14
Temporal lobe epilepsy	1 in 16*
Congenital deafness	1 in 8

* excluding febrile conclusions.

studies are normal, then the empirical risk of recurrence is only 1–2 per cent.

It has recently become clear that only 15–20 per cent of couples who have a recognisable risk for having a severely handicapped child actually receive genetic counselling. This is largely a failure of doctors, either to appreciate the risk, or to explain it to the couple concerned, or to search out other relatives who might be at high risk. A population study in Birmingham on the heterogenous condition of retinitis pigmentosa, demonstrated that almost all couples who had symptoms by the time of marriage would have liked to have known the genetic implications of their condition. In autosomal dominant disorders and X-linked disorders there are often high risks for relatives outside the nuclear family and some follow-up system, like that provided by genetic registers, is needed. The conclusion is, inevitably, that many more people than at present would like to have, and should be offered, genetic counselling.

Linkage analysis using probes for DNA polymorphisms

A potentially very helpful aid to counselling in single gene disorders is the use of DNA probes to detect DNA polymorphisms and indirectly to detect genes which are located near the polymorphisms. This technique was developed because DNA can be cut into fragments by bacterial enzymes known as endonucleases or restriction enzymes, because these fragments can then be incorporated into bacterial plasmids or phages (a technique known as recombination) and reproduced or cloned in the bacterial host, and because subsequently the fragments can be made radioactive with ^{32}P. These synthesised radioactive fragments can be used to identify complementary fragments of DNA obtained from the white blood cells of individuals to be investigated. They are called probes because of their value as investigative tools.

These DNA probes are useful because they enable recognition of the polymorphic variation that exists in DNA from different individuals. These polymorphisms occur because the endonucleases (referred to above) cut DNA at specific sites. If a specific site is not present in an individual, because of a variation in DNA structure at that point, then the enzyme will cut the DNA at a later site and a fragment of DNA that is longer than usual will be formed. Thus, the polymorphisms recognised through DNA probes are different lengths of DNA that are secondary to altered DNA structure.

For example, there is a probe called L 128 which is complementary to a stretch of DNA that is situated on the short arm of the X-chromosome. This stretch of DNA is released when the DNA is split by the endonuclease called Taq1, and occurs in two forms: a long (called C1) and a short (called C2). A male, having only one X chromosome will have either C1 or C2 but a female, with two X chromosomes could be C1, C1; C2, C2; or C1, C2. Family studies have shown that this C1/C2 polymorphism is near to the locus for Duchenne and Becker muscular dystrophy and also to the locus for X-linked retinitis pigmentosa.

Using linkage analysis in families that are informative for the relevant polymorphism it will soon be possible to identify gene carriers before symptoms and signs have appeared and to offer prenatal diagnosis through analysis of fetal DNA obtained from trophoblasts or fetal blood cells. There will however be difficulties in knowing which of the isolated cases of X-linked recessive diseases are new mutations. Although there are many technical difficulties to be overcome with these techniques, the hopes for the future are very promising. The reader is referred to a clear account by Weatherall (1982).

FURTHER READING

Blyth H & Carter C O 1969 A guide to genetic prognosis in paediatrics. Spastics International Medical Publications, London

British Medical Bulletin 1976 Human malformations 32: no 1

British Medical Bulletin 1978 The HLA system 34: no 3

Carter C O 1969 An ABC of medical genetics. Lancet Ltd, London

Emery A E H 1976 Methodology in human genetics. Churchill Livingstone, Edinburgh

de Grouchy J & Turleau C 1977 Clinical atlas of human chromosome John Wiley & Sons, New York, Chichester, Brisbane, Toronto

Roberts D F, Chavez J & Court S D M 1970 The genetic component in child mortality. Archives of Disease in Childhood 45: 33–38

Weatherau D J 1982. The new genetics and clinical practice. The Nuffield Provincial Hospitals Trust. London.

11

Behaviour disorders and child psychiatry

Few children will admit that they are disturbed by their thoughts and feelings; they show their upset by disturbed behaviour. The Isle of Wight survey showed that 6 per cent of 10-11 year olds had a psychiatric disorder requiring treatment or further assessment; one-third of these children had problems at home and at school; of the remainder, one-half showed problems only at school and the other half only at home.

Disturbed behaviour in a child must be assessed in relation to the stage of development, if it is to be understood; the child who shows his frustration by lying on the floor and kicking may be considered normal at 2 years of age, but disturbed at 12 years old. The pre-verbal child has few outlets for his feelings and any upset is usually shown by some disturbance in sleep, eating habits or bowel and urinary function. Older children may be able to discuss their feelings; but an objective description from parents and teachers is important.

Once a child can speak he may show disturbance by negative behaviour such as refusal to speak, refusal to go to bed alone, or separate from mother. Habits may develop such as nail biting or withholding of faeces. This negative behaviour is part of the usual behaviour of toddlers, often described as the 'terrible twos'. Parents who are worried about their child's behaviour, can be reassured that it may be a passing phase, but should it persist treatment may be required.

Children over the age of 3 may show these symptoms mentioned above or, more commonly, failure in toilet training, enuresis or encopresis. Problems are common in children of this age; if the phobia becomes incapacitating, it requires treatment. Somatic symptoms in the form of headaches, abdominal pain or vague aches and pains,

may also develop. If a positive medical diagnosis cannot be made, then a positive psychiatric diagnosis should be sought, but these sysptoms should not be over-investigated. Adolescence poses its own problems.

Common problems in childhood are outlined in Table 11.1.

Table 11.1 Common problems in childhood

Birth — 1 year	Difficulty in going to sleep or waking Poor feeding or vomiting Restlessness
1–3 years	Refusal to separate from mother Refusal to go to bed alone Nightmares Constipation Nail biting
Over 3 years	Clinging behaviour Encopresis Phobias Abdominal pain or headaches Delayed or incoherent speech

PSYCHOLOGICAL ASSESSMENT IN CHILDREN

This should be based on school reports, a detailed history from the parents or guardians, and interview with the child and psychological tests if indicated.

A school report gives an indication of whether the child shows disturbance in relationships with adults or children, or whether there is any learning difficulty.

The history

Both parents should be seen if possible, as they

may have different views of the child. It also allows the interviewer to make some assessment of the marital interaction. Questions should be asked concerning the following matters:

1. *Current problem.* The parents will describe this and some questions can be asked as to possible precipating factors such as separation or illness

2. *The pregnancy and birth.* Was this baby planned and how did the mother feel during the pregnancy? Was there any separation following delivery?

3. *Feeding.* Was the baby breast or bottle fed and was this easily established. Were solids accepted? Has there been any feeding disturbance or food fads?

4. *Toilet training.* How was this introduced and established? Have there been any relapses?

5. *Sleep.* What has been the child's sleep pattern and has this altered in any way? Does the child have nightmares or talk about dreams?

6. *Speech development.* Has speech developed appropriately or is it delayed?

7. *Habit disorders.* Does the child have any mannerisms or tics or disorders such as thumb sucking, nail biting or head banging

8. *Motor development.* Is the child coordinating?

Interview with the Child

This must be geared to the age and stage of development of the child. It is important to reassure the child that you are not going to give him an injection or hurt him, and some explanation that you are there to listen to any worries he may have will be reassuring. Younger children will want to use toys. They will also be able to draw and give you associations to the pictures.

If a child has difficulty in talking then questions may help, but may only produce monosyllabic answers. A child's three wishes will also give insight into his areas of anxiety.

The child should be seen together with his parents and also separately.

Information gained from interviewing the Child alone includes: appearance; motor development; attention span; speech; manner of relating; emotional state; atitudes to home, school, parents; and feelings about his problems.

Psychological Tests

These are used to measure IQ and levels of achievement, while projective tests will highlight areas of difficulty. It is important to know whether school failure is due to low IQ or to anxiety, as the treatment differs. Educational psychologists or clinical psychologists attached to the Child Guidance Clinics will be qualified to adminster these tests.

CHILDREN IN HOSPITAL

Inevitably some young children have to be admitted to hospital either for short or long-term treatment. The effects on the child may be two-fold:

1. Separation from mother and his familiar surroundings
2. The effects of pain and medical and surgical interventions.

1. Separation

Children under the age of 4 years are entirely dependent on their parents and have an especially close relationship with their mother, or primary caretaker. Separation from mother should be gradual and only for a few hours in the beginning; children may start at a half-day playgroup or nursery from the age of 3 years. If the child has to go into hospital it is best that his mother stays with him and, if this is not possible, that she is allowed free visiting during the day in order to minimise the effects of separation, such as the feeling of deprivation of love and security. Children under 4 years of age are too young to understand that they are ill or have to be separated from their parents. Despite preparation for admission, and the presence of the mother, many children still show sleep disturbance, temper tantrums and may be insecure even 6 months after a stay in hospital.

Prolonged hospital admission may lead to serious impoverishment of the personality. Children who are in hospital for a long time may be 'promiscuous' in their behaviour and latch on to any adult in their search for affection.

2. Effects of medical and surgical treatment

Although the taking of blood by venepuncture may seem relatively insignificant to doctors, children perceive it as extremely traumatic. It may be viewed as an assault and the 'stealing' of something important. Children in hospital have to passively accept ministrations of nurses and to hand over ownership of their own body. Thus, a child who is toilet trained and proud of it, may suddenly be required to urinate or defaecate in front of a strange adult — if he complies this may lead to a regression once he returns home and an inability to maintain bowel and bladder control. Children may make more fuss over apparently minor interventions than over major surgery, and may even deny it is going to happen.

Before any procedure, an age-appropriate explanation should be given to the child. This may simply be that the prick of the needle will hurt for a second, but there will be no lasting pain. It is not worth trying to con a child that a procedure will be painless because he will never believe you again.

3. Chronic illness and death

Children who are subjected to chemotherapy will develop coping strategies, but these do no always meet with medical and nursing approval. It is natural for a child to be angry when he is ill and it is healthy to express this anger. The anger however, is often directly towards adults who are trying to help the child and they may find it hard to accept. From the child's point of view it is worse to turn the anger inwards and become depressed, but from the parent's and staff's viewpoint it may be easier to manage. No child should be forced to acknowledge that he is dying if he does not want to know; sensitive handling of questions will often allow parents, staff, siblings and the dying child to share feelings which allow the child to die peacefully instead of fighting and struggling.

It is remarkable that children frequently choose the most junior nurse or medical student to ask 'will I ever get better?' or 'am I going to die?' Perhaps they sense that the inexperienced will be more honest. These questions, however, need not be answered directly nor avoided, but the subject can be opened up by replying 'what has made you think that?' The child can then share his experiences and understanding of the treatment and perhaps make more realistic plans for the future.

DEVELOPMENTAL AND HABIT DISORDERS

In these conditions there is a delay in acquiring control of a function or functions or the body, or there is a regression to earlier modes of behaviour.

Enuresis

(see Chapter 15)
The cause may be physical or emotional; emotional disturbance is usually seen as regressive behaviour after bladder control has been established. Stresses leading to regression may be a death in the family, including death of a pet, birth of a sibling, or separation due to parental or the child's own illness, and hospitalisation.

Treatment

1. Exclude a physical cause
2. An active interest in the child is important; the family may be very angry with the child, but often the mother is surprisingly compliant with the child's symptom. A carrot, not a stick, is the basis of treatment but it is unrealistic for the mother to wash sheets daily with no comment and possibly the child and mother should change the bedding together
3. Reward systems may be valuable. A simple star chart or payment for a dry night may encourage the child
4. Explanations may also be important to the child and parents, particularly if bedwetting is associated with nightmares. It usually occurs in stage 4 rapid eye movement sleep, but may have a meaning to the child, if this is explored in an interview
5. Drug treatment: tricyclic antidepressants
6. Conditioning with a pad and buzzer. The child's bed is made with two aire gauze sheets separated by a cotton sheet and connected to

a bell or buzzer. As the child starts to wet the bed he completes the electric circuit and the buzzer wakes him. Gradually he wakes before the alarm goes off, as the feeling of a full bladder is associated with waking. This is not suitable under the age of 8 years

7. Psychotherapy may be indicated if there are clear emotional precipitants. Depending on the clinical assessment, this may be aimed individually at the child, or in a family setting to elucidate the interactions. Formal psychotherapy should be with a trained therapist.

Encopresis

This usually presents as soiling the underclothes on the way to or from school, although occasionally soiling occurs at night. It may also be associated with smearing of faeces or defaecating in unusual places. Soiling is more frequently seen in boys than girls.

1. Continuous soiling may be due to lack of toilet training and may occur in children who are generally ill cared for

2. Regressive soiling may be associated with secondary enuresis and the precipitating factors are similar

3. Aggressive soiling. This is seen in children who feel oppressed by parental demands to be clean and tidy and to perform well at school.

Treatment depends on the cause, but retraining and removal of impacted faeces may be necessary. In regressive and aggressive soiling, psychotherapy or family therapy may be indicated.

Nightmares and pavor nocturnus.

Many children recount their dreams and will talk freely about nightmares, these are usually related to anxiety or wishes which they know are unacceptable in the daytime. Nightmares often have a precipitant, such as the birth of a sibling, and if the child can talk about his anger and feelings of displacement, the nightmares will disappear. Where nightmares occur in REM sleep, pavor nocturnus occurs in stage 4 sleep and children have no memory of the disturbance. Parents describe the child as calling out in his sleep, sitting bolt upright and staring. The child does not

appear to hear the parents' calming words but within a few minutes he lies down and continues to sleep.

Reassurance is usually sufficient for both parents and children. If pavor nocturnus persists the child might need a small dose of a tricyclic antidepressant at night to make sleep lighter, and break the pattern.

Other habit disorders

These include feeding disorders, nail biting, speech defects and sleep disorders. All of these may reflect poor training and poor mother-child interaction. Treatment is aimed at helping the child to develop normally and helping the parents to be consistent in their handling of the child.

CONDUCT DISORDERS

By definition these disorders cover the group of children whose behaviour is antisocial. It is usually society and not parents who complain about the child, and juvenile courts, probation officers or social workers are often involved. Although parents may complain of the child's behaviour, the parents themselves are often antisocial. They may be inconsistent and rejecting towards the child. Symptoms include lying, stealing, truancy, physical aggression and vandalism.

Truancy

As with other conduct disorders, this is more common in boys than girls. There may be a family history of truancy, although the parents are not aware that the child is truanting. He will leave for school in the morning and return home at the appropriate time in the evening, but during the day he will be involved in petty crime. These children are usually not highly intelligent and find school unrewarding. Truancy is more common in the older age groups.

Treatment must be aimed at both the family and the individual and may involve social change. Some children have to be removed from home to boarding school or residential placements. Other children can be helped via the parents, who receive social help, or encouragement to set consistent limits.

NEUROTIC DISORDERS

Neurotic children suffer from their symptoms. The symptoms are persistent and incapacitating in some areas of life.

Common symptoms are depression, anxiety, obsessional rituals and somatic symptoms. Although some anxiety is common in response to new situations, neurotic children respond out of all proportion to the stimulus.

School refusal

This is an extremely common condition, although it may not be obvious to the general practitioner, paediatrician or even school. The child may appear physically ill, or present with complaints of headache, stomach-ache, or general malaise. There may be a genuine physical illness initially, from which the child fails to return to school. Sometimes lengthy physical investigations reveal no illness and it is only then that anxiety and panic are recognised.

Table 11.2 Non-attendance at school

	School refusal	Truancy
Age	5–11 years	Over 12 years
Parents	Collude with child over non-attendance	Unaware of problem
Achievement	High with high goals	Non-academic, with only practical goals
Treatment	Insight therapy	Structural change

The child often expresses the wish to go to school but is unable to leave home, or if he does he cannot enter the classroom. However, once he returns home he appears perfectly well. Girls outnumber boys in primary school age, but in adolescence this becomes more of a problem for boys. Although the child may say a specific teacher or subject is what he is trying to avoid, this is usually a rationalisation and the real problem is that of leaving mother. Mothers of these children often have phobic symptoms or excessive anxiety and the mother and child become locked into a mutually clinging relationship.

Treatment

The child must be given a date to return to school and the father or educational welfare officer, or other outside agent should be involved in actually taking the child from home to school, this helps child and mother.

The child should not be allowed to change school or have home tuition as this colludes with his problem. Physical examination is necessary to rule out physical illness, but long investigations should not be embarked upon. The teachers will need information about the child and how to manage him when he says he feels ill. Diazepam may be helpful as a single dose on waking in the morning, but should not be used long term.

Ongoing work with the family, aimed at helping them to adjust in a more healthy manner, will be necessary if the symptom is not to recur.

Other forms of anxiety

As a child develops it is important that he develops *signal anxiety*. This means that he does not rely on the presence of adults to warn him of danger, but can recognise when he needs to avoid danger. An example of this is that children learn to judge the speed of cars when crossing the road.

As this signal anxiety is developing it may appear to be exaggerated at times, almost to phobic proportions. Thus it is common to see children who are phobic of dogs or other animals. This may be a developmental phase but if it persists it may need full investigation, as it may represent a displacement of anxiety from a deeper irrational fear to something which seems to have a rational basis.

Depression

Children may show symptoms of depression, tearfulness, listlessness, inability to concentrate, poor appetite, excessive sleepiness and hopelessness. It may be clear that the child is reacting to a family disturbance or loss of a parent, but sometimes there seems to be no precipitating cause. The child may develop obsessional behaviour as a defence against depression. This is usually seen in ritual behaviour where the child must do things in a particular order, and he believes this will prevent his feeling sad.

Treatment

Treatment is usually based on psychotherapy for the child, to help him to understand his feelings and therefore to react differently. Family therapy may be indicated if there are tensions which are not being openly discussed.

CHILDHOOD PSYCHOSIS

Psychotic children have an altered contact with reality and are attempting to adapt to a subjectively distorted concept of the world. In young children, the diagnosis can be made from the behaviour which includes a failure to make normal emotional contact with people. It is important to try to distinguish psychotic behaviour from that of the intellectually subnormal child. It is also important to rule out any other organic pathology.

1. Acute toxic conditions

In these children there is a diffuse impairment of cerebral function with a state of delirium or confusion. Common causes are systemic infection, intracranial infection, metabolic disturbances, chemical intoxications including drugs, and brain injury.

2. Chronic organic causes

a. Lead encephalopathy

Lead encephalopathy may present as a behaviour disorder with symptoms or irritability, restlessness, inability to concentrate and loss of interest

b. Cerebral lipidoses

The onset of symptoms is usually between 3 and 5 years of age and the child's condition deteriorates rapidly. Although neurological signs are usually present the child may present as psychotic.

3. Psychoses of mixed aetiology

a.   Infantile psychosis or autism
b.   Late onset psychosis or childhood schizophrenia

A distinction may be made between the two following conditions (Table 11.3) and also between them and mental subnormality.

a. Infantile psychosis.

Kanner in 1943 described three features of autistic children: a lack of awareness of people and an avoidane of contact; delay or absence of speech with abnormalities such as echolalia, where the

Table 11.3 Comparison of early onset and late onset psychosis

	Early onset (autism)	Late onset (childhood schizophrenia)
Age of onset	Before 3 years	After 5 years
Speech	Delayed or echolalia	No abnormality
Schizphrenic symptoms	Absent	Auditory and bodily hallucinations, thought insertion and withdrawal and broadcast delusions
Motility	Steotypies	Loss of volition. Apathy
Incidence of schizophrenia in relatives	Lower than average	Above average
Drug treatment	Symptomatic relief only	Phenothiazines useful

child merely repeats what is said to him, and an obsessional desire for sameness, differences causing a catastrophic reaction. Parents may describe the baby as 'very good' and able to entertain himself. However, this usually means he is avoiding social contact and prefers objects, often a hard object, to people. The parents may also describe rituals which the child has developed, or stereotyped behaviour. Autistic withdrawal and speech delay, or absence of speech development usually lead parents to seek advice during the child's second year, but they usually describe problems from birth. The incidence is 4–5/10 000, with four boys to one girl. The incidence appears to be higher in social classes one and two but some people argue that intelligent parents push harder for action than less intelligent parents.

Treatment. All forms of treatment have been tried with mixed claims of success.

(i) Institutional care. Some families are unable to care for their autistic child, either because of violence, other children or the parents suffer too much. There are a few specialised institutions offering skilled teaching and handling

(ii) Behaviour therapy is aimed at rewarding acceptable behaviour and punishing unacceptable behaviour. A programme must be worked out for each individual child

(iii) Psychotherapy is very time consuming and not always rewarding, although it can lead to breakthroughs in communication

(iv) Drugs may be needed to treat symptoms such as violence or sleeplessness, but are not curative.

b. Late-onset psychosis

Children appear to be developing normally and then after the age of 5 years the parents or teachers notice abnormalities of behaviour and a falling off the academic performance. The symptoms are similar to those adult schizophrenic symptoms described by Schneider. These include hallucinations, delusions, thought withdrawal, thought insertion, and loss of volition. In talking to these children the clinician will know that the child is psychotic because of his apparent chaos and misunderstanding of the world. The parents of this group of children have a significantly higher rate of schizophrenia than the general population. They also tend to be isolated, which is attributed to their personalities. This contrasts with parents of the infantile psychosis group, whose social isolation is secondary to their child's illness.

Treatment of these children also varies. The *infantile psychosis* group pose severe difficulties in day-to-day handling and often have to be admitted to day units or residential units for behaviour modification or long-term psychotherapy, the parents also need long-term counselling.

The *late-onset* group respond well to phenothiazine tranquillisers or haloperidol, although short-term hospital admission may be necessary. Supportive psychotherapy for the child and parents may also be beneficial and some families benefit from family therapy. The course of the illness is usually progressive and insitutional care may be necessary eventually.

ADOLESCENCE

Adolescence is a time of turmoil and can cause distress to both the adolescent and those who have contact with him.

The task for each adolescent is to leave behind his childhood dependency on his parents and to begin to function more as an independent person. He must be able to risk parental disapproval without feeling that he must give in to parental demands. This may be in the area of sexuality, friendships or work. The parents have to allow their adolescent son or daughter to make mistakes and to be different from parental ideals. This is not always easy and many parents, especially mothers who may be menopausal, find it hard to allow their children free expression of sexuality.

The adolescent also has to come to terms with his or her sexually maturing body. He must feel in control of his body and find acceptable outlets for sexual and aggressive feelings. This involves changes in types of relationships with friends of the same and the opposite sex. The demands and expectations of these friends will be more adult.

The problems of adolescence are numerous, but there are two serious conditions, anorexia nervosa and drug addiction.

Anorexia nervosa

The condition occurs mainly in girls although it has been described in boys. The onset is usually soon after puberty in a girl who is overweight and starts to diet. She finds herself unable to stop and becomes emaciated. Her periods cease, if they have commenced, and the girl becomes determined to keep her weight at pre-pubertal levels. These girls have an unrealistic perception of themselves and believe they are fat when, in reality, they are thin; their perception of other people is not distorted. The girl herself is often active and cheerful and it is her parents who seek help.

Once recognised this conditions requires specialist help. This usually means inpatient treatment in a special unit with therapy available both for the adolescent and her family. Untreated these girls survive on the brink of death and may die while still denying their problem.

Drug addiction

Drug addiction is increasing in our society. In its widest definition it covers smoking, drinking, the use of diazepam, sniffing solvents through to the abuse of LSD and heroin. Adolescence is a time of experimentation and many young people test for themselves the effects of alcohol and tobacco. They may also take various tablets and cannabis without becoming dependent on them. However, the dividing line between experimenting and addiction is very narrow. The adolescent who becomes dependent on drugs is usually one who is depressed and may have had early losses in his or her life. These adolescents are disillusioned with life and may be on the fringe of criminal activity, drug addiction forces them further into crime because they have to finance the habit.

If an adolescent is suspected of drug abuse because of erratic or other changes in behaviour, clinical examination and an objective history are essential. This may reveal altered pupil size or reaction, injection sites or infected injection sites. In solvent sniffers there may be inflammation and sores around the mouth and nose. Urine can be analysed for the presence of drugs and once the diagnosis is confirmed treatment at a drug addiction clinic is usually indicated.

THE ROLE OF THE DOCTOR

It will be clear from these descriptions of both the physically ill children who respond to stress with behaviour problems, and those children under stress who have somatic symptoms, that the general practitioner will be the first doctor whom the parents consult. In order to sort out the physical and emotional problems the doctor will have to spend time taking a history and listening carefully to the child, the family and their worries.

Once a diagnosis has been reached much of the treatment can be managed by the GP or a paediatrician. If a referral to a child or adolescent psychiatrist is made, the reasons must be carefully explained to the child and family. Too often, the family feel that the doctor has given up or become 'fed up' with them, and is therefore handing them over. Joint management of a family can be extremely rewarding.

Individual therapy must be given by a trained therapist but marital therapy and family therapy are often given by two therapists, one of whom may be a doctor and the other a psychotherapist or social worker.

Children attend school and their teachers are often concerned with day-to-day management, so that regular communication is vital if they are to complement treatment. It is also important to involve community social workers and probation officers, who already know the family, when planning a treatment programme. The multidisciplinary approach can be destructive if it is used merely to dispel anxiety of the professionals and allows no one to take responsibility for helping a child and his family. If used properly the involvement of different professionals can be most rewarding.

FURTHER READING

Barker P 1971 Basic child psychiatry. Staples Press, London
Earle E M 1979 Psychological effects of mutilating surgery in children and adolescents in the psychoanalytic study of the child. 34:

Freud A 1973 Normality and pathology in childhood. Penguin, Harmondsworth

Kahn J 1981 Unwillingly to school. Pergamon Oxford

Kolvin I 1971 Studies in childhood psychoses. British Journal of Psychiatry 118: 341–419

Laufer M 1975 Adolescent disturbance and breakdown. Penguin, Harmondsworth

Robertson J 1975 Young children in hospital, 2nd edn. Tavistock, London

Rutter M L 1975 Helping troubled children Penguin, Harmondsworth.

Graham P J 1966 Psychiatric disorders in ten to eleven year old children. Proceedings of Royal Society of Medicine 59: 382–87

Winnicott D W 1964 The child, the family and the outside world. Penguin, London

12

Infectious diseases

Infections are the commonest reason for children to be brought to their general practitioner. Infections of the upper and lower respiratory tracts, gastrointestinal and urinary tracts, bone, joints and central nervous system are described in other chapters. This chapter will focus on some of the common infectious diseases seen in children in this country. How these infections may affect the fetus and newborn infant is also described. A guide to the clinical diagnosis of the rashes caused by the major acute infectious diseases in children is included at the end of the chapter.

COMMON INFECTIOUS DISEASES OF CHILDHOOD

In the UK there has been a dramatic reduction this century in the morbidity and mortality from infectious diseases. Many factors are responsible for this change, including improved housing conditions, sanitation and nutrition, and the introduction of vaccines. The role of medical treatment and the widespread use of antibiotics is more difficult to determine. Some of the infectious diseases are kept under surveillance (Table 12.1) and preventive measures taken in the community, when appropriate, to avoid the spread of infection. In industrialised countries many of these infectious diseases of childhood have become more of an inconvenience than serious illnesses. However, the loss of time from school for the child, and from work for their parents, both during the illness and until the child can return to school, can be significant (Table 12.2). Although they are uncommon, there are still serious complications of these infectious diseases and they have also taken on a renewed importance in children who are immunocompromised.

Measles

The measles virus is transmitted by direct contact or droplet spread with respiratory secretions and is highly infectious. The illness is so common in children that it tends to be regarded as a normal event of childhood. This is unfortunate as it is an unpleasant, potentially serious and is preventable. Since the introduction of measles immunisation, the incidence has declined somewhat but it

Table 12.1 Notifiable infectious diseases, England and Wales 1981

Acute encephalitis	Leprosy*	Relapsing fever
Acute meningitis	Leptospirosis	Scarlet fever
Acute poliomyelitis	Malaria	Smallpox
Anthrax	Marburg disease	Tetanus
Cholera	Measles	Tuberculosis
Diptheria	Ophthalmia	Typhoid fever
Dysentery	neonatorum	Typhus fever
Food poisoning	Paratyphoid fever	Viral haemorrhagic
Infective jaundice	Plague	fever
Lassa fever	Rabies	Whooping cough
		Yellow fever

* Data collected centrally in confidence by departments of health

Table 12.2 Incubation period and period of exclusion from school of the common infectious diseases

Illness	Incubation period (days)		Minimum period of exclusion from school*
	Range	Usual period	
Measles	7–14	10	7 days from the onset of the rash
Chickenpox	10–24	14	6 days from the onset of the rash
Rubella	14–21	18	4 days from onset of the rash
Mumps	12–31	18	Until swelling has subsided (7 days minimum)
Hepatitis A	15–50	28	Until clinical recovery and not before 7 days from onset of jaundice

* This is based on the 'Guidance on the exclusion of children from day schools on account of infectious diseases' issued by the Inner London Education Authority Area Health Authorities' School Health Service, 1980.

continues to be widespread as the acceptance rate for immunisation is only around 50 per cent or less. This contrasts with the USA where the incidence has fallen dramatically as their immunisation acceptance rate is much higher.

Clinical features

The incidence of measles is highest in the pre-school child. Since the introduction of measles immunisation, an increasing proportion of affected children are of school age.

The incubation period of around 10 days is followed by a prodromal illness of fever and widespread congestion of the mucous membranes, with coryza, conjunctivitis and cough. The prodromal illness lasts 3–4 days, during which the child is very miserable and anorexic. Bronchitis is part of the illness as the involvement of the mucous membranes includes the epithelium of the bronchi and bronchioles and crepitations can usually be heard on auscultation of the chest. Observing Koplik's spots is helpful in making the diagnosis at this stage as they are pathognomonic of measles. They may be difficult to detect and are tiny white spots, like grains of salt, on the inflamed buccal mucosa and are best seen opposite the second molar teeth. They are visible 2–3 days before the onset of the rash and then fade when the rash appears. They are sometimes still visible a day or two after the rash has emerged. The rash starts behind the ears, and spreads to the forehead and then to the face and down the body. It is initially a dull red, maculopapular rash but becomes confluent and blotchy. The rash and fever are usually maximal a day after the onset of the rash. In the week following the disappearance of the rash staining of the skin may be quite marked in some patients. The rash starts to fade by the third day in the same sequence as it appeared.

Complications

Complications arise from extension of the inflammation caused by the virus or from superadded bacterial infection. They are most likely in those who have a severe attack and in infants and young children. The commonest complications are respiratory, especially bronchopneumonia, otitis media and laryngotracheitis, but these are seen only infrequently in well-nourished children. Children with leukaemia or who are immunocompromised may develop a severe giant-cell pneumonia which is usually fatal.

Febrile convulsions may occur during the prodromal illness and during the first 2 days of the rash. Post-infectious encephalitis has been reported to occur in up to one in 1000 cases. Approximately 7–10 days after the onset of the illness the child develops a headache, vomiting and drowsiness which may progress to coma and be accompanied by convulsions. The course is unpredictable; 60 per cent recover completely, but as many as 25 per cent have permanent brain damage and in 15 per cent it is fatal. A rare late complication, occuring in one in 100 000 cases, is subacute sclerosing panencephalitis.

Treatment

There is no specific treatment. Regular paracetamol will assist in reducing the fever and may make the child feel less miserable. Antibiotics are only required for bronchopneumonia or otitis media. Children with encephalitis or significant upper airways obstructions from laryngotracheitis will need to be closely monitored in hospital.

Measles in the developing countries

Measles remains a serious illness in the developing countries where it carries a high morbidity and mortality. This is primarily related to the socio-economic conditions and it is an especially serious illness in areas where the diet is deficient in protein. The rash in these malnourished children may be confluent and become deep red, purple or even haemorrhagic, and then desquamate. There is a high incidence of secondary bacterial infection with otitis media and bronchopneumonia. These children often have a very sore mouth and severe diarrhoea resulting in a marked loss of weight, which may take many weeks to be regained. It is important to ensure that these children do not become dehydrated and to maintain their nutrition both during and after the illness.

Chickenpox and shingles

Chickenpox (varicella) and shingles (zoster) are caused by the varicella-zoster virus. Chickenpox, the primary infection, is highly infectious and is transmitted by droplet spread or direct contact, either from lesions in the mouth and respiratory tract or, less commonly, from vesicles on the skin. Shingles cannot be contracted directly from a patient with chickenpox but results from reactivation of the virus which lies dormant in a dorsal root ganglion. It is a source of infection to those who have not had chickenpox.

Chickenpox

Chickenpox is characteristically a mild illness in children. The incubation period usually lasts 14 days and may be followed by a short prodromal stage of malaise and a low grade fever but, more often, the onset of the illness is marked by the appearance of the rash. This begins as red macules which progress rapidly to papules and vesicles. The vesicles then dry to form crusts which form scabs and these fall off without leaving scars. The lesions are itchy and premature removal of the scabs or secondary infection may result in scar formation. The lesions appear in crops, so that all the stages are visible even over a small area. There are often 2 or 3 successive crops of lesions over the first few days, but this varies widely from a handful of lesions to 5 or more successive crops. The rash starts in the hair and has a centripetal distribution, with the lesions most densely grouped on the trunk and decreasing in density on the limbs and face, although they may spread as far as the palms and soles. Lesions are usually present on the mucous membranes where they take the form of shallow ulcers as the roofs of the vesicles are removed.

Complications

Occasionally lesions become secondarily infected, usually with *Staphylococcus aureus* or streptococci. Other complications are very uncommon in healthy children. In encephalitis, symptoms and signs develop 3–10 days after the appearance of the rash, and ataxia from cerebellar involvement is common. The prognosis is much better than in measles encephalitis, and at least 80 per cent recover completely. Adults with chickenpox tend to experience a more severe form of the disease, and are more likely to develop chickenpox pneumonia. In contrast to normal children, chickenpox in an immunocompromised host may cause pneumonia and be very severe or even fatal. This includes children with leukaemia or lymphomas, and those on cytotoxic drugs or high doses of corticosteroids. When any of these children first present, the state of their immunity to varicella should be assessed so that their parents can be alerted to the potential danger of chickenpox. The patients should try to avoid contact with infected children but this is difficult and should it occur, zoster immune globulin should be given as soon as possible, preferably within 48 hours. Haemorrhagic chickenpox, which has a high mortality, is fortunately rare. Occasionally, children develop Reye's syndrome shortly after they have had chickenpox. Aspirin ingestion has been implicated in the pathogenesis of Reye's syndrome and although their true relationship is still unclear, in the USA it has been recommended that aspirin be avoided in children with chickenpox.

Diagnosis

It is seldom necessary to have laboratory confirmation of the clinical diagnosis. The virus can be demonstrated by electron microscopy of vesicular fluid, by culture or fluorescent-antibody staining. Infection can also be confirmed serologically by a four-fold rise in antibody.

Treatment

In most cases no specific treatment is necessary, but calamine lotion may be soothing. If the pruritus is troublesome, an oral antihistamine, such as trimeprazine tartrate (Vallergan), can be given. Acyclovir (Zovirax), an antiviral agent which acts as a competitive inhibitor of the viral DNA polymerase, appears to be effective against varicella-zoster infections and to have low toxicity. A course of acyclovir needs to be considered in immunocompromised children and those with serious complications. There is now an experimental vaccine, which has been used in children with leukaemia.

Shingles

Herpes zoster is much less common than chickenpox in childhood but is occasionally seen even in infants and young children. It is usually confined to the skin supplied by the sensory nerves of one or two dorsal root ganglia. Unlike adults, itching, burning or pain rarely precede the lesions,

and it is usually a mild illness causing little discomfort and without postherpetic neuralgia.

Herpes simplex infections

Herpes simplx infections are caused by the viruses Herpes hominis, types 1 (HSV 1) and 2 (HSV 2). HSV 1 is mainly associated with infection of the mouth and lips, eyes, skin and central nervous system, whilst HSV 2 causes mostly genital and neonatal infections.

Type 1 infection is common in childhood. Primary infection with clinical symptoms occurs in less than 10 per cent of infections, so, in most instances, the infection is not apparent. By adulthood 70–90 per cent of people have antibodies to the herpes simplex virus. Sometimes the virus remains latent and produces recurrent clinical symptoms.

Primary infection causes gingivostomatitis, vulvovaginitis, keratoconjunctivitis, or encephalitis. Acute gingivostomatitis (Fig. 12.1) is much the commonest. It affects children between 1 and 3 years old, who develop a high fever, irritability and sore throat resulting in refusal to eat or drink. The gums become swollen, red and friable. White plaques or shallow ulcers appear on the buccal

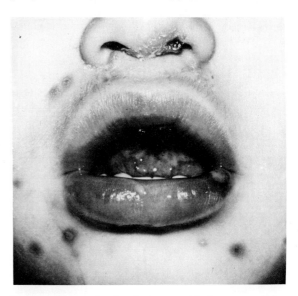

Fig. 12.1 Herpes simplex gingivostomatitis (by prepermission of the Board of Governors, The Hospital for Sick Children, London)

mucosa, tongue, palate and fauces. Saliva drools from the mouth and may result in satellite skin lesions around the mouth and anterior chest. The anterior cervical lymph nodes may be enlarged and tender. The severity of the illness varies, but in severe cases the illness lasts 10–14 days. The child may become dehydrated from refusing to eat or drink. Vulvovaginitis sometimes results from transfer of the organism from the mouth with contaminated fingers. In children with eczema, the infection may become extensive or even generalised (Fig. 12.2). Superadded bacterial infection (Staphylococcus aureus or streptococcal) is common. The illness may be very severe or even fatal from viraemia, septicaemia, shock from plasma loss or disseminated intravascular coagulation. Keratoconjunctivitis is uncommon, but dendritic ulcers may proceed to scarring and loss of vision. Herpes simplex encephalitis is a serious condition but is fortunately rare.

The diagnosis is usually made from the clinical appearance. It can be confirmed, if necessary, by

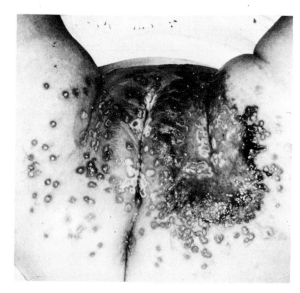

Fig. 12.2b Severe herpes simplex vulvovaginitis in the same child (by permission of the Board of Governors, The Hospital for Sick Children, London)

culture, electron microscopy of vesicular fluid, microscopic examination for inclusion bodies, or serologically.

Treatment of the gingivostomatitis is mainly supportive and the child's state of hydration must be kept under review. Topical treatment with idoxuridine is only partially effective and most children find any interference with the lesions very unpleasant; it is best avoided. In severe herpes simplex infections, treatment with intravenous acyclovir will need to be considered. In eczema herpeticum, the topical steroids used to treat the eczema should be stopped and systemic antibiotics and antiviral therapy with acyclovir may be required. Keratoconjunctivitis should be managed by an ophthalmologist. Topical acyclovir has recently become available for the treatment of ocular lesions.

Rubella

Rubella or German measles is caused by the rubella virus and is transmitted by close and repeated contact with the respiratory secretions of an infected person. Rubella is common in young children but is also seen more often in older children and adolescents than the other childhood exanthematous diseases. The incubation period is

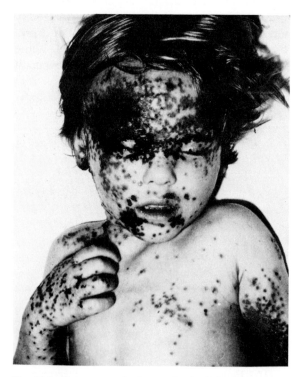

Fig. 12.2a Severe extensive herpes simplex infection in a child with eczema (Kaposi's varicelliform eruption) (by permission of the Board of Governors, The Hospital for Sick Children, London)

about 18 days; with a range of 14–21 days. In children, it is usually a very mild illness and symptoms before the appearance of the rash are uncommon. The infection is often subclinical. The pale pink macular or maculo-papular rash starts on the face and behind the ears and spreads down the body. It has usually started to disappear from the face by the second day and faded completely by the third day. It often loses its discrete appearance and can become scarlatiniform. There may be generalised lymphadenopathy especially involving the suboccipital, postauricular and cervical lymph nodes. Coryza, conjunctivitis and sore throat, if present are minimal. In the adolescent or young adult there may be a mild prodromal illness, with a slight fever, malaise, a few swollen and sometimes tender lymph nodes and they often have arthralgia or arthritis, mainly affecting the joints of the hands and feet, 2–3 days after the onset of the rash. The complications of rubella, encephalitis and thrombocytopenic purpura, are extremely rare.

Hepatitis

Two causes of viral hepatitis have been identified, viruses A and B. A further relatively common agent or group of agents has been designated non-A, non-B, but has not been identified. In patients with hepatitis in whom infection from the hepatitis A and B viruses, the Epstein-Barr virus and cytomegalovirus have been excluded, a diagnosis of infection by the non-A, non-B virus can be made.

Hepatitis A virus infection

Hepatitis A is the commonest form of hepatitis seen in children. The hepatitis A virus is an enteric virus, transmitted through close contact by the faecal-oral route, often on contaminated fingers. The infection is commonest when the living conditions are overcrowded and inadequate and the standard of hygiene poor. Most children in these conditions have antibodies to the hepatitis A virus by late childhood, whereas the frequency of antibody in children of high socioeconomic status is low. There has been a marked decrease in the incidence of hepatitis A in the UK over the last few years. The virus can be identified in the stools of infected persons by electron microscopy 1–2 weeks before, and usually a few days after, the onset of jaundice, and infectivity is maximal during this period.

The incubation period is between 15–50 days with an average of 28–30 days. Three to 5 days before the onset of jaundice, the patient becomes anorexic with nausea, vomiting and there may be dull abdominal pain especially over the right hypochondrium or epigastrium. There may be a fever and mild diarrhoea. Just before the icteric phase the urine may become dark from the presence of bilirubin and the stools may become pale. The jaundice lasts for several days. The liver may be enlarged and tender on palpation and there may be mild enlargement of the spleen and lymphadenopathy. In young children the infection is mostly subclinical or mild. They often remain anicteric. If they become jaundiced it is usually only for a day or two. The vast majority of affected children recover completely.

The liver function tests are abnormal with a rise in the serum aminotransferases. The bilirubin may or may not be raised. Investigations will be required in children with hepatitis when the illness is atypical, especially severe or protracted. Other causes of jaundice will then need to be considered, especially hepatitis B, the hepatitis of infectious mononucleosis or cytomegalovirus, chronic active hepatitis and Wilson's disease. In obstructive jaundice, the alkaline phosphatase level is markedly elevated, whereas it rarely rises above one and half times normal in hepatitis A infection. A definite diagnosis of hepatitis A can be made by detecting a rise in antibodies such as hepatitis-A-specific IgM.

There is no specific treatment. Children who are feeling unwell will restrict their activities accordingly and bed rest need not be enforced.

No special diet is required, but dietary fat may be restricted if it is found to cause nausea. Hands must be washed diligently and a high standard of personal hygiene maintained to prevent spread of the disease to others. In hospital, these patients are isolated and nursed with enteric precautions. An injection of pooled immunoglobulin following exposure may prevent or modify the illness and is recommended as soon as possible for household and institutional contacts. (The standard dose of immunoglobulin is 500 mg in those over 10 years and 250 mg in those less than 10 years). Children with hepatitis A infection can return to school 7 days after the onset of jaundice if they have recovered clinically. Prophylactic immunoglobulin is recommended for travellers to countries where hepatitis A infection is endemic if they may stay in areas where the personal hygiene and sanitation are poor.

Hepatitis B virus infection

Hepatitis B is a relatively uncommon illness in children in industrialised countries, but the incidence is much higher in countries where the carrier rate of the hepatitis B surface antigen (HBsAg) is high. In Northern Europe and North America the carrier rate is low, around one in 1000 adults, but it is much higher in the Far East and Africa. Children at special risk for hepatitis B are babies born to mothers who are HBsAg carriers, those who live in institutions, or are immunocompromised. Those who receive multiple blood transfusions or blood products are also at increased risk but this can be minimised by screening all blood for HBsAg.

The clinical features are similar to those of hepatitis A but the prodromal phase of malaise tends to be longer and the jaundice may be more prolonged. Adolescents and young adults may have arthralgia, usually of several small joints, and prodromal skin rashes. Most patients make a complete recovery. Some become chronic carriers of the HBsAg but are perfectly healthy, and a few develop chronic persistent hepatitis or chronic active hepatitis and cirrhosis. In countries where the carriage rate of HBsAg is high, it is associated with primary liver cancer in adult life. Special precautions must always be taken when drawing blood samples or handling the blood of these patients to avoid self-inoculation and, if it occurs, anti-hepatitis B immunoglobulin should be given immediately. Children with hepatitis B can return to school when they have recovered clinically. Those who become carriers should not be excluded from school, but this information must be provided for any dental or surgical procedures. A hepatitis-B vaccine has recently been developed from fully purified formalin-inactivated HBsAg particles derived from the plasma of chronic carriers of the antigen. With this vaccine it should become possible to offer protection to those at increased risk of infection. As well as the infants of mothers with HBsAg this would include health care and laboratory staff and patients and staff in institutions for the handicapped.

Scarlet fever

Scarlet fever is caused by the erythrogenic toxin of the group A haemolytic streptococcus. The severity of the illness has waned considerably and fortunately it is now a mild illness with very few complications. There have also been marked changes in the post-streptococcal diseases, rheumatic fever and glomerulonephritis. Rheumatic fever has become very rare in the UK, although it remains of considerable importance in many developing countries. Post-streptococcal glomerulonephritis has become much less common and the illness is less severe.

The incubation period is 2–4 days and starts with tonsillitis, fever, headache and malaise. In most cases the child has a sore throat and the tonsils are red and congested, usually with a white exudate. The rash develops in 12–24 hours and is a punctate erythema, with tiny pin-head size puncta against an erythematous background, which blanches on pressure. It is most profuse on the trunk and limbs, with reddish discolouration in the lines of skin creases especially in the ante-cubital fossae and groin. On the face, the skin is only flushed with sparing of the area around the mouth giving circumoral pallor, but this appearance may also be seen in other febrile conditions, especially lobar pneumonia. There is a thick white coating of the tongue through which the inflamed papillae project, giving the white strawberry tongue. By the third to fifth day, the coating disappears leaving the papillae prominent, the strawberry tongue. The rash fades after a few days and this may be followed by desquamation, especially of the palms and soles. Although in the past this desquamation was often dramatic it tends now to be very slight with perhaps a small area of desquamation around the nails. Occasionally, scarlet fever is seen as a complication of infected wounds and burns.

It is usually possible to identify the organism

from a throat swab, or a streptococcal infection can be demonstrated from a raised antibody titre to streptolysin O (ASO), or other streptococcal antibodies. In practice, most children in whom a clinical diagnosis of scarlet fever is made do not have any investigations but are given a course of penicillin. This may modify the illness if severe, but probably has little or no effect on the mild illness seen today. In countries where rheumatic fever is prevalent, prolonged prophylactic treatment with penicillin is important.

Infectious mononucleosis

Infectious mononucleosis (glandular fever) is caused by the Epstein-Barr (EB) virus. It is transmitted by close contact. The virus is excreted in nasopharyngeal secretions during the illness whether symptomatic or asymptomatic and may continue for some months afterwards. It is also excreted intermittently by healthy individuals who are seropositive for EB virus antibody and who must often be the source of infection as few patients are aware of recent contact with an affected person.

Clinical disease from infectious mononucleosis has a peak incidence in adolescents and young adults. It usually has a gradual onset with malaise, anorexia and a fever. Most have a sore throat and tender swollen glands. On examination of the throat, petechiae may be visible on the palate and sometimes the tonsils are enlarged and covered with a thick white exudate. Peritonsillar oedema may be severe and cause difficulty in swallowing and breathing. There may be generalised lymphadenopathy especially affecting the cervical lymph nodes and there may be splenomegaly. Some patients have a maculo-papular rash, which is especially florid if ampicillin has been taken. Only a small percentage of patients are jaundiced although over 80 per cent have abnormal liver function tests. Cranial nerve palsies and other central nervous system abnormalities are very rare. Infectious mononucleosis is not uncommon in young children, especially in those of lower socioeconomic circumstances, but the clinical course is often much milder with much less prominent pharyngeal symptoms.

Differential diagnosis

The differential diagnosis depends on the mode of onset. Where there is exudative tonsillitis, streptococcal tonsillitis and diphtheria need to be considered. Prominent lymphadenopathy will need to be differentiated from other causes especially leukaemia and lymphoma, cytomegalovirus and toxoplasmosis.

Diagnosis

The blood film shows atypical mononuclear cells affecting more than 10 per cent of the total. They are not specific for infectious mononucleosis but may also be seen in other viral infections especially cytomegalovirus, adenovirus and also in toxoplasmosis. The diagnosis can be confirmed by showing heterophile antibodies with the Paul-Bunnell or 'Monospot' tests. Heterophile antibody is present in 85–90 per cent of affected adolescents and adults but many children do not produce heterophile antibodies at any stage of the illness. A definitive diagnosis of infectious mononucleosis in young children requires detection of antibody to the EB virus.

Treatment

In virtually all cases the disease is self limiting and only symptomatic treatment is necessary. Sport is often restricted if the spleen is enlarged to reduce the small risk of splenic rupture. Very severe pharyngeal oedema causing respiratory obstruction or severe hepatitis will usually respond to a short course of corticosteriods.

Mumps

Mumps is caused by a paramyxovirus. It is transmitted by droplet spread or direct contact with the saliva of an infected person. The incidence of infection is highest in school-age children.

The incubation period is 16–18 days which ends in fever, anorexia and malaise. The next day a parotid gland may enlarge and this progresses over the next 1–3 days. The child may complain of ear ache which is made worse by movement of the jaw, especially eating. The gland is painful and tender, but this gradually subsides over the next 3–7 days. Within a couple of days the other parotid gland usually becomes enlarged, but in one-quarter of cases the parotid enlargement is unilateral. The submaxillary and sublingual salivary glands are occasionally involved. In around one-third of cases the infection is subclinical.

The illness is mostly localised to the parotid glands. When making the diagnosis the enlarged parotid has to be differentiated from enlarged cervical lymph nodes. If the parotid gland is enlarged the ascending ramus of the mandible cannot be palpated. Mumps is an important cause of aseptic meningitis, which usually develops 3–7 days after the parotitis, but may also precede the parotitis or the parotitis may be absent. Recovery is usually uneventful, although very occasionally the patient has a unilateral or bilateral sensorineural hearing deficit. Epididymo-orchitis is rare before puberty and pancreatitis is a well recognised but rare complication.

Investigations are not usually required, but infection with mumps can be identified either serologically or by isolating the virus from saliva, urine or cerebrospinal fluid. The serum amylase is elevated in two-thirds of cases of mumps parotitis. There is no specific treatment.

Roseola infantum (exanthem subitum)

The causative agent is presumed to be a virus but it has not been identified. Infants between 6 months and 4 years of age, particularly those around one year old are most commonly affected. The infant suddenly develops a high, sustained fever which lasts for 3–4 days. During this period the infant may have a febrile convulsion, but otherwise does not seem as ill as one would expect from the high fever. There are few abnormal physical signs other than the fever, perhaps a slightly injected pharynx and some lymphodenopathy. There is a dramatic fall in the fever to normal and simultaneously, or shortly afterwards, a widespread rose-pink maculopapular rash develops first on the trunk and then spreading to the face and extremities. The diagnosis can only be made after the appearance of the rash and is entirely clinical as laboratory tests do not help. There is no specific treatment.

THE PERINATAL PERIOD

The fetus may be exposed to maternal infection throughout pregnancy and at delivery. Rubella and cytomegalovirus in the mother are important infections which may result in damage to the fetus. Toxoplasmosis is rare in the UK but may also cause severe fetal damage. Exposure of the fetus to herpes simplex, chickenpox and hepatitis B are less common, but all may cause serious disease in the newborn infant. There is no consistent evidence that mumps, the enteroviruses (coxsackie or echovirus) or influenza cause damage to the fetus.

Congenital rubella

The outcome for an individual fetus when a pregnant woman has rubella is difficult to predict. There is a risk of damage to the fetus when the mother has a primary rubella infection but not if she has reinfection. The stage of pregnancy at which the infection occurs is critical. Infection in the first 4 weeks of pregnancy may result in spontaneous abortion whilst the risk of fetal damage in this period may be as high as 50 per cent falling to 25 per cent at 5–8 weeks and 8 per cent at 9–12 weeks with a small risk of deafness following infection at 13–20 weeks gestation. Some infected babies are normal at birth but subsequently develop deafness and developmental delay later in childhood.

A wide range of defects is seen in infants and children with congenital rubella (Table 12.3). Most affected infants are small for gestational age and fail to thrive in early life. There is often damage to the eye (cataracts, glaucoma and pigmentary retinopathy), the heart (especially patent ductus arteriosus), the ear (perceptive deafness) and there may be damage to the central nervous system (microcephaly, mental retardation and cerebral palsy). Other manifestations in early infancy include thrombocytopenic purpura, hepatitis, hepatosplenomegaly, myocarditis and pneumonitis.

Diagnosis

The diagnosis can be made by culturing the virus

Table 12.3 Features of congenital rubella

	Approximate incidence in confirmed cases (per cent)	Type of defect
Growth	80	Small-for-gestational-age, failure to thrive
Ears	75	Perceptive deafness
Heart	50	Patents ductus arteriosus, ventricular septal defect, and peripheral pulmonary stenosis
Eyes	40	Cataract, glaucoma, microphthalmia pigmentary retinopathy
CNS	35	Microcephaly, mental retardation, cerebral palsy
Other	30	Thrombocytopenic purpura, hepatitis, hepatosplenomegaly, pneumonitis, myocarditis, osteopathy, translucency of metaphyses of long bones, especially distal femur and proximal tibia

in the urine or from the nasopharynx, or by demonstrating IgM specific antibodies to rubella in the blood in the first few months of life. Affected infants may excrete virus for many months and they then have the potential to transmit infection to other susceptible individuals.

Rubella during pregnancy

Around 10–15 per cent of pregnant women are found on serological testing to be susceptible to rubella. Rubella infection during pregnancy may be suspected from a rash or if the woman comes into contact with an affected person, usually a child in the family (Table 12.4). Many rubelliform

Table 12.4 Clinical history of mothers of children with congenital rubella

Clinical history	Per cent
Clinical rubella	46
Rash (not diagnosed)	13
Contact: no illness	16
No illness or contact	25

rashes are caused by other virus infections, and an early and accurate diagnosis of rubella is essential if proper management of the pregnancy is to be offered to the mother. Investigation is required as soon as possible after exposure. The most widely used serological test is for haemagglutination-inhibiting (HAI) antibodies.

The diagnosis of a recent rubella infection is made in conjunction with the clinical history and, in particular, after considering the time between exposure and testing. If the first blood sample is taken within 10 days of exposure, which is well within the incubation period and shows no antibody the patient is susceptible to rubella and further antibody tests should be done after 10 and 20 days. A seroconversion on paired samples indicates a recent infection. Alternatively, a recent infection can be identified by detecting rubella-specific IgM antibodies, as they are usually detectable for only a few weeks after rubella infection.

Antibody detected within the incubation period suggests previous exposure to rubella and that the patient is immune. This is best confirmed with a second specimen taken after the end of the incubation period, when there should not be a significant change in antibody titre. If the first specimen is taken after the incubation period and antibodies are present, the patient may be immune or have had a recent infection. A recent infection can then be identified by finding rubella-specific IgM antibodies.

The routine screening test for HAI antibodies performed in the antenatal clinic only indicates whether the person is susceptible or immune to rubella and whether immunisation should be recommended postnatally. If antibody is present it does not indicate the time when the infection occurred and although this is usually before pregnancy, it may have been recent. Rubella immunisation of 11–13-year-old girls began in 1971 in the UK and the number of pregnant women who are susceptible to rubella should decrease.

Women should avoid becoming pregnant within 3 months of receiving rubella immunisation. The inadvertent administration of rubella vaccine to a susceptible pregnant woman may result in fetal infection in about 20–25 per cent cases. No evidence of damage has been documented in these cases but the numbers are relatively small.

Cytomegalovirus

Cytomegalovirus (CMV) is the commonest known infection of the fetus. In industrialised countries it can be isolated from about one in 300 newborn infants.

Between 20 and 60 per cent of pregnant women do not have antibody to cytomegalovirus. Almost all mothers who acquire CMV during pregnancy are asymptomatic, although occasionally an illness resembling influenza or even glandular fever occurs. Congenital infection may occur after primary infection in the mother or from recurrent infection which is usually due to reactivation of latent virus.

Congenital abnormalities are seen more frequently in infants born after primary maternal infection than in those born after recurrent maternal infection. Their precise frequency is unknown. Most babies from whom CMV is isolated are asymptomatic. Only 10 per cent or less have clinical evidence of damage at birth, but it is estimated that some form of damage is detectable during infancy or childhood in 20–30 per cent of all babies with congenital CMV infection. Some affected babies are small for gestational age and may have hepatosplenomegaly, hepatitis, thrombocytopenic purpura and occasionally pneumonitis. Some have neurological damage with microcephaly, mental retardation and deafness. There may also be a retinopathy and cerebral calcification on a skull radiograph. Congenital CMV is thought to be a significant cause of mental retardation and hearing loss.

The virus can best be identified by isolation in tissue culture preferably from urine or from a throat swab. IgM-specific antibody to CMV in the blood is unfortunately not always present in infected infants. No specific treatment is available and excretion of the virus by affected infants may extend for several years. Although transmission of infection to susceptible contacts is extremely rare provided normal levels of hygiene are maintained, a seronegative pregnant woman should avoid caring for an infant known to be excreting the virus.

Chickenpox and shingles

Chickenpox infection during pregnancy is uncommon. Shingles does not affect the fetus but chickenpox may. The effect will depend on the period of pregnancy when the infection occurs. Infection during the first 4 months does not usually affect the fetus but a very few infants have been described with a characteristic pattern of malformations. This has been named the congenital varicella syndrome and includes scarring of the skin, muscular atrophy, hypoplastic extremities, atrophic digits and cerebral cortical atrophy with microcephaly and mental retardation. The babies of women who have chickenpox 1–3 weeks before delivery often have mild chickenpox. If chickenpox occurs within 4 days of delivery there is insufficient time for the fetus to receive maternal antibody and the newborn baby may develop severe generalised chickenpox (Fig. 12.3). This has a mortality of up to 30 per cent and the infants

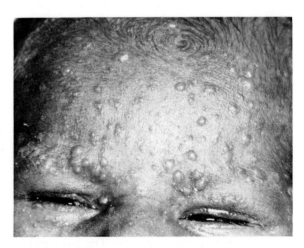

Fig. 12.3 Chickenpox in a neonate (by permission of the Board of Governors, The Hospital for Sick Children, London)

should be given zoster immune globulin at birth. Treatment with the antiviral agent acyclovir looks promising.

Herpes simplex virus

Infection of the newborn infant with herpes simplex virus usually occurs from the maternal genital tract at the time of delivery. The genital type 2 (HSV 2) strain of virus is slightly more common as the pathogen than the type 1 strain (HSV 1).

Neonatal herpes may be localised or disseminated. When disseminated, the infant may be jaundiced, have purpura and develop respiratory distress and shock. The central nervous system may also be involved with meningitis and encephalitis. The mortality is extremely high, 80 per cent of these infants die and one-half of the survivors have permanent damage. The infection may be confined to the central nervous system, or localised to the skin, eyes and mouth. At present infection in this country appears much less common than in the USA.

When active maternal genital herpes occurs at the time of delivery, exposure of the baby can be minimised by delivering the baby by Caesarean section, preferably before or within 4 hours of rupture of the membranes. However, in most cases of neonatal herpes infection there is no history of genital herpes in the mother. Results of treatment of infected infants with acyclovir are encouraging.

Newborn infants may become infected from herpetic lesions of attendants although this is very uncommon. It is advisable for all those with primary or recurrent herpes simplex lesions to avoid nursing newborn babies.

Hepatitis A and B

Maternal infection with hepatitis A during pregnancy has been associated with premature onset of labour, but there is no definite evidence of fetal damage. Should a pregnant woman come into contact with hepatitis A, it is generally advised that she should be given immunoglobulin.

Vertical transmission of the hepatitis B virus from mother to baby mostly occurs at delivery or within the first few weeks of life. Most pregnant women who are HBsAg positive are chronic carriers and often come from South-East Asia or Africa. Those who also carry the e antigen (an internal component of the core) in their blood are often of Chinese origin and have an increased risk of transmitting HBsAg to their babies. Other mothers with an increased risk of carrying HBsAg are those who are drug addicts, have received transfusions of blood or blood products or been tattooed. Primary clinical infection of the mother is uncommon, but when it occurs in the third trimester, the infant has a high risk of acquiring HBsAg. The baby is exposed by the ingestion of maternal blood at delivery or from inoculation through abrasions in the skin.

Most infants who acquire HBsAg are asymptomatic, but they may well become chronic carriers and a few may develop serious liver disease and be at increased risk of primary liver cancer in adult life.

The management of babies born to mothers who are HBsAg carriers is still controversial. Normal pooled immunoglobulin is not of any value, but there is evidence that hepatitis-B immunoglobulin administered within 48 hours and at regular intervals during the first few months markedly reduces the acquisition of the HBsAg. It has also been suggested that the blood of these infants be checked for HBsAg periodically and that those who become HBsAg positive during this period should be kept under surveillance. Long-term protection can be achieved with the newly developed hepatitis B vaccine.

Toxoplasmosis

Toxoplasmosis is caused by the protozoon *Toxoplasma gondii*. Infection in pregnant women is almost always asymptomatic, but sometimes is similar to mild 'flu or glandular fever. The incidence of primary infection during pregnancy varies widely in different countries. In the UK it is rare, with an incidence of congenital infection of only one in 20 000 live births. Most babies born with congenital toxoplasmosis are asymotomatic but up to 20 per cent have clinically recognisable damage. The severely affected infant may be small-for-gestational-age and have jaundice, hepatosplenomegaly, anaemia, thrombocytopenia, convulsions and hydrocephalus or microcephaly. There is a characteristic chorioretinitis and there may also be intracranial calcification.

The most widely used diagnostic test is the toxoplasma dye test. The diagnosis can be confirmed by demonstrating a persistently raised or rising titre. IgM antibodies to toxoplasma can also be detected using immunofluorescence.

Drugs used to treat a pregnant woman or affected infant include pyrimethamine, sulfadiazine or spiramycin.

RASHES

There is considerable overlap in the rashes caused by different infections. In arriving at a diagnosis, additional information is needed. A particular infection may be prevalent at the time within a community, the organism may have been identified and the natural history of the illness known. There may be a history of contact with an infected person. The patient's past history of infection needs to be known although this is notoriously unreliable for some infections, e.g. rubella. The immunisation history may be more helpful, although it should be remembered that inoculation is not synonymous with immunity. Other factors are the length and clinical features of the prodromal period. In addition to the appearance of the rash, there is its distribution and the sequence in which it appeared and disappeared. Associated symptoms and signs are often helpful. A definite diagnosis may not be possible from the clinical features when the child is first seen, but may become apparent from the subsequent course of the illness. Laboratory investigations are sometimes required to identify the cause of the illness.

Petechial and purpuric rashes

Petechiae or purpura are important to identify in an unwell child as they may be caused by meningococcal septicaemia, which is likely to be fatal within hours unless treated. Initially, there may be only a few petechiae, sometimes only evident on the conjunctivae in a febrile and unwell child. The lesions may become widespread, variable in shape and size and may subsequently develop a necrotic

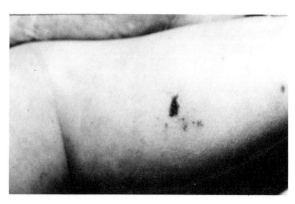

Fig. 12.4 Typical skin lesions in a child with meningococcal septicaemia

centre (Fig. 12.4). The septicaemia may progress so rapidly that the meninges remain unaffected. The child becomes shocked and in severe cases there is disseminated intravascular coagulation. Similar skin lesions are also seen, although much less frequently, in *Haemophilus influenzae* and pneumococcal infections, and in Rocky Mountain spotted fever and arbovirus infections in endemic areas.

Any child in the community who develops a petechial or purpuric rash and is febrile and unwell should be presumed to have meningococcal septicaemia and immediately given a large dose of penicillin parenterally. Although this may prevent the organism from being identified by culture, the antigen can still be positively identified, and it may be life-saving. The child must be transferred urgently to hospital.

Petchiae or purpura are seen in many other conditions. The cause may be thrombocytopenic or non-thrombocytopenic. They are seen in the non-thrombocytopenic vasculitis of Henoch-Schönlein purpura where the purpuric rash has a characteristic distribution over the buttocks, legs and elbows, often with arthritis, gastrointestinal pain and renal involvement. Important causes of thrombocytopenic purpura include idiopathic thrombocytopenic purpura, leukaemia, the haemolytic-uraemic syndrome, disseminated intravascular coagulation and congenital infection from rubella, cytomegalovirus or toxoplasma.

A guide to the clinical diagnosis of the rashes seen in the major acute infectious diseases is given in Table 12.5.

Table 12.5 Clinical diagnosis of the rashes seen in the major acute infectious diseases

Rash	Causes	Comments
Erythematous Scarlatiniform	Scarlet fever	Post group-A streptococcal infection of the throat or skin. Associated features — tonsillitis or infected skin lesion, characteristic appearance of the tongue. Punctate erythema, spreading from neck downwards avoiding the face which is flushed and has circumoral pallor. Desquamation
	Viruses	Scarlatiniform rashes are seen in a number of viral illnesses, e.g. adenovirus
	Chickenpox	Transient scarlatiniform rashes sometimes before the vesicles appear
	Drugs and other allergic reactions	Wide variety of allergens, e.g. antibiotics
	Kawasaki's disease (mucocutaneous lymph node syndrome)	First described in Japan, but seen increasingly in Europe and North America. Erythematous rash on the trunk. Other diagnostic features of the illness are: spiking fever lasting 5 or more days; bilateral conjunctivitis; dry, cracked, red lips with erythematous nasopharyngeal oedema; reddening of the palms and soles on day 3 to 5 with desquamation by the second or third weeks and enlarged cervical lymph nodes; 1 per cent mortality from thrombosis and aneurysms of the coronary arteries
Morbilliform (measles like)	Measles	Rash is dusky-red, blotchy and becomes confluent. Spreads from behind the ears and back of the neck then to the face, trunk and limbs. Staining of skin. Koplik's spots are pathognomonic but may not be visible. If conjunctivitis, coryza, or cough are not present, it is unlikely to be measles
	Adenovirus } Coxsackie }	Morbilliform rashes may be seen in other viral infections
Rubelliform	Rubella	Rash, even with postauricular and occipital lymphadenopathy not specific to rubella. In a pregnant woman, diagnosis of rubella or exposure to possible rubella must always be confirmed serologically
	Adenovirus } Echovirus } Coxsackie }	Can all cause a rubelliform rash
	Roseola	Rose-pink rash, starts on trunk and appears when fever subsides
	Allergic reaction	Allergic reactions to drugs and many other allergens. Wide range of rashes, including scarlatiniform, moblliform and rubelliform rashes. Extensive and sometimes confluent rash in patients with infectious mononucleosis especially after taking ampicillin
	Collagen vascular disorders	Rash in systemic jevenile chronic arthritis appears with the fever, dissapears in a few hours. Often localised, mainly on the trunk and proximal limbs
Papulosquamous	Pityriasis rosea	Rose-coloured papules with white scales on the surface. Herald patch on trunk. Lesions mainly on the trunk and may assume Christmas tree like configuration as they may follow a diagonal pattern from the spine following the ribs. May be itchy
	Psoriasis	Lesions are chronic

Table 12.5 (continued)

Rash	Causes	Comments
Vesicular	Chickenpox	Variable number of vesicles. Even if there are only a few lesions, more can usually be found on the scalp and mucous membranes. Lesions first appear on the trunk.
	Shingles	Confined to sensory nerve dermatome
	Smallpox	Now eradicated
	Herpes simplex	Usually gingivostomatitis with lesions on tongue and buccal mucosa and some satellite lesions around the mouth, or vulvovaginitis or cutaneous lesions
	Eczema herpeticum	Herpes infection on eczematous skin. Lesions may become widespread (Kaposi's varicelliform eruption) and the patient may become severely ill
	Hand, foot and mouth disease	Shallow ulcers in the mouth, vesicles on the hands and feet, and on the buttocks in infants. Usually caused by coxsackie A16 virus
	Herpangina	Vesicles or ulcers on fauces and mucous membranes of posterior part of mouth. Fever, anorexia and dysphagia for 2–5 days. Mainly caused by coxsackie virus infection
	Impetigo	The vesicles are usually around the mouth and become pustular and crust. Mostly caused by *Staphylococcus aureus*, also streptococci
	Viruses	Vesicular rashes are sometimes seen in a number of viral infections e.g. coxsackie, echovirus
Erythema multiforme	Allergy to food, drugs, etc	Discrete circular macules, often with central clearing to form a target lesion, mostly on the upper limbs. May be a wide variety of lesions, with macules, papules, urticaria, and bullae and several different types of lesions present at once. A severe form of the disease, with mucous membrane involvement of the mouth, conjunctivae and genitalia is the Stevens-Johnson syndrome
	Viral infection — herpes simplex, coxsackie, *echovirus*	
	Bacterial infection — Group A streptococcus	
	Mycoplasma	
	Collagen vascular disorders	
	Cause often not identified	
Urticaria	Allergic reaction (causes as for erythema miltiforme)	Raised lesions, variable size and shape. White lesions on surrounding erythematous base. Itchy and evanescent. Sometimes accompanied by angioedema of eyes and face and, rarely, tongue and upper airways which may be life threatening
Erythema marginatum	Rheumatic fever	Erythematous rash with a pale centre. The margin is sometimes raised and it migrates across the skin
Bullous	Bullous impetigo	Caused by *Staphylococcus aureus* and less commonly by streptococcal infection of the skin. Roof of a bullous lesion may be readily removed and lesions then resemble scalds (scalded-skin syndrome)
	Herpes simplex Chickenpox Erythema marginatum Stevens-Johnson syndrome	Some of the lesions in these acute illnesses may be bullous. Bullae may also be seen in ammoniacal napkin rashes, burns, and in a number of rare, chronic skin conditions

Allergic and other immunological disorders

Descriptions of allergic disorders appeared in many ancient texts, but it was not until 1906 that von Pirquet introduced the term allergy. Lucretius (94–55 BC) observed that 'One man's meat is another man's poison', which must be the most concise definition of allergy, if we add that the reaction is immunologically mediated. The terms allergy and hypersensitivity can be used interchangeably; and atopy is used to describe several associated diseases such as asthma, eczema, perennial allergic rhinitis, pollenosis, acute urticaria, gastrointestinal allergy and anaphylaxis.

PRINCIPLES OF ALLERGY AND IMMUNITY

An allergic state depends on prior exposure to substances known as allergens or antigens, resulting in altered reactivity on subsequent exposure. The management of allergic disease in the past has, therefore, focused on identifying the offending agent so that avoidance or attempts at induction of tolerance (immunotherapy) could be used. Recent studies have given clinical allergy a much firmer scientific basis.

The types of allergic reaction can be divided into four categories:

Type 1 Immediate hypersensitivity or anaphylactic reactions

The reaction occurs within minutes of exposure to the allergen, which combines with reaginic antibody (immunoglobulin E), fixed on the surface of mast cells and basophils, resulting in the release of vasoactive amines such as histamine and prostaglandins. An example is allergic rhinitis.

Type 2 Cytotoxic reaction

A reaction of varying rapidity of onset, where antibody is directed towards a cell component or an antigen fixed to cells, with damage resulting from an interaction of complement and mononuclear cells, e.g. autoimmune haemolytic anaemia.

Type 3 Arthus or antigen-antibody complex reaction

A reaction which develops over a few hours and is produced by soluble toxic complexes which are a combination of antibody, antigen in excess and activated complement. Neutrophil polymorphs are also involved in the reaction. Examples of the reaction are extrinsic allergic alveolitis and serum sickness.

Type 4 Delayed or cell-mediated reaction

A reaction taking at least 24 hours to develop and mediated by sensitised thymus-derived lymphocytes (T-cells) which, in contact with an antigen, release lymphokines. This results in inflammatory changes and cellular infiltration by lymphocytes and macrophages. Examples include contact dermatitis and the tuberculin reaction.

While these four subdivisions help in understanding the immunological reaction, they are not mutually exclusive, but an intergrated series of inter-relating and interdependent systems. This can be illustrated by the sequence of events which occurs when an antigen or allergen presents at a mucosal or epithelial surface.

The mechanical barrier offered by the skin and mucous membranes provides the first line of defence. Mucociliary clearance mechanisms provide additional protection in the respiratory tract. Lysozymes in sweat, tears, saliva and mucus are bactericidal, whilst iron-binding proteins such as lactoferrin in breast milk are bacteriostatic by depriving bacteria of the essential substrate, iron. Once antigen has penetrated into tissues a complex cooperation system involving T-cell complement and macrophages results in ingestion of the antigen. First, the macrophage migrates to the site, a process known as chemotaxis, and is then presented with the antigen in an ingestible form by opsonisation, a function of the alternative pathway of complement. In the case of microorganisms, these are then killed by various intracellular lysozymes. The bursa-derived lymphocytes (B-cells), with the mediation of T-cells, are transformed into plasma cells, which then produce specific antibodies against the antigen. Antibody production is modulated by some subsets of T-cells, designated helper cells which trigger and suppressor cells which suppress responses. Each reste of plasma cells produces only one antibody type of the five classes of immunoglobulin.

Immunoglobulins

IgG is the major class of immunoglobulin in normal serum which, because it is of relatively low molecular weight, is also present in interstitial fluids such as breast milk, and is transferred across the placenta. It is the predominant antibody produced in response to secondary antigenic challenge. There are four sub-types labelled IgG_{1-4}.

IgA is the second most abundant antibody in the serum but is the main antibody of secretions. It is found in significant amounts in tracheobronchial, gastrointestinal and genito-urinary secretions. It is particularly important in reducing the amount of free antigen absorbed through epithelial surfaces. There are two sub-types labelled IgA_{1-2}.

IgM consists of a large molecule which is virtually restricted to the intravascular space and is synthesised largely during the primary immune response.

IgE is present in only trace amounts in normal serum but rises during parasitic infestation. It binds to mast cells and basophils and, when two bound IgE molecules are linked by antigen, the mast cell degranulates releasing vasoactive amines which mediate the type 1 hypersensitivity response. IgG_4 may function in a similar way.

IgD exists in low concentration in normal serum but its physiological role is unclear. It may act as a B-cell antigen receptor modulating the humoral response.

It can be seen from Figure 13.1 that IgG and IgM both activate and bind complement to form complexes with an antigen and aid its elimination.

The complement system

The complement system consists of several components which, when activated, undergo a series of reactions, similar to the coagulation cascade, and produce cell lysis, increased vascular permeability and enhanced phagocytosis. Two pathways of activation are recognised; the classical, which follows a sequence involving complement components 1, 4, 2, 3, 5, 6, 7, 8, 9 sequentially, and the alternative pathway, which bypasses the early components by activating the third component (C3) directly.

IMMUNODEFICIENCY DISORDERS

Gross forms of immunodeficiency leading to excess infection are rare and usually obvious. Subtle and mild defects are, however, more common and may lead to the development of atopy which occurs in at least 15–20 per cent of the population and, possibly, also predispose to the later development of lymphoreticular malignancy and autoimmune disease. Transient defects also occur; these may be due to delayed maturation in infancy or secondary phenomena, which are much commoner then primary defects. Table 13.1 lists the primary immunodeficiency disorders, dividing them into those predominantly associated with defects of humoral immunity, cellular-immune function, combined defects, special syndromes, phagocyte defects and finally complement defects. Impairment of immune responses may occur secondary to a variety of factors including malnutrition; protein loss, such as occurs in nephrotic syndrome and protein-losing enteropathy; virus infections, such as measles, producing temporary impairment of delayed hypersensitivity; congenital virus infec-

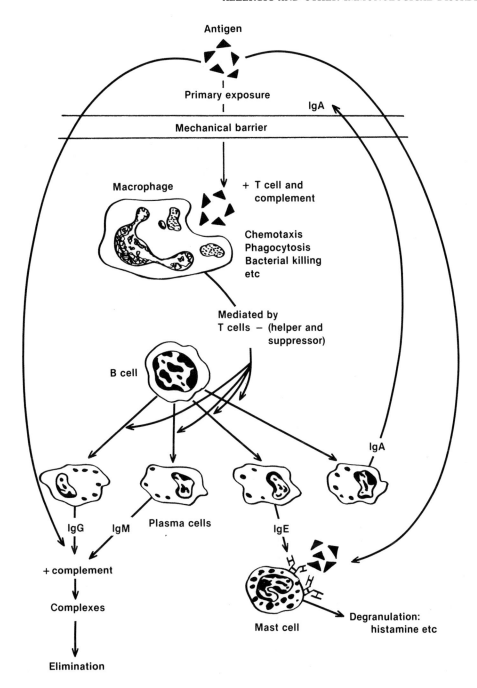

Fig. 13.1

tions; malignant disease; drugs such as steroids and immunosuppressants; and splenectomy.

Diagnosis of immunodeficiency

A thorough history is important in the clinical assessment of a patient with possible defects in immune function; details of the family history, health in pregnancy and the neonatal period are important. Congenital virus infection can produce immunodeficiency; prematurity results in less maternal IgG transfer and, therefore, a transient

Table 13.1 Immunodeficiency disorders

Group	Disease	Associated features and complications
Humoral defects	Panhypogammaglobulinaemia (X-linked or recessive)	Pyogenic infection; polyarthritis
	Selective IgA deficiency (1 : 700 population)	Asymptomatic pyogenic infection; atopy
Predominantly cell-mediated defects	di George syndrome	Thymic hypoplasia & absent parathyroids Hypocalcaemia; cardiovascular defects; FTT candidiasis
	Mucocutaneous candidiasis	Sometimes iron deficient: *Candida* infection
Combined defects	Severe combined immunodeficiency	Diarrhoea; FTT Infections: pyogenic; fungal; pneumocystis
	Reticular dysgenesis	Fatal in early infancy
Special syndromes	Ataxia-telangiectasia (recessive)	Low IgE and IgA Ataxia; Dementia; telangiectases
	Wiskott-Aldrich syndrome (X-linked)	Combined immunodeficiency Eczema; thombocytopenia; infection
Phagocyte defects	Chronic granulomatous disease(X-linked)	Pyogenic infection; abscesses & fistulae
	Shwachmans syndrome	Pancreatic insufficiency; FTT; steatorrhoea; neutropenia; infection; short stature
Complement defects	Familial angio-oedema (dominant)	C1-esterase inhibitor deficiency Recurrent angio-oedema
	Opsonisation defect (1 : 20 population)	Asymptomatic; FTT; pyogenic infection; dermatitis; atopy

hypogammaglobulinaemia. Small-for-dates babies are more susceptible to infection probably because of intrauterine malnutrition. Most patients, even with severe immunodeficiency disorders, remain well for the first few months of life because of maternally-derived protection. Children with di George syndrome, however, often have associated major congenital heart disease and neonatal hypocalcaemia and this gives the clue to diagnosis. Family history may highlight some of the X-linked recessive disorders, and other types of immunodeficiency are associated with an increased likelihood of relatives having autoimmune disease, lymphoreticular malignancy or atopy.

Physical examination may reveal signs of damage due to past recurrent infections, such as bronchiectasis. Failure to thrive is a common feature in immunodeficient children and, therefore, accurate records of weight and height plotted on standard charts will be valuable. Infants with severe immunodeficiency sometimes lack palpable lymph nodes and the tonsils may be small or absent. Characteristic defects may be seen in children with special syndromes such as ataxia telangiectasia and di George syndrome.

A careful microbiological and viral screen is necessary as the various disorders sometimes predispose to particular infections. A lateral radiograph of the upper airway reveals the presence or absence of adenoidal tissue whilst a chest radiograph in infancy should show a thymus and may reveal the presence or sequelae of recurrent respiratory tract infection. Specific tests of immunity include a full blood count, emphasising the differential count and film, measurement of immunoglobulin concentrations, and tests for the presence of specific antibodies such as isohaemagglutinins (IgM antibody), anti-streptolysin O titre (IgG antibody), and antibodies which should have been produced by previous immunisation. Lymphocyte T and B-cell numbers can be estimated. Skin tests using candida, trichophyton or tuberculin antigens show the presence of normal delayed hypersensitivity (type 4). Various components of the complement cascade can also be measured. A reduction in C3 indicates activation of the classical pathway, and C4 the alternative pathway. The ability of the patient's serum to opsonise yeast particles for phagocytosis by polymorphs obtained from a healthy subject, can also be tested. Various aspects of phagocyte function including chemotaxis, organism killing and nitroblue tetrazolium

(NBT) reduction, defective in chronic granulomatous disease, will also be indicated in certain situations. The atopic subjects can be distinguished by prick skin testing using a range of common inhalants and ingestant allergens.

Treatment of immunodeficiency

Avoidance of pathogens and vigorous treatment of established infection form the basis of much of the management of these disorders. The range of specific therapies available for the primary immuno deficiency disorders is limited. Replacement of non-antigen specific factors by fresh blood transfusion, such as in the opsonisation defect, can sometimes be of benefit. Specific immunoglobulin replacement produces dramatic improvements in the panhypogammaglobulinaemias, but is not without complications such as allergic reactions. Bone marrow transplantation thymus grafts and administration of heat labile extracts of lymphocytes (transfer factor) are used in the cellular and combined immunodeficiencies. As the understanding of humoral factors which influence immune responses extends, pharmacological approaches to these disorders may become possible. Levamisole has several effects on immune mechanisms and has been used with some success in patients with chemotactic defects. Many other drugs of this variety are likely to become available over the next decade.

Immunodeficiency patients are susceptible to infection by attenuated microorganisms and live virus such as those used for immunisations and, therefore, these vaccines should not be given.

Atopy

Atopy is probably the commonest manifestation of immunodeficiency. It occurs in 15–20 per cent of the population and amounts to one-third of all chronic diseases of childhood. The immunological abnormalities most commonly associated with atopy include IgA deficiency, either as a transient maturational or persistent defect, an opsonisation defect and low C2. Atopy also occurs more frequently in patients with cystic fibrosis and there is some suggestion that it may be more frequent

in cystic fibrosis heterozygotes (carriers). It must be emphasised that the atopic status is not synonymous with atopic disease; positive prick skin tests have been found in up to 30 per cent of asymptomatic school children and allergic disease can occur in non-atopic individuals exposed to very high concentrations of a particular allergen, as in certain industrial environments. Environmental influences play an important role in influencing the manifestations of atopy; factors such as month of birth, infant feeding practices, sex, age; emotion and intercurrent viral infection have been suggested as important influences.

Prevention

As temporary immunologic maturational defects in early infancy may predispose to the development of later atopy, it should be possible to protect such individuals during their susceptible period and thus prevent disease. The first major foreign protein to which infants are exposed is cow's milk. A reduced incidence of atopic disease in infants of allergic parents occurs if they have been fully breast fed for at least 3 months and with avoidance of highly allergenic foods until 6 months. Breast feeding reduces exposure not only to cow's milk allergens but also to bacterial endotoxin. E. coli bacteria colonise the intestinal tract of bottle-fed children and the endotoxin released acts as an adjuvant to enhance immunological reactions and, therefore, promotes the development of sensitivity to any allergen. Breast milk actively inhibits gut colonisation by this organism. Divergent results have been produced by using alternative milk preparations such as soya or goat's milk for the prevention of atopic disease. This merely substitutes one foreign protein with another. Sensitisation to allergens can, unfortunately, occasionally occur in fully breast-fed infants. Whole food protein is absorbed through the gastrointestinal tract and can appear in breast milk; this has led to the suggestion that breast-feeding mothers should also avoid common food allergens. Until the value of this practice is established it cannot be generally recommended. Other factors may predispose to the development of atopy later in childhood, these will not be influenced by infant feeding practices.

Established atopy

Atopy may cause a wide spectrum of complaints including diarrhoea, vomiting, failure to thrive, urticaria, angio-oedema, eczema, allergic rhinitis, conjunctivitis, and asthma. A wide variety of substances, usually proteins, are known to cause reactions. Table 13.2 gives the common agents

Table 13.2 Classification of allergens

Inhalants	
House dust mite	*Dermatophagoides pteronyssinus*
Grass pollens	Timothy, cocksfoot etc
Tree pollens	Silver birch, plane etc
Animal danders	Cat, dog, feathers etc
Mould spores	Cladosporium, Aspergillus etc
Ingestants	
Cow's milk	B lactoglobulin etc
Egg	Albumen
Fish	
Nuts	
Food colouring	Tartrazine etc
Contactants	
Antibiotic creams	
Rubber	
Dyes	
Injectants	
Drugs	
Antisera	
Immunisations	
Physical agents	
Temperature	
Humidity	

classified by mode of contact. The type of allergy, its clinical manifestations and the allergen variety can occur in any combination and this may be multiple, making classification by allergy alone or by sytem involved, pointless. Classification is usually by commonly accepted terms rather than functional. The classical and obvious include anaphylaxis, urticaria and angio-oedema, all of which occur within minutes of exposure, often to foods or drugs. Asthma, rhinitis, and eczema are all recognised to be associated with and caused by allergy, though sometimes timing between exposure and reaction may be prolonged. Diarrhoea, vomiting, failure to thrive and abdominal colic are accepted as sometimes being due to food allergy. The rather more dubious conditions which have been associated with allergy include sudden infant death syndrome and behaviour disturbances. It remains to be established whether these conditions are ever really caused by, or are only sometimes associated with, allergy. Finally, there are non-existent allergies, sometimes resulting in misplaced treatment. There have been reports of frankly malnourished infants on unsupervised and unnecessary allergy avoidance diets.

Diagnosis

An accurate diagnosis of allergy must always precede any therapeutic recommendations and again, clinical history and examination take precedence. The general paediatric history should be supplemented by details of possible allergen exposure timed in relation to symptoms. Such features as infant feeding and timing of weaning may provide useful background information in relation to the onset of symptoms. Specific questions on known allergen exposure such as to pets should always be asked and the association of symptoms with physical agents such as temperature, humidity, tobacco smoke, sprays and other fumes sought. The type of housing may also influence allergic disease. Such factors include age of property, proximity to waterways, type of heating, carpeting, furniture and bedding. A careful dietary history is important and a particular note should be made of those foods for which the child has specific likes or dislikes. The family history should include both indirect and direct questioning, particularly for allergic disease and other disorders associated with immunodeficiency. In considering the environment of the child it should be remembered that he or she will spend an appreciable time during the day at school or out of doors. Timing of symptoms in relation to such locations will be important. Reactions to drugs and immunisations may also be relevant. In eliciting information about specific disorders it should be remembered that there is a great deal of lay confusion between such terms as dermatitis and eczema; catarrh, chronic sinusitis and rhinitis; bronchitis and asthma. The physical examination should be thorough. A particular note should be made of the child's facies; the allergic patient may have discolouration and swelling of the eye-lids, a transverse nasal crease due to the nose constantly being rubbed up and down and evident mouth breathing due to rhinitis obstructing the nasal airway. The nasal mucosa can easily be examined using an auroscope and the pale swollen inferior turbinates due to allergic rhinitis, easily seen. Serous otitis media with a conductive deafness is a quite frequent association of allergic rhinitis. Red, runny eyes with blepharitis and a cobble-stone conjunctiva indicates allergic conjunctivitis. Bowed sternum, spinal kyphos and Harrison's sulci may all be signs of chronic asthma. The skin should be carefully examined, particularly the flexures and the scalp. Hypopigmentation may indicate areas of previous skin disease. Occasionally, allergic children manifest dermatographism.

Investigation

The presence of the atopic status can be confirmed by finding a raised differential white count for eosinophils (greater than $4 \times 10^9/l$, increase of total serum IgE and allergy skin tests. There are several techniques to detect immediate skin hypersensitivity including prick, scratch and intradermal methods. Prick tests are preferred as scratch tests give an increased number of non-specific positive results while intradermal tests are more likely to produce a constitutional reaction. The skin is punctured and lifted slightly using a 23 gauge needle held at 45° through a drop of the allergen extract on the skin surface. The range of allergens used will depend on the problem but a

typical screen might inlcude a negative control 0.5 per cent phenol in normal saline, a positive control histamine 1 mg/ml, house dust extract, house dust mite *Dermatophagoides pteronyssinus*, cat fur, cow's milk, egg albumen, grass pollen, tree pollen, *Cladosporium herbarum* and *Aspergillus fumigatus*. The reaction is assessed after 15 minutes and the diameter of weals recorded in millimetres. A weal of 2 mm diameter or greater is considered positive. It is also valuable to re-examine the site of skin tests 3 or 4 hours later to see whether a late reaction with erythema and induration has developed. Serum IgE antibody measurements can be made using the radioallergosorbent tests (RAST).

Unfortunately, there is no consistently reliable diagnostic test for specific allergies. The above tests provide useful confirmatory evidence but can be negative even in obvious cases and positive in symptomless atopic patients. Immunological mechanisms other than those mediated by IgE may sometimes be involved. Circulating immune complexes and complement consumption have occasionally been demonstrated during reactions and, if present, can provide an additional objective aid to diagnosis. Where gastrointestinal symptoms predominate, small intestinal biopsy may show a mucosal change such as partial villous atrophy or cellular infiltration of the lamina propria. If specific allergy diagnosis is considered essential then direct challenge of the organ involved with

Table 13.3 Useful investigation in immunological disordes

	Asthma/eczema rhinitis	Infections Severe	Unusual	Autoimmune disease
Full blood count	+	+	+	+
X-ray for lymphoid tissue	−	+	+	−
IgG, A, M	(±)	+	+	+
Antibodies	−	+	+	−
Auto-antibodies	−	(±)	(±)	+
T and B cell membranes	(±)	+	+	−
T cell responses	−	+	+	−
Delayed hypersensitivity tests	−	+	+	+
Organism killing	−	(±)	+	−
Complement studies	(±)	+	−	+
Opsonisation	(±)	+	−	(±)
Allergy prick skin tests	+	+	(±)	(±)
Serum IgE	+	(±)	(±)	(±)
IgE antibodies	(±)	−	−	−
Direct organ challenge	(±)	−	−	−

+ = necessary
− = unnecessary
(±) = may be useful in certain cases

appropriate controls and allergen is necessary. Even these are open to misinterpretation as other intercurrent events may cause a reaction. In the case of food allergy this has led some authorities to suggest that a minimum of three challenges must be performed and that food allergy can only be diagnosed if the symptoms are identical in type and timing after each challenge. The other alternative is to use a double-blind challenge technique, where symptoms are recorded during periods on the offending food or a suitably disguised dummy product.

Specific Allergic Disorders

Atopic Dermatitis

This is a chronic recurring skin disorder usually manifest in early infancy. The skin goes through phases of erythema, macules, papules, vesicles, oozing, scaling and crusting. Later, pigmentary changes and chronic lichenification occur. At times the skin is intensely itchy and children frequently scratch to the point of bleeding.

Three to 5 per cent of all children suffer from this disorder; 80 per cent of infants with eczema have a clear family history of atopy and 50 per cent subsequently go on to have other manifestations of atopic disease such as asthma or allergic rhinitis. By 3 years of age 70 per cent resolve completely and of the remaining 30 per cent, half have minor flexural problems thereafter, whilst the other half have severe persistent eczema. The condition must be distinguished from seborrhoeic dermatitis, impetigo, napkin dermatitis and ichthysiform erythroderma.

The underlying pathological mechanisms are still not fully understood but eczema is usually associated with clear evidence of atopy, with high serum IgE levels, blood eosinophilia and positive skin tests. There is increasing evidence that food allergy is particularly important in causing exacerbations of eczema. Patients with this condition are particularly prone to generalised infection with herpes simplex and vaccinia viruses, as well as to bacterial infection.

Simple treatment consists of the use of non-perfumed soap or emulsifying ointment for baths, the avoidance of irritant clothing and bedding, attention to emotional factors which may exacerbate the problem, and the use of topical steroid preparations, preferably in a dilute form, such as 1 per cent hydrocortisone. During severe exacerbations secondary bacterial infection should be considered and, after taking appropriate swabs, both local and systemic antibiotics should be used. Extensive use of topical steroids can lead to tolerance or tachyphylaxis, that is a diminution of pharmacological response with increasing requirement for the drug. Prolonged topical corticosteroid, particularly of high potency, can lead to systemic absorption with subsequent adrenal suppression and growth failure. Local side effects include thinning of the skin, telangiectasia and striae. If there is any evidence to suggest food as a cause the use of oligo-allergenic diets may be indicated. If significant improvement occurs on the diet, single foods can be reintroduced at weekly intervals to determine which produce reactions. This can subsequently be validated by double-blind challenge. Oligo-allergenic diets are nutritionally incomplete and should only be used with appropriate dietitian's advice.

Contact dermatitis

Contact dermatitis is an inflammatory response in the skin due to a type 4 allergic reaction following contact with an external agent. The skin changes are very similar to eczema but localised to areas of contact. The commonest type occurring in infancy is napkin dermatitis produced by prolonged contact with urine, faeces, antiseptics, soap and detergents in the nappy. Other common causes include chemicals used in dyes for clothing, nickle compounds, rubber compounds, preservatives in various creams, medications and cosmetics. Diagnosis can be achieved by patch testing, with the offending allergen held in contact with the skin for 48 hours and the site examined 20 minutes after removal, for erythema, oedema and vesicles. Treatment consists of avoidance and a short course of topical corticosteroids to the affected area.

Urticaria and angio-oedema

Urticaria (hives) is a transient eruption of weal-and-flare reactions of varying sizes lasting from minutes to days. It occurs due to release of vaso-active substances in the superficial dermis. Angio-oedema is a similar reaction confined to the deeper dermis and subcutaneous tissue. Both are extremely common problems throughout life but chronic urticaria persisting for months is more a problem of young adults than children. The major causes include infections, particularly beta-haemo-lytic streptococci, viruses, and parasite infes-tations, drugs such as antibiotics, foods, insect bites, non-infectious systemic illnesses such as the autoimmune disorders, psychological factors, physical agents such as cold, light, heat and exer-tion, and finally hereditary disorders such as the very rare C_1-esterase inhibitor deficiency leading to hereditary angio-oedema, a dominantly inherited condition.

The treatment involves avoidance of the precipi-tating cause and the use of an appropriate anti-histamine of the Hl-blocking variety. Recently, it has been suggested that H2-blocking agents such as cimetidine may be of value if H1-blockers have not produced a satisfactory response on their own. One should beware of the patients with a tartrazine sensitivity who, when treated with chlorphenira-mine preparation containing tartrazine, have continuing problems. Thus colouring-free prep-arations are preferred. Ketotifen, a new antihis-tamine with possible other anti-allergenic properties, is worthy of trial in resistant cases. Cyprohepta-dine is sometimes more effective in patients with urticaria induced by extremes of temperature. In life-threatening cases of angio-oedema with upper airways obstruction, treatment with adrenaline (1: 1000) by deep subcutaneous injection is essen-tial. Hereditary angio-oedema due to C1-esterase inhibitor deficiency can be treated specifically with non-virilising androgen preparations such as oxymetholone danozol or stranozol, which increase the level of C1-esterase inhibitor.

Allergic rhinitis and conjunctivitis

Allergic problems involving the upper respiratory tract are probably grossly under-diagnosed. The incidence in childhood has been quoted as anything between 2 and 20 per cent. The problem can be perennial or seasonal. Seasonal symptoms tend to be acute and relatively severe with episodes of sneezing and itching of the nose. There is a watery nasal discharge and partial or complete nasal obstruction. Patients quite frequently also have sore, red, itchy eyes with swollen eyelids. Perennial symptoms tend to be less acute and less severe, with relatively less involvement in the eyes, but may be associated with recurrent headaches, sore throat and repetitive cough. Quite frequently, patients with allergic rhinitis also have serous otitis media with reduced hearing and signs of fluid in the middle ear.

Clinical history and timing of symptoms will provide the most useful guide to the specific allergy diagnosis. Knowledge of tree pollen, grass pollen and mould spore counts may help delineate specific allergies which can then be confirmed by skin testing, IgE antibodies and nasal provocation testing. The commonest cause of perennial prob-lems is allergy to house dust mite, and here, a history of profuse sneezing on arising in the morn-ings with progressive improvement of symptoms during the day is typical. Apart from the usual diagnostic tests, examination of the nasal discharge for eosinophils will aid diagnosis of nasal allergy.

The differential diagnosis of allergic rhinitis includes hypertrophy of the adenoids, so-called vasomotor rhinitis, which is really perennial rhin-itis for which no allergic cause can be found, nasal foreign body, recurrent sinus infection and nasal polyps, the latter two being sometimes associated with cystic fibrosis.

Simple avoidance measures are usually impos-sible both for perennial and seasonal rhinitis. Nasal sympathomimetic agents which produce vasocon-striction are not to be recommended for regular use as rebound occurs requiring increased doses and, also, nasal mucosal atrophy may be produced. Antihistamine therapy will decrease the severity of symptoms but drowsiness is a frequent side effect and may be sufficient to interfere with schooling. Nasal sodium cromoglycate, provided that it is taken at least four times daily, may be effective but, in distinction to its use in asthma, results in allergic rhinitis have been disappointing. The use of local nasal corticosteroid in the form of beclo-methasone dipropionate aerosol has improved the management of this disorder considerably but must be used regularly between two and four times daily. Systemic corticosteroids produce a dramatic, though brief, relief of symptoms. Such therapy is only very occasionally justified for a short period in patients with severe problems, who are facing an important event such as major school examinations. If all else fails it may be worthwhile considering immunotherapy.

Asthma

Asthma is a condition characterised by intermittent attacks of cough, breathlessness and wheezing due to reversible narrowing of airways caused by bronchial smooth muscle spasm, mucosal oedema and increased secretions. It must be remembered that whilst asthma is the commonest cause of wheezing, any condition which produces narrowing of intrathoracic airways such as an inhaled foreign body, tuberculous lymph glands or bronchiolitis, will produce similar symptoms. At least 10 per cent of all children have asthma and, for most, it is a relatively mild condition. It is the cause of one-fifth of all school absences. A small number of children, 5.3 per 100 000 children between the ages of 5 and 14 years, die each year because of the condition. Thus, children with asthma may range from the very mild cases, with only occasional episodes of minimally distressing wheeze which will settle even without treatment, to the very severe chronic asthmatics with frequent attacks of distressing wheeze, limited exercise tolerance, stunted growth and deformed chest. Approximately 5 per cent of the whole child population will require some form of treatment to control their asthma whilst 0.5 per cent of the population will have chronic severe and persistent problems. As a general rule, those children with an early age of onset, less than 2 years, and frequent attacks in the first year after onset, tend to have more severe and persistent problems. Those who have a few episodes of wheezing in mid-childhood are likely to improve with age. Overall, about 40 per cent of asthmatic children ill become symptom free, 34–35 per cent improve, 24 per cent remain unchanged, 1 per cent deteriorate and 0.5 per cent die. There is no magic age at which children grow out of their asthma and furthermore, as many as 50 per cent of children who lose their symptoms may redevelop the problems in late adolescence or early adult life.

Over 90 per cent of asthmatic children can be shown to be allergic on simple allergy skin testing with the commonest positive reaction being to house dust and house dust mite, closely followed by cat fur and grass pollens. Asthma, however, can be precipitated by many factors often acting simultaneously and in a variety of combinations. Even in clearly allergic asthmatics, attacks may be produced by intercurrent viral infection, exercise such as running in cold weather, emotional disturbance, non-specific irritant dusts or fumes and changes in humidity or temperature. In up to 90 per cent of cases a simple 6-minute, free-running exercise test will produce significant airflow limitation, that is, a greater than 10 per cent fall in peak expiratory flow rate, within 10 minutes of completing the exercise. In other words, most childhood asthmatics will have both easily demonstrable allergy and bronchial lability.

Some attacks such as those after exertion are short lived and will subside spontaneously but others may last for hours or days and require treatment. During attacks children frequently have a productive cough with apparently purulent sputum, which usually contains eosinophils, Charcot-Leyden crystals and Curschmann's spirals. As a result of impaired ventilation, hypoxia develops and the resultant hyperpnoea initially produces hypocapnoea. During very severe attacks, however, particularly in young children respiratory failure with hypercapnoea may develop. Treatment will depend on the severity and frequency of symptoms. A careful record of symptoms from day-to-day on a diary card with a note of possible associations such as exposure to pets or development of infection will aid decisions in management. It is worthwhile issuing a peak flow meter to record peak flow rates twice daily at home, on the diary card.

Avoidance of precipitating factors is the cheapest and most ideal treatment, but life in an allergen, infection and exercise-free environment would be an unbearable and probably impossible. Simple avoidance recommendations are worthwhile, particularly if the family pet is involved. House dust mite elimination techniques may help but are often inadequate. These include the use of synthetic materials for bedding, the removal of soft toys from the bed, regular vacuum cleaning of the mattress, which should be enclosed in a plastic cover. As emotion plays an important role in potentiating problems, it is imperative that the child and family should be helped to gain a realistic understanding and acceptance of the condition. This can usually be achieved by the paediatrician but, occasionally, specialist family psychotherapy may be needed.

Drug therapy falls into three main categories. The first is bronchodilators, which can be either beta-sympathomimetic agents such as salbutamol, terbutaline, fenoterol; xanthine derivatives such as theophylline, aminophylline, choline theophyllinate; or parasympatholytic agents such as ipratropium bromide. Beta-sympathomimetics can be administered as a syrup, tablet, pressurised aerosol, nebulisable solution or injection. Inhalation is rather more effective than oral medication and during severe attacks parenteral therapy may be necessary. In general, these drugs are used to control acute episodes of wheezing though occasionally they are used regularly. Unfortunately, beta-sympathomimetics are often ineffective in infants under 18 months of age but the other two varieties of bronchodilator may be active in younger patients. Xanthine derivatives may be given orally or parenterally. Sustained-release preparations have recently become available which have a prolonged effect for up to 12 hours, necessitating only a twice daily dosage. When these preparations are used, such as Phyllocontin or Slophylline, dosage should be adjusted by measuring either plasma or saliva theophylline levels (the therapeutic range is between 10 and 20 mg/l). Ipratropium bromide is available as a pressurised aerosol or a nebuliser solution.

The second form of drug therapy is sodium cromoglycate (Intal). It is a prophylactic preparation which apparently stabilises mast cells, thus preventing mediator release. It is taken by inhalation of a powder and must be administered at least three times daily. Most failures of this treatment are due to incorrect use of the inhaler, which is quite common in small children. Physiotherapists can play an important role in training children

to use the inhaler correctly. In young children it can be administered by nebuliser.

Finally steroids may be used in severe asthmatics, where sodium cromoglycate and bronchodilators have been ineffective. The use of potent topically active preparations, such as beclomethasone dipropionate, betamethasone valerate or budesomide by inhalation, have dramatically improved the management of severe asthma. Only a very small number of cases require regular systemic steroids, preferably as prednisolone, given on alternate days.

Specific allergy therapy at the present rests with immunotherapy. This consists of a graded series of increasing doses of allergen, usually administered by subcutaneous injection. This should be reserved for those allergic factors which cannot be eliminated and can be demonstrated to play a major role in producing asthma. Patients controlled on simple and safer conventional therapy should not be considered for immunotherapy. In practice, only pollen and house mite immunotherapy have been convincingly shown to have any beneficial effect and these only in very carefully selected patients.

Acute exacerbations of asthma presenting at hospitals should initially be treated with nebulised salbutamol or terbutaline. If response to this therapy is poor then parenteral therapy is required. A loading dose of intravenous aminophylline (maximum 5.6 mg/kg) is normally given slowly over 20 minutes but should be avoided if the child has been given xanthine in the previous 6 hours or 12 hours in a slow-release formulation. Thereafter, a continuous infusion (0.9 mg/kg) should be maintained. Alternatively, intravenous salbutamol in a dose of 10 μg/kg/hour or more may be given. If there is no immediate response, intravenous hydrocortisone and subsequently oral prednisolone will also be necessary. Oxygen should be given to all patients requiring parenteral therapy. A small number of patients with severe respiratory failure ($PaCO_2$ rising above 65 mmHg or 8.5 kPa) may require ventilation. This emergency procedure is summarised in Figure 13.2.

The aim of treatment should be to allow children to attend normal school with minimal absences, and to participate in all normal activities.

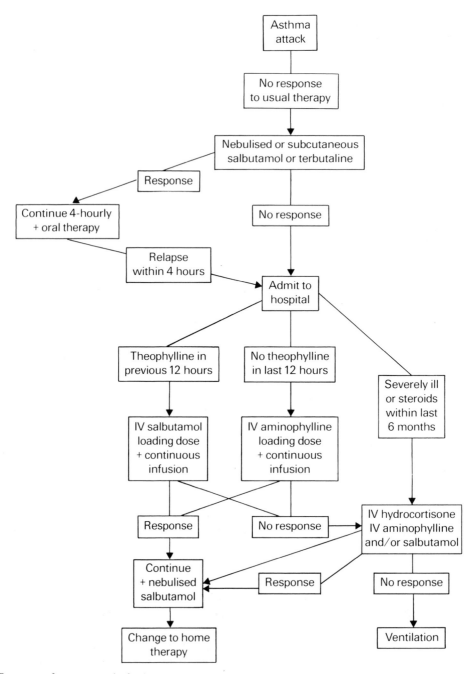

Fig. 13.2 Treatment of an acute attack of asthma

If their activities are being inhibited then treatment should be adjusted accordingly.

Anaphylaxis

Anaphylaxis is a systemic reaction which is poten-tially life-threatening. It usually occurs within minutes of provocation and, without treatment, is rapidly progressive. Symptoms may involve virtually any system. The skin shows flushing, pruritus, urticaria and angio-oedema; the respir-atory tract, stridor, hoarseness and wheezing leading to respiratory failure; the cardiovascular system, rapid weak pulse, hypotension and shock; and the gastrointestinal system, dysphagia, nausea, vomiting and diarrhoea. There may also be sweating, incontinence and very occasionally convulsions. The commonest cause is probably antibiotic sensitivity followed by reaction to insect stings, foods and other drugs. It is also a very real risk during immunotherapy.

The key to treatment is adrenaline administered by deep subcutaneous injection in doses of 0.2–0.5 ml of a 1: 1000 aquaeous solution. It should be repeated at 10–15 minute intervals as required. Intravenous antihistamines may also be given and oxygen administration may be essential. Intravenous aminophylline, hydrocortisone and cardiovascular and respiratory support may also be necessary.

Patients known to have anaphylactic reaction to unavoidable agents such as insect stings, should be supplied with emergency medication kits. They can be instructed to administer adrenaline themselves and may also use an adrenaline pressurised aerosol prior to gaining medical attention.

Insect Allergies

Reactions to insect stings may range from mild local erythema with swelling and pain, to urticaria, angio-oedema or even anaphylaxis. The acute treatment of generalised reactions is described above. Approximately 40 per cent of patients who have a second sting, particularly if it is within 2 weeks or more than 5 years after the first reaction have a diminished response. Only 10 to 20 per cent are likely to have a worse reaction. It is now possible to assess the likelihood of a subsequent major reaction by skin testing with venom extracts and measuring venom-specific IgE antibodies. Recent evidence suggests that immunotherapy with venom extract is effective in reducing subsequent reactions, though the questions of optimal therapy and duration of treatment have not been resolved.

Gastrointestinal Allergy

Virtually any ingested substance can produce an allergic reaction in the gastrointestinal tract, leading to vomiting, diarrhoea, abdominal pain or failure to thrive. Cow's milk sensitivity is of major importance in infants. It contains a vast number of allergens of which five have been fully characterised, betalactoglobulin, casein, alphalactalbumin, bovine serum albumin and bovine gammaglobulin. Betalactoglobulin is by far the commonest cause of sensitivity and for this reason it is sometimes possible to use a milk substitute which contains hydrolysed casein, such as Nutramigen or Pregestimil. If casein also produces a reaction it may be necessary to use a soya-protein-based milk such as Prosobee, Wysoy or Velactin. Soya, however, is becoming more widely used in infants' feeds so that the incidence of allergy to this product has also increased. Egg and cow's milk allergy is probably the most common combined sensitivity and a dietician can provide lists of foods free from these dairy products.

Where food allergy has been diagnosed it is wise to keep the patient off the offending foods for at least one year after the last symptomatic contact. Children with previously clearly identified food allergies are often able to tolerate the offending foods, at least in small quantities, after one to 2 years.

There is some evidence that regular administration of large doses of sodium cromoglycate orally may protect the child from the gastrointestinal manifestations of allergy. It is likely that orally active, systemically absorbed compounds will be developed. There is currently no place for immunotherapy in gastrointestinal allergy.

FURTHER READING

Bierman C W & Pearlman D S 1980 Allergic disease of infancy, childhood and adolescence. W B Saunders Co, Philadelphia

Clark T J H & Godfrey S 1983 Asthma. Chapman & Hall Medical, London (2nd edition)

Hayward A R 1977 Immuno-deficiency, Current topics in immunology no 6. Edward Arnold Ltd, London

Kuzemko J A 1978 Allergy in children. Pitman Medical, Tunbridge Wells

Lessof M H (ed) 1984 Immunological and Clinical Aspects of Alergy. John Wiley & Sons, Bristol

Soothill J F, Hayward A R & Wood C B S 1983 Paediatric Immunology. Blackwell, Oxford

14

Gastrointestinal disorders

Young children frequently complain of gastrointestinal symptoms. These are commonly secondary to disorders outside the alimentary tract while many diseases of the gut are associated with few specific signs. It is, therefore, essential to carry out a full general examination and to elicit a clear history remembering that there is a great variation in the way in which many parents use words such as diarrhoea, vomiting, appetite or constipation.

VOMITING

Some of the important causes of vomiting in infancy are shown in Table 14.1. The timing, frequency, volume, and content of the vomitus should all be noted as these may give clues as to the diagnosis and to progress. Projectile vomiting must be distinguished from posseting or rumination.

Gastro-oesophageal reflux and hiatus hernia

Effortless regurgitation of stomach contents is often seen in healthy babies in the first few months of life. It usually attributed to gastro-oesophageal reflux. Most of the infants concerned have a normally placed gastro-oesophageal junction and yet have a tendency to regurgitate gastric contents into the lower oesophagus. Present evidence suggests that effective lower oesophageal closure is brought about by the combined action of an intrinsic muscle sphincter, the presence of an intra-abdominal segment of oesophagus subject to abdominal pressures, and the mucosal arrangement at the junction which acts as a choke. In many babies it would appear that the integration

Table 14.1 Vomiting in Infants

Feeding problems

Infection
  enteral
    oral candidasis
    gastroenteritis
  parenteral
    respiratory tract
    otitis media
    urinary
    central nervous system
    septicaemia
Gastro-oeseophageal reflux
  hiatus hernia

Intestinal obstruction
  congenital malformations
  pyloric stenosis
  intussusception

Malabsorption
  coeliac disease
  cow's milk protein intolerance
  lactose intolerance

Cerebral
  birth trauma
  hydrocephalus
  meningocephalitis
  intracranial space-occupying lesion

Metabolic disorders
  galactosaemia
  idiopathic hypercalcaemia
  aminoacidaemias

Endocrine
  adrenogenital syndrome

Renal
  renal tubular acidosis
  uraemia

of these factors is inadequate, and reflux occurs. This causes no distress, except to the mother, weight gain is generally satisfactory and, in the majority of infants, the symptoms have resolved by the age of 6 months. Simple measures that may be taken include keeping the infant in a sitting position and adding a thickening agent such as Nestargel to the feeds.

More severe reflux may be associated with an abnormal position of the gastro-oesophageal junction, as in a partial thoracic stomach or hiatus hernia. Oesophagitis is then more likely to develop, causing blood to be seen in the vomit and in some cases failure to thrive and stricture formation. Aspiration pneumonia may also occur. If any of these features are seen, further investigation is required.

A barium swallow and meal by an experienced radiologist is necessary to demonstrate the presence of pathological reflux or a sliding hiatus hernia, and oesophagitis can be assessed endoscopically. If a hernia is present the infant should be nursed continuously at an angle of at least 60° to the horizontal. The volume of individual feeds may be reduced by increasing their frequency, preparations containing alkalis may give symptomatic improvement. Anticholinergic drugs may reduce gastro-oesophageal tone and should be avoided. Surgery is only indicated for those who continue to fail to thrive, become anaemic or develop a stricture. There remains a group of infants whose growth appears to be compromised by marked regurgitation but in whom no organic lesion is demonstrated. They will usually respond to the symptomatic treatment described above.

Hypertrophic pyloric stenosis

In this condition gastric emptying is disturbed as a result of hypertrophy of the pyloric musculature. It is not present at birth but develops during the neonatal period. It occurs in approximately three infants per 1000 in the UK. The aetiology is obscure but is probably multifactorial, involving both genetic and environmental factors. It is more common in first-born children and males are affected four times more frequently than females. There is an unexplained association with unconjugated hyperbilirubinaemia, and various congenital abnormalities of the gut such as oesophageal and duodenal atresia and ano-rectal anomalies.

Clinical features

Vomiting after feeds usually commences in the second or third weeks of life. The vomit is never bile stained but it occasionally contains blood. It becomes increasingly copious and eventually projectile. The infant is hungry and will readily take another feed but, in due course, he will become wasted, dehydrated, constipated and miserable. On examination the crucial physical signs to elicit are visible gastric peristalsis and a palpable pyloric tumour. These are best observed while the infant is feeding cradled in his mother's arms with his head supported on her left. A peristaltic wave should appear as a rounded lump passing slowly from left to right across the epigastrium. Gentle and patient palpation of the right upper quadrant of the abdomen should be carried out with the tips of the fingers of the left hand. A firm smooth olive-sized mass may be felt just lateral to the right rectus muscle between the costal margin and the umbilicus. It is most easily located after a vomit and its consistency should alter as the muscle contracts and relaxes.

Management and prognosis

Radiological investigation is not usually necessary, however, if a pyloric tumour is not definitely palpable, barium studies may confirm elongation and narrowing of the pyloric canal with indentation of the antrum and duodenal cap. A hypochloraemic, hypokalaemic alkalosis accompanies the loss of gastric secretions, this together with dehydration must be corrected before surgery. Other coincidental causes of vomiting such as a urinary infection should always be considered. The treatment of choice is pyloromyotomy (Ramstedt's operation which is curative. Post-operative complications are few, oral feeding may be resumed within 4 hours, the infant being rapidly regraded onto a full strength milk. Medical treatment with atropine methonitrate (Eumydrin) or dicyclomine hydrochloride (Merbentyl) is rarely indicated.

Vomiting in older children

Some of the main causes of vomiting in older children are given in Table 14.2.

Recurrent vomiting in the absence of a recognisable pathology, and occuring in the middle years of childhood, forms part of what is known

Table 14.2 Causes of vomiting in the older child

Infections
Acute appendicitis
Drug ingestion
Cyclical vomiting
Diabetic ketosis
Migraine
Motion sickness
Peptic ulceration
Intestinal obstruction
Dietary indiscretion

as the periodic syndrome. It may be related to emotional stress and form part of a family pattern of psychosomatic disorders. The attacks may be mild but, in some patients, there are sudden bouts of retching and vomiting often preceded by abdominal pain or headache. There may be sufficient dehydration and acidosis to necessitate the administration of intravenous fluids while intramuscular chlorpromazine helps to alleviate the vomiting. Recovery is rapid and complete. The frequency of symptoms is usually variable although often described as cyclical. The role of psychological factors remains unclear. The attacks tend to diminish with age although some children later develop migraine.

Haematemesis

Prolonged severe retching for any cause may result in blood staining of vomit. The most common source of bleeding in childhood haematemeses is the nasopharynx where a history of epistaxis and swallowed blood is relevant. More serious causes are coagulation disorders, oesophagitis, oesophageal varices, gastric erosions duodenal ulceration and acute poisoning.

DIARRHOEA

Although many parents take a great interest in their infant's bowel function, stool-gazing is an overrated occupation. The range of normality is wide, and most changes of stool frequency, colour or consistency are of no serious significance. Observations which are useful diagnostic pointers include the onset of watery diarrhoea, or the presence of blood or oil. The former is seen in gastroenteritis, carbohydrate intolerance, and in

such rare disorders as ganglioneuroma or chloride-losing diarrhoea. The commonest causes of bleeding are a rectal mucosal tear or infection, a Meckel's diverticulum or colitis must also be considered. Oily stools denote gross steatorrhoea, as may be seen in pancreatic insufficiency. Small bowel malabsorption with lesser degrees of steatorrhoea may coexist with clinically normal stools. It is important to establish the chronological development of the stool abnormality, relating it specifically to birth, the dietary introduction of gluten-containing cereals, cows' milk, or sucrose, and to emotional disturbances in the family or environment.

Persistence after an acute onset should be identified. A suspicion of associated failure to thrive should ideally be confirmed by plotting the growth pattern on a centile chart. Some of the important causes of diarrhoea are discussed below, and a list indicating the range of possible aetiologies is shown in Table 14.3.

Toddler diarrhoea

Most toddlers whose mothers say that they are

Table 14.3 Causes of diarrhoea in childhood

Toddler diarrhoea
 irritable bowel syndrome

Gastrointestinal infection
 bacterial ⎫
 viral ⎬ gastroenteritis
 tuberculosis ⎭
 amoebiasis
 giardiasis

Extra-intestinal infection
 Upper respiratory tract
 pulmonary
 urinary

Malabsorption syndromes
 small bowel enteropathy
 carbohydrate malabsorption
 pancreatic insufficiency
 bile acid deficiency

Inflammatory bowel disorders
 ulcerative colitis
 Crohn's disease

Miscellaneous
 overfeeding in infancy
 chronic constipation with overflow
 antibiotic therapy
 endocrine disorders
 gut resections

passing loose, frequent, bulky or offensive stools have no definable abnormality. Characteristically, they are gaining weight, developing normally and have no abdominal distension. They may well have a prominent abdomen secondary to a normal lordotic posture. Such children may be described as having non-specific diarrhoea or the irritable colon syndrome. They often pass three to six mucus-containing loose stools every day; the stools sometimes contain undigested vegetables but, in some, the stools are in fact manifestly normal most of the time and in other chidren the stool changes are secondary to respiratory infections, or may reflect the emotional climate of the family. There may be a preceding history of an apparent gastroenteritis. The diagnosis is supported by the normal results of such simple investigations as stool and urine microscopy and culture, stool pH and reducing substance analysis, haemoglobin and white blood cell count. In the management extensive investigation or dietary manipulation should be avoided but rather concentrate on explanation and reassurance that this is a benign, self-limiting disorder, usually resolving by school age. The physiology of the condition continues to be studied and although the sensitivity of the childhood alimentary tract to emotional stress is well recognised, no consistent pathogenic mechanism has yet been identified.

Gastroenteritis

Infective diarrhoea and vomiting chiefly affects children under 2 years of age. Overcrowding, poverty, and malnutrition all increase the incidence of epidemics. Symptoms follow actual invasion of the bowel wall by pathogens, or adherence of toxin-secreting organisms to the small bowel mucosa, stimulating fluid and electrolyte movement into the lumen. The major pathogenic bacteria involved include enteropathic *Escherichia coli*, salmonellae, shigellae, staphylococci, *Yersinia enterocolitica*, *Campylobacter* and *Vibrio cholerae*. Viruses of importance are rotavirus, coronavirus and adenoviruses.

Clinical features

The illness often begins with vomiting, and progresses to watery diarrhoea within 24 hours. Blood in the stool may be seen particularly in campylobacter and shigella infections. The most important clinical features are consequent upon dehydration and electrolyte disturbance. These result in loss of skin turgor, dry mucous membranes, reduced intra-ocular tension, acidotic breathing and, in infants, a sunken fontanelle. In mild dehydration (up to 5 per cent loss of body weight) these signs are minimal, but the child is symptomatic and pyrexial. In moderate dehydration (10 per cent) the infant is drowsy and oliguric, with sunken eyes and a definite reduction in skin turgor. In severe dehydration (10–15 per cent) the child is semi-conscious, acidotic and in shock, with cold clammy and mottled skin. If, despite clear evidence of considerable fluid loss there are no signs of circulatory collapse, hypernatraemic dehydration should be suspected; here the skin has a doughy feel to it and often neurological signs, including convulsions, occur.

Management

The cornerstone of treatment is the correction of dehydration by water and electrolyte replacement. Solids and milk should be discontinued. Patients with moderate and severe dehydration require intravenous fluid while those with mild dehydration may be rehydrated with oral solutions* at home provided vomiting is not too severe. After 12–24 hours of rehydration, quarter-strength milk is reintroduced and graded up to full strength over 1–2 days.

Sometimes there is sufficient damage to the jejunal mucosal border to impair lactase activity. This temporarily causes lactose malabsorption (see page) and a recurrence of diarrhoea on reintroducing cow's milk.

Stool examination should include microscopy, microbiological culture and electronmicroscopy for virus particles. The routine use of antibiotics is not advised. There is no good evidence that they reduce mortality or morbidity and they may, in fact, cause harm by promoting a carrier state and the proliferation of resistant organisms. On the

---

*The oral fluid should be water to which electrolytes and glucose are added, often as an commercially available powder. Glucose is important not only as an energy source, but also as a driving force for the absorption of fluid and electrolytes.

other hand, bacteraemia and septicaemia, e.g. typhoid fever, should always be treated with an antibiotic to which the organism is sensitive. Drugs which reduce gut motility or which absorb fluid from the stool offer only symptomatic relief and do not alter the course of the illness.

MALABSORPTION

Malabsorption is suggested clinically by the triad of failure to thrive, abdominal distention and diarrhoea. Some of the causes in childhood are listed in Table 14.4. The major group is that which causes small bowel mucosal enteropathies. Such patients will eventually show additional signs and symptoms relating to reduced absorption of iron, folic acid, and vitamin D and K, and some become hypoproteinaemic.

If malabsorption is suspected clinically, screening tests for xylose and fat absorption should be performed together with a full blood count and stool microscopy and culture. If on jejunal biopsy villous atrophy is found (Figs 14.1 and 14.2), a specific diagnosis must be established. Any damage to the mucosal brush border will impair

Table 14.4 Some causes of malabsorption

Small bowel mucosal abnormality
Morphological
  non-specific
    coeliac disease
    cow's milk protein intolerance
    giardiasis
    post-gastroenteritis
    protein energy malnutrition
    tropical sprue
    immunodeficiency states
  specific
    intestinal lymphangiectasia
    abetalipoproteinaemia
Functional
    lactase deficiency secondary to morphological changes
    primary lactase deficiency
    sucrase-isomaltase deficiency
    glucose-galactose malabsorption
    chloride-losing diarrhoea

Intraluminal abnormalities
Exocrine pancreatic insufficiency
    cystic fibrosis
    pancreatic achylia and cyclic neutropenia
Altered bile acid enterohepatic circulation
    hepatic immaturity in preterm infant
    cholestasis
    cirrhosis
    blind loop syndrome
    ileal resection
    Crohn's disease of ileum

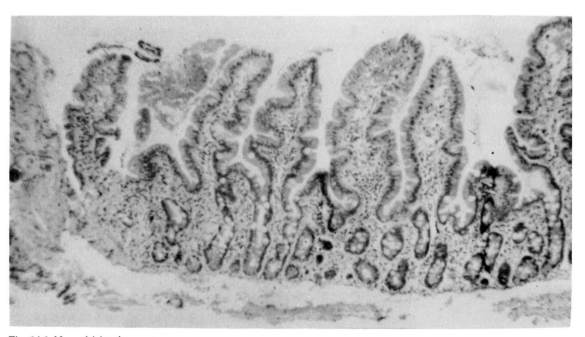

Fig. 14.1 Normal jejunal mucosa

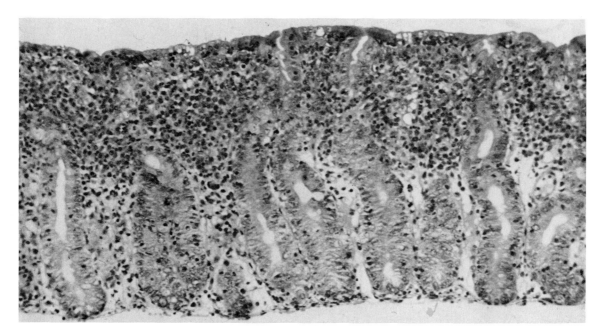

Fig. 14.2 Subtotal villous atrophy of the jejunum

disaccharidase activity, lactase being the most vulnerable enzyme. Clinical lactose intolerance is a frequent secondary phenomenon which should resolve as the cause of the villous atrophy is treated.

Coeliac disease

In coeliac disease the protein, alpha-gliadin which is present in gluten in wheat and other cereals, causes mucosal damage characterised by complete atrophy of the villi, predominantly in the proximal small bowel. (The population incidence of coliac disease in the UK is approximately one in 2000, with some familial clustering.) There is a tissue-typing association with HLA-DR3, DR7 and HLA-B8 and the disorder is commoner in girls. The pathogenic mechanisms have not been elucidated. No abnormality of alpha-gliadin digestion has been shown. Various immunological disturbances have been demonstrated but whether these are of primary or secondary significance has not been determined.

Clinical features

The typical child with coeliac disease presents around the age of one year with poor weight gain, diarrhoea, abdominal distention and anorexia. Vomiting and irritability may be notable. On examination there is abdominal distension, hypotonia, and muscle wasting, with flattening of the buttocks (see Figs. 14.3 & 14.4). An accurate dietary history relating to gluten intake must be obtained. Older children may have less obvious clinical features, growth impairment may not be marked, diarrhoea is not invariable; abdominal pain and anaemia may be present and rickets is seen, particularly in Asian children.

Management

Withdrawal of gluten from the diet results in total clinical and histological remission. Intolerance is permanent and may be confirmed by an oral challenge carried out in relation to changes in jejunal histology. A mucosal biopsy taken on a gluten-free diet is compared with one taken 3 months later after the daily addition of 10–20 g of gluten to the diet. In children under the age of 2 years in whom it was not possible to completely exclude other causes of an enteropathy on presentation, a formal gluten challenge must subsequently be carried out. The long term prognosis on a gluten-free diet is excellent. It is well recognised that patients whose coeliac disease has been diagnosed in adult life

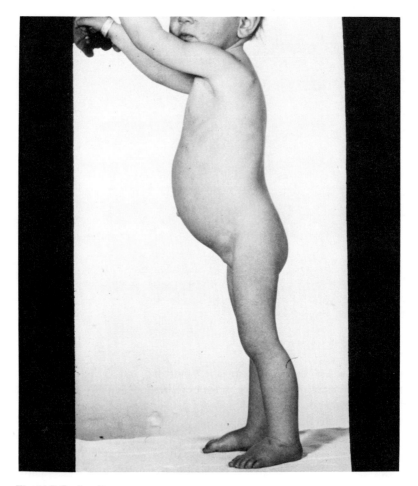

Fig. 14.3 Coeliac disease

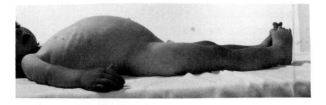

Fig. 14.4 Coeliac disease — abdominal distension still evident when child recumbent

have an increased susceptibility to malignancy. There is no evidence to date that individuals treated from childhood are similarly at risk.

Food allergy
(See also Chapter 13)

The normal immunological response of the gut to oral antigen is to produce humoral or cellular immunity, or tolerance. Local IgA or circulating IgG or IgM antibodies are assumed to have a protective role; cellular responses are currently poorly defined. Immunological tolerance is an active state of immunoregulation in which cellular and humoral responses are not demonstrable. If a situation develops in which tolerance is broken or different classes of immunoglobulin antibody such as IgE are produced in excess, immunological reactions may occur which cause local tissue damage. These are termed hypersensitivity reactions and may be recognised in the gut as allergies. Since the gastrointestinal tract is a major lymphoid organ, not only containing many lymphocytes in the lamina propria, but also being the site or extensive cell traffic involving circulating lymphocytes, immunocompetent cells may be distributed all over the body and be triggered into activity by the ingestion of oral antigen. Factors which predispose to the development of hypersensitivity reactions include luminal conditions, such as the nature of the antigen and the presence of adjuvants, and mucosal conditions, which affect the presentation of antigen to lymphocytes.

In the healthy gut, antigen enters via the Peyer's patches. If an enteropathy is present, antigen will gain access to the mucosa in unusual concentrations and at unusual sites. In addition, there are clearly genetically determined aspects of immunoreactivity. The food proteins which most commonly provoke hypersensitivity reactions are contained in cow's milk and eggs.

Cow's milk protein intolerance

Clinical features

Two main groups of affected children are seen. The first have an unequivocal reaction to small volumes of cow's milk which provoke immediate symptoms such as local oedema, vomiting, wheezing, rashes, or diarrhoea containing blood. In the second group of patients the onset of symptoms is more insidious with failure to thrive predominating. They may also have diarrhoea and vomiting and on examination show evidence of weight loss and, on occasion, abdominal distension.

The first group often show other features of allergy and appear to have symptoms on their first exposure to cow's milk having previously been breast fed. The second group have often tolerated cow's milk initially and have developed their hypersensitivity following an episode of mucosal damage due to a condition such as gastroenteritis.

Management

It is very easy to assume a causal relationship if an infant's symptoms resolve on exclusion of cow's milk from the diet. Since this may be a coincidental improvement any association must be confirmed by subsequent challenge, having excluded the possibility of lactose intolerance.

In the first group of patients a challenge must be carried out with care, starting with 5 ml of cow's milk and gradually increasing the volume given over 48 hours. Clinical observation remains the best way of monitoring the response since none of the various immunological parameters so far suggested have proved to be diagnostic.

The second group of infants have evidence of malabsorption and require a jejunal biopsy while on a normal diet. If an enteropathy is present it must be shown that exclusion of cow's milk is associated with histological improvement and that subsequent challenge provokes a relapse.

The most practical treatment is to replace cow's milk with soya milk or a hydrolysed cow's milk protein formula (chapter 8). A few patients will become sensitised to the protein which is substituted into the diet; if goat's milk is used folic acid supplements must be given.

Many, but not all, of the first group tolerate cow's milk by the age of 2 years, most children in the second group recover within a few months of diagnosis.

Lactose malabsorption

Lactose is split into its component monosaccharides, glucose and galactose, by the disaccharidase enzyme lactase. This is present in the microvillus brush border of the columnar epithelial cells which line the intestinal mucosa. When small intestinal lactase activity is deficient, lactose passes on to be metabolised in the caecum and colon by the normal gut flora. Water is drawn into the bowel from the osmotic effect of the lactose load while the increased hydrogen ion concentration attendant on the accumulation of lactic acid impairs water absorption in the colon; the stools are fluid and the stool water is acid and contains glucose.

Lactase activity may be secondarily impaired in any disorder associated with a small bowel enteropathy. In such cases normal activity will return as the lesion resolves. Lactase levels rise to normal at or just after birth so that some newborns show a temporary deficiency. A primary lactase deficiency present from birth does occur but it is very rare and is recessively inherited. An acquired isolated lactase deficiency develops in many non-Caucasians with late childhood onset. Some authorities even regard the presence of lactase in Caucasian adults as abnormal, its persistence is thought to have given a genetic advantage in cattle-rearing communities.

Note that lactose malabsorption does not always result in lactose intolerance. This will depend on the lactose load given and the length of bowel in which lactase is deficient.

Clinical features and management

The passage of watery stools with a pH less than 5.5 and containing reducing substances as demonstrated by Clinitest tablets is suggestive of lactose malabsorption. The patient also experiences colicky abdominal pain, abdominal distension and increased flatus.

Lactose intolerance is confirmed if lactose exclusion from the diet relieves the symptoms and subsequent challenge using lactose, 2 g/kg body weight in a 10 per cent solution, causes a recurrence. Normal lactose absorption may be confirmed by demonstrating a rise in blood glucose after an oral lactose load, absence of a rise may reflect malabsorption or variations in the rate of gastric emptying. If lactose has reached the colon and been metabolised by bacteria, hydrogen will be produced and may be measured in expired breath after a lactose challange. Lactase may be measured directly in a mucosal biopsy specimen which also allow histological examination to demonstrate an enteropathy.

Treatment with a lactose-free milk in infants will control symptoms. The formulae available are discussed in Chapter 8. It is unusual to have to exclude all dairy products in older children. When lactose intolerance is secondary to acute gastro-enteritis it is usually possible to reintroduce cow's milk after 2–4 weeks. Clearly, the distinction between cow's milk protein intolerance and lactose intolerance is important.

Carbohydrate malabsorption

Sucrose and starch are also hydrolysed by brush border disaccharidases. Sucrase, maltase and isomaltase activities are less vulnerable than lactase, and reductions are only seen in severe enteropathies. There is a rare recessively-inherited deficiency of sucrase and isomaltase which causes watery stools after a sucrose or starch load. If Clinitest tablets are used to test for undigested sucrose in stool water, acid must first be added to hydrolyse the sugar. Such patients are symptomatic in early childhood and respond to a reduction in dietary sucrose and starch, but they will usually tolerate increasing amounts as they grow older. Monosaccharide intolerance may be seen in association with severe enteropathies, particularly in infancy.

Giardiasis

Giardia lamblia is a flagellate protozoon which is transmitted in water or food. The trophozoite inhabits the duodenum and jejunum, and cysts are periodically passed in the stools. Its distribution is worldwide.

Clinical features and management

The symptoms vary from mild diarrhoea in a perfectly well child to frank malabsorption with chronic diarrhoea, vomiting, abdominal pain and failure to thrive. The latter group are likely to have a jejunal enteropathy. The diagnosis can only be finally excluded by histological examination of a duodenal aspirate or mucosal biopsy. An association with IgA deficiency has been reported, however, in practice this is rarely encountered. The drug of choice is metronidazole. Repeated courses may be necessary, alternative drugs are mepacrine and nimorazole.

Cystic fibrosis
(See Chapter 17)

CONSTIPATION

Constipation may be defined as difficulty or delay in the passage of stools. In babies the application or this definition may not be straight forward. It was wise to regard acute and chronic constipation as being different problems and to differentiate them from soiling (the passage of loose stools in clothing) and encopresis (the passage of normal stools in abnormal places).

The breast-fed baby may initially open his bowels after each feed and then quite normally pass unformed stools once a week. The bottle-fed baby's stools are usually drier and harder and may be passed with difficulty. Neither infant is necessarily constipated and an accurate history must be elicited. If there is concern, and particularly if abdominal distension is present, several disorders should be borne in mind. These include an anal stenosis, malposition or other anomaly, a spinal abnormality, Hirschsprung's disease, hypothyroidism, or malabsorption causing such bulky stools that defaecation is difficult.

The toddler's acute problems may originate in the anxious circumstances of potty training, following febrile illnesses, or changes in diet or environment which have resulted in a reduced food intake. If the subsequent passage of a hard stool causes a rectal mucosal abrasion or fissure, blood may be seen on the stool and defaecation may become painful and infrequent. Most acute episodes improve spontaneously, but in children who are prone to constipation a high residue diet, with or without a short course of laxatives is advisable.

Chronic constipation is associated with abdominal distension and large faecal masses are readily palpable per abdomen. There is often a history dating back to infancy, with delay in the passage of stool lasting 3 weeks or more interspersed with intermittent leakage of faecal fluid. Physical examination should exclude obvious anal and spinal abnormalities; rectal examination reveals a ballooned rectum with stool close to the anal verge. Laxatives should not be commenced if enormous, rocky

faecal masses are present, the lower bowel should first be emptied using an enema. A regular bowel habit should then be established by combining an oral intake of sufficient bulk with the use of a stimulant laxative. Since many patients are anorexic at this stage a bulk purgative is useful initially, but it should not be necessary to repeat the enema. Relapses are common, so laxatives may be needed for several months after a normal pattern has been regained in order to cover the period during which the dilated lower bowel with its diminished sensation is returning to normal. Behavioural problems commonly fade away as bowel control returns. Children who fail to respond to treatment or who relapse rapidly require further investigation.

Hirschsprung's disease

Hirschsprung's disease is characterised by a congenital absence from the bowel wall of the intrinsic autonomic ganglion cells which form Auerbach and Meissner's plexus. There is a concomitant hypertrophy of the extrinsic autonomic nerves supplying the affected gut. The resulting lack of propulsive activity causes chronic constipation and gross dilatation of the proximal bowel.

The original descriptions were of lower colonic and rectal involvement, however, it is now recognised that there is a wide range of abnormality from ultrashort segments to changes in the entire large and small intestine. The general population incidence is estimated to be about one in 5000 with familial clustering.

Clinical features

The majority of patients present in the neonatal period with evidence of lower bowel obstruction with delay in the passage of meconium and vomiting. Abdominal distension can be sufficient to cause respiratory embarrassment. In older children, failure to thrive may be noted and the history of intractable constipation precedes potty training. Rectal examination reveals an empty rectum while the sphincter may be tight but distensible. A serious complication of the condition is enterocolitis.

Management and prognosis

The diagnosis is confirmed by barium enema, ano-rectal pressure studies (manometry) and mucosal suction biopsy.

In a patient without bowel preparation the radiological appearances include a narrow agan-glionic segment and immediately proximal to it, with a transitional or cone zone dilated proximal bowel. Anorectal manometry shows a failure of relaxation of the internal sphincter. Rectal histology reveals absence of the submucosal ganglion plexus, hypertrophy of nerve fibres, and there is increased acetylcholinesterase activity in the lamina propria.

The principles of treatment are the relief of obstruction, usually by colostomy, with eventual excision of the aganglionic segment and anasto-mosis of ganglionic bowel to the anal canal. Most children thereafter have satisfactory control of defaecation, while a minority continue to suffer from constipation or fail to achieve continence. The major mortality occurs in the neonatal period, particularly if enterocolitis supervenes.

ABDOMINAL PAIN

Recurrent pains, over a period of months, are common in childhood, and of these abdominal pain is the commonest. Most conditions (see Table 14.5) can be identified from the history and clinical examination and by simple tests such as screening of the urine.

Recurrent abdominal pain typically makes the child stop playing and want to lie down, he often looks pale and may vomit. He points to the umbilicus or near it, when asked where it hurts. On examination there is vague tenderness but no guarding or rigidity, the descending colon may be palpable, but this is found in many normal children. Recovery is complete within an hour or two and the child returns to normal activities. It is always wise for the doctor to consider organic conditions while exploring the more likely emotional causes. It is necessary to come to an understanding of the child, and his family and school background. This takes time, but is essential if parental fears are to be explored, traumatic situations in the child's life identified and, as confidence is built up, if practical advice is to be formulated and accepted. The family should not be left in a diagnostic vacuum nor should reliance be placed on placebo drug therapy.

Colic

Babies are often said to have colic or wind when they draw up their legs and scream. This should never be assumed without careful consideration. Even if the interpretation is correct, no precise cause may be found. Some infants may be observed to be swallowing large quantities of air during feeding, in others, one may be led to the conclusion that they are reflecting parental anxiety or depression. Improvement occurs with an anti-cholinergic drug or simply a brief placement in the atmosphere of a well-run children's ward. Res-olution by 3 months of age is the general rule.

Appendicitis
(See Chapter 23)

INFLAMMATORY BOWEL DISEASE

Ulcerative colitis

Ulcerative colitis is characterised by diffuse inflammation and ulceration of the mucosa of the rectum and colon proximal to it. It is rare in child-hood (4 in 100 000) and affects both sexes equally. The peak incidence periods are the first year of life and between 8 and 9 years of age. The aetiology is unknown but probably reflects an interaction between infective, genetic and immunological factors.

Table 14.5 Causes of recurrent abdominal pain of childhood

Gastrointestinal	Extra-gastrointestinal
Gastroenteritis	Renal infections
Appendicitis	Renal calculi
Mesenteric adenitis	Pneumonia
Henoch-Schonlein purpura	Diabetes mellitus
Intestinal obstruction	Sickel cell disease
Malabsorption syndromes	Lead poisoning
Inflammatory bowel disease	Porphyria
Peptic ulcer	Epilepsy
Pancreatitis	Referred from spine,
Hepatitis	ovaries, testes, pelvis
Tuberculosis	

Clinical features

Most children present with bloody diarrhoea, lower abdominal pain, weight loss, lack of energy, nausea and a low-grade fever. Abdominal examination generally reveals non-specific tenderness. Extra-intestinal manifestations occur and include erythema nodosum, arthritis, mouth ulcers, and pyoderma gangrenosum. Occasionally, life-threatening fulminating toxic dilatation of the colon occurs.

Management and prognosis

Bacterial (Shigella, Salmonella, Campylobacter, *E. coli*) and amoebic infections must first be excluded. A double-contrast barium enema shows proctitis and an abnormal colonic mucosal pattern, with loss of haustration, pseudopolypi formation and disordered motility. A typical X-ray is shown in Figure 14.5. Endoscopy should be done and biopsies taken to confirm the diagnosis.

Any fluid and electrolyte disturbance or anaemia needs to be corrected and the diet must contain adequate protein and calories. Opiates and anticholinergic drugs should be avoided since they predispose to the development of toxic megacolon. Specific therapy includes oral and rectal steroids, and sulphasalazine. Prednisolone is eventually given on an alternate day regimen, gradually being withdrawn to leave the patient on daily maintenance sulphasalazine.

The clinical course is chronic with relapse and remissions. Surgery is indicated if acute symptoms do not respond to intensive medical care, if presisting gut activity leads to chronic ill health and delay in growth or puberty, or if local complications such as perforation occur. There is an increased incidence of malignancy which is related to the duration and extent of the disease. Patients who present in childhood are at great risk in adult life since after 10 years of active disease 20 per cent develop cancer during each subsequent decade.

Crohn's disease

Crohn's disease causes inflammation of the whole thickness of the bowel wall. Histologically, there is in addition granuloma and fissure formation. The terminal ileum or the colon is particularly affected, although any part of the alimentary tract may be involved, with normal bowel in between and with sparing of the rectum. It, too, is rare in childhood (1 in 100 000), the aetiology is obscure.

Clinical features

The diagnosis is rarely made at an early stage. The significance of anorexia and abdominal pain is often missed; the astute physician is alerted by the presence of growth failure or weight loss, an abdominal mass, painless perianal fissures, anaemia, finger clubbing or an unexplained fever.

Nutritional deficiences are common and are caused by malabsorption and loss of protein and blood from the gut. Extra-intestinal lesions are less common than in ulcerative colitis.

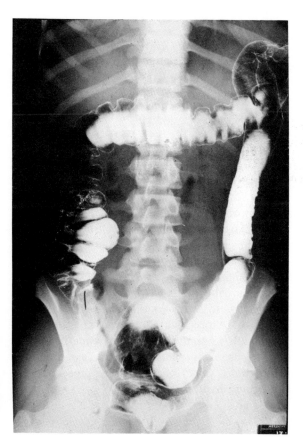

Fig. 14.5 Descending colon in ulcerative colitis

Management and prognosis

Barium studies of both small and large bowel are necessary. Oedema, spasm and fibrosis cause narrowing ('string sign'), patchy involvement is seen (skip lesions), fistulae may be demonstrable and, in the colon eccentric lesions and 'rose thorn' spikey ulcers are seen. A typical X-ray is shown in Figure 14.6. Endoscopy and biopsy should be performed, the classical macroscopic appearance includes aphthous ulcers and a 'cobblestone' mucosal pattern.

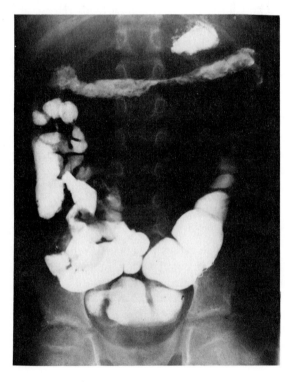

Fig. 14.6 Barium enema showing Crohn's disease of the colon

Unfortunately, there are no specific curative drugs available but general supportive measures, such as maintenance of nutrition are important. Steroids, sulphasalazine and azothiaprine may be effective in inducing a remission but do not prevent a subsequent relapse. If bacterial overgrowth is present metronidazole is useful.

Surgical resections of the affected bowel must be regarded as palliative since the recurrence rate in children is high. Chronic indications include growth retardation, delayed puberty, recurrent

obstruction, fistulae and extra-intestinal complications. Acute indications include perforation, severe haemorrhage and acute obstruction.

Parasitic infections

Threadworms (*Enterobius vermicularis*)

Enterobius vermicularis is a common parasite in school children throughout the world. The entire life cycle is completed in man. It is usually spread within families. The worms' habitat is the caecum and appendix from where they migrate to the lower rectum and eggs are laid on the perianal skin. Following scratching with the fingers, eggs are reingested and the cycle continues. The usual symptom is perianal irritation. The worms may be demonstrated by microscopic examination of a piece of transparent adhesive tape placed on the skin near the anus. The whole family should be treated with a drug such as mebendazole, piperazine or thiabendazole.

Roundworms (*Ascaris lumbricoides*)

Ascaris lumbricoides is principally harboured by young children both in the tropics and in areas extending well into the temperate zones. The eggs develop in moist soil contaminated with faeces. Following ingestion, larvae hatch into the small intestine, pass through the bowel wall to the liver, and thence travel to the lungs where they remain causing a local inflammatory reaction. They then move up the bronchial tree to the pharynx where they are swallowed and mature into adult worms in the small intestine.

Most patients are asymptomatic. Larval migration through the lungs causes cough, dyspnoea and wheezing. Abdominal symptoms depend on the worm load. In heavy infestations frank malnutrition may be precipitated, particularly in undernourished communities and sometimes the physical mass of parasites may cause intestinal obstruction. The treatment is piperazine or bephenium hydroxide.

Toxocariasis (visceral larva migrans)

Toxocara canis and *Toxocara catis* undergo a similar

life cycle in dogs and cats to that of ascaris in man. Infection is, widespread. If children ingest the eggs, larvae emerge in their intestine, however, their subsequent migration is disturbed in the human environment and they lodge in various organs, becoming encysted and causing a local inflammatory response. The liver lungs, eye, brain, kidneys, heart and muscle may all be affected. Children of pre-school age are typically infected. They may show anaemia, failure to thrive, hepatosplenomegaly, eosinophilia and respiratory symptoms. Neurological and ophthalmological signs may also occur. Diethylcarbamazine is used in treatment, the household pet should be dewormed using piperazine.

Taeniasis

Taenia solium and *Taenia saginatum* are tapeworms which have as their intermediate host, the pig and cow, respectively. The worms develop in the human intestine following ingestion of cysts in infected beef or pork. The symptoms include abdominal pain and diarrhoea, and segments of proglottides may be seen in the stools. *T. sagninatum* larvae on emerging from cysts in man, lodge in various tissues causing local inflammation with calcification in muscle, (cystercicosis); if in the brain, convulsions may follow. Treatment with niclosamide causes expulsion of the worms.

LIVER DISORDERS

Hepatomegaly

The liver is normally palpable in infancy and early childhood. There are numerous causes of pathological enlargement. They may be broadly classified as follows:
1. Hepatitis — acute, chronic
2. Infiltration or deposition of fat, mucopolysaccharides, glycogen
3. Venous congestion — right ventricular failure, tricuspid incompetence
4. Space-occupying lesions — abscess, cyst, tumour
5. Chronic haemolysis — thalassaemia.

The presence of splenomegaly suggests infection, a metabolic disorder or occasionally portal hypertension. Biochemical assessment of hepatic function may be followed by liver biopsy if the diagnosis remains obscure.

Jaundice

The differential diagnosis of neonatal jaundice is discussed in Chapter 7. In older children the commonest aetiology is viral hepatitis (see Chapter 12), although many other infectious agents are recognised. Other causes of jaundice include chronic active hepatitis, biliary cirrhosis and haemolysis which may be due to hereditary spherocytosis, haemoglobinopathies, or G6PD deficiency.

Hepatocellular failure

Acute liver failure may complicate viral hepatitis, follow drug ingestion such as paracetamol, or represent the end stage of a chronic hepatic disorder such as cirrhosis. The syndrome provokes a complex disturbance of fluid and electrolyte balance, with a bleeding diathesis, increasing jaundice and a progressive encephalopathy terminating in coma and death. Intensive care is necessary and should be carried out in a specialised unit. Any precipitating causes should be corrected if possible. The general supportive measures include the maintenance of respiration and an adequate circulation, control of hypokalaemia, hypoglycaemia and haemorrhage, reduction of blood ammonia levels by sterilisation of the gut and control of protein intake, and provision of adequate calories and vitamins.

Reye's syndrome

This syndrome consists of an acute encephalopathy and fatty degeneration of the liver and other organs such as the kidneys and pancreas. A wide range of viruses and toxic agents have been implicated, however, the mechanism of injury is unknown. Most patients are under the age of 2 years. After a short prodromal illness, vomiting, delirium, convulsions and coma supervene. Hepatomegaly occurs, the serum transaminases are elevated but few children are jaundiced initially. The main management problems are persistent hypoglycaemia and cerebral oedema; the mortality is high.

Chronic hepatitis

An on-going hepatitis persisting for more than 2 or 3 months may be regarded as chronic. Histological assessment is essential to distinguish between chronic persistent and chronic aggressive hepatitis. The former is characterised by inflammatory infiltrate confined to the portal tract. In aggressive or active hepatitis the hepatocytes are swollen, and there are perilobular changes with inflammatory cells spreading out from the portal tract giving the appearance of piecemeal necrosis. These changes are non-specific with respect to aetiology.

Clinically, persistent hepatitis carries a good prognosis and requires no treatment. Chronic aggressive hepatitis is more serious. Its presentation may be acute with fever, anorexia, and jaundice but, in some patients, it is insidious with arthralgia, fever, colitis or erythema nodosum. These children require treatment with steroids to which azothiaprine is added if a biochemical remission is not obtained.

Cirrhosis and portal hypertension

The histological definition of cirrhosis includes destruction of the normal lobular architecture of the liver with areas of nodular regeneration of hepatocytes surrounded by fibrous tissue. Some of the causes are listed in Table 14.6. The clinical features vary according to the aetiology, they are minimal early in the disease but all will, in due course, show the signs of portal hypertension. Ascites, splenomegaly and hypersplenism, oesophageal varices, anaemia, finger clubbing, spider naevi and liver palms should all be looked for. Malabsorption will eventually occur.

Investigations are directed towards assessment of the degree of liver injury and to identification of the underlying pathology. Wilson's disease must always be excluded. If specific therapy is unavailable treatment is aimed at the prevention of

Table 14.6 Some causes of cirrhosis

Post-hepatitis
  viral hepatitis
  chronic active hepatitis
  hepatitis due to drugs or
  toxins

Metabolic
  Wilson's disease
  galactosaemia
  alpha-1-antitrypsin deficiency

Storage disease
  glycogenosis III and IV
  Gaucher's disease
  mucopolysaccharidoses
  Niemann-Pick disease

Biliary cirrhosis
  biliary atresia
  cystic fibrosis
  ulcerative colitis
  familial intrahepatic cholestasis

Indian childhood cirrhosis

Venous congestion
  congestive cardiac failure
  constrictive pericarditis
  Budd-Chiari syndrome
  veno-occlusive disease (Jamaica)

complications. Genetic counselling may be appropriate. Steatorrhoea is lessened by giving the dietary fat as medium chain triglycerides, fat soluble vitamin supplements may be given parenterally, and cholestyramine relieves pruritus. Ascites should be treated with diuretics including aldosterone antagonists, rather than by paracentesis. Anaemia should be corrected. Complications include haemorrhage, septicaemia and the development of hepatoma.

FURTHER READING

Anderson C M, Burke V 1975 Paediatric gastroenterology. Blackwell Scientific Publications, Oxford
Walker-Smith J A, Hamilton J R, & Walker W A 1983 Practical Paediatric Gastroenterology. Butterworths, London
Mowat A P 1979 Liver disorders in childhood. Butterworths, London

15

Disorders of the kidney and urinary tract

THE DEVELOPMENT OF RENAL FUNCTION

The changes that take place in renal function during the first few days and weeks of life are important in the clinical management of sick infants. In reviewing these changes, it is useful to consider the major processes in urine formation, namely:
1. Filtration (in which the major determinant is renal blood flow)
2. Tubular reabsorption
3. Tubular secretion.

Each of these functions is an essentially independant process, but each is directed by the homeostatic requirements of the individual.

The formation of urine commences in the glomerular capillaries by a process of ultrafiltration, which results in the reduction of a protein-free, cell-free filtrate of blood. Renal blood flow is the major determinant of glomerular filtration and maturational changes in filtration rate are accompanied by similar changes in renal blood flow. In infancy the glomerular filtration rate (GFR) is low compared with the adult, achieving adult values at about one year of age. The renal fraction of cardiac output in the newborn baby is calculated as approximately 5 per cent in the first 12 hours of life. This value reaches approximately 10 per cent during the first week but these figures are less than the adult values of 20–25 per cent. In addition to these haemodynamic changes, other characteristics of the immature kidney are important. One is a marked degree of heterogenicity, so that from nephron to nephron, there is more variability within the kidney both in structure and in function than one finds later in life. Another characteristic is that the kidney develops in a centrifugal fashion, so that deeper structures are the earliest formed containing the most mature glomeruli and receive the highest rate of blood flow.

The pattern in the adult kidney is of a higher rate of blood flow to the outer cortex than to other cortical areas. This is in striking contrast to the newborn in which the lowest rate of flow is to the outer cortex and the highest to the deeper cortex. During periods of hypoperfusion there is probably a change in intrarenal blood flow away from the outer cortex into the inner cortex and juxtamedullary areas which could be a factor in the neonatal kidney predisposing to cortical necrosis.

The renal tubules selectively reabsorb about 98 per cent of the glomerular filtrate. The final composition of the urine depends not only on reabsorption but on secretion as well. The transport processes involved maybe active or passive. Active transport requires energy and sodium reabsorption accounts for a major proportion of the oxygen consumption by the kidney. Passive transport does not require a direct expenditure of energy and is dependent upon concentration or osmotic gradients. The fractional reabsorption of sodium in infants is comparable with that of adults (greater than 90 per cent). Under normal conditions the infant can handle a variable salt diet. However, under conditions of salt loading the neonatal kidney may lack the capacity to excrete the excess sodium with resultant increases in extracellular fluid volume, weight gain and oedema. Possible factors that may be involved in this lack of naturiuresis may include a low intrarenal blood flow distribution. The latter would result, as described above, in the preferential perfusion of inner cortical glomeruli with long loops of Henle (salt-retaining). The newborn kidney would therefore appear to be better suited to conditions of salt deprivation than to salt loads.

Another explanation of the avidity of salt by the neonate may rest in the renin-angiotensin system. Strikingly high levels of renin and aldosterone have been demonstrated in young infants enhancing distal tubular reabsorption of sodium and favouring vasoconstriction of the superficial cortical blood vessels.

It is recognised that the newborn kidney does not concentrate urine to the same extent as the mature kidney. The response of the adult kidney to the stimulus of dehydration is to excrete a urine with an osmolality in the range of 1000–1200 mosmol/kg water as compared with the newborn 700–800 mosmol/kg water. This led to recommendations concerning the dietary management of the infant, suggesting a need for an abundant source of water and a relatively low solute load in the diet. Another of the cortical functions of the kidney is to maintain systemic acid-base balance. In the course of metabolism, and particularly with growth, hydrogen ions are released into the extracellular fluid and must be buffered and then excreted by the kidney. Early studies suggested that the immature kidney performed this function very poorly, the kidney function being unable to acidify urine and unable to excrete much acid. This characteristic has subsequently been shown to occur only during the first few days of life and it is recognised that the infant can acidify urine in response to an acid load. Children have lower plasma bicarbonate levels up to about one year of age probably due to the lowered threshold for bicarbonate reabsorption in the proximal tubules and higher plasma phosphate levels which may be in part related to the low GFR.

Renal function tests

The two most commonly used tests for making a gross estimate of glomerular function are plasma urea and creatinine concentration. Many factors will influence urea synthesis; urea production rises with an increased protein intake, gastrointestinal bleeding, infection, burns, muscle trauma or corticosteroid therapy. Production of urea falls when protein intake is reduced or the liver has been damaged. The normal range of plasma urea in children appears to be between 4.0 and 6.0 mmol/l and is somewhat less in infants.

Creatinine is formed in muscle at a relatively constant rate from creatinine phosphate; its daily production is proportional to muscle bulk. Since mass increases faster than surface area with growth, and since GFR is proportional to surface area, the normal plasma creatinine rises with age. Normal values for plasma creatinine in relation to age are known and for children values within the range of 30–80 μmol/l are considered normal.

Measurement of GFR is the best method of assessing the amount of functioning renal tissue. Bearing in mind that the excretion of any substance found in both urine and blood can be expressed as a clearance; it follows that a substances clearance which is equal to GFR must fulfill certain requirements. These are:

1. The concentration of the substance in glomerular fitrate must be identical to that in plasma, i.e. the substance is freely filtered
2. It must not be secreted by the tubules
3. It must neither be reabsorped by the tubules nor leak through them.

If these requirements are met, it follows that filtrate rate and excretion rate must be identical. Since the filtration rate of any freely filtered substance is equal to the GFR multiplied by its plasma concentration (P), and the excretion rate is expressed by urinary concentration (U) multiplied by urine flow (V) it follows that:

$$GFR \times P = U \times V$$

(where P = plasma concentration, U = urinary concentration and V = urinary volume/minute) dividing both sides by P:

$$GFR = \frac{U \times V}{P}$$

Endogenous substances such as creatinine have been used to measure GFR by clearance method. Creatinine clearance gives a somewhat overestimated GFR, due to some secretion of creatinine by the proximal tubule and is also dependent on a reliable 24-hour urine collection which is frequently difficult to obtain in children. In recent years exogenous substances such as chromium-51-labelled EDTA, have been used for measuring clearance without urine collection. This method involves analysis of the rate of disappearance of the chemical from the plasma.

Testing the kidney's ability to concentrate the urine is the simplest means of assessing tubular function. The most reliable clinical measure of concentration is given by the osmometer which measures the freezing point of urine with great accuracy. For a normal child, a simple concentration test involving no fluids for at least 12 hours, usually overnight, and eating meals without liquids, followed by the testing of an early morning urine sample (having previously emptied a full bladder if necessary), will produce a urine with a specific gravity of 1.025 or an osmolality of greater that 800 mosmol/kg water.

Tests of urinary acidification will reveal the two main causes for acidosis accompanying renal disease, which may be either an inability to excrete hydrogen ions due to reduced ammonia production (distal or type 1 renal tubular acidosis) or, the inefficient reabsorption of bicarbonate ions by the proximal tubule (type 2 renal tubular acidosis). However a random urine of pH of 5.5 or less suggests a normal ability to acidify urine.

URINARY TRACT INFECTION

Pathogenesis

The sequelae or urinary tract infection (UTI) in childhood are more serious than those in the adult. It is now well recognised that there is impairment of renal growth and renal scarring in children where infections are associated with vesicoureteric reflux. The scarring is seen at the site of intrarenal reflux, that is, where urine is extravasated into renal tissue by the back pressure of urine applied to the renal pelvis during micturition. Vesicoureteric reflux is found in 30–50 per cent of children with UTI, irrespective of whether they are symptomatic and attending hospital, or asymptomatic and attending hospital, or asymptomatic and are found on school survey. It is, therefore, likely that reflux may cause renal damage in association with the ascent of organisms into the kidney, the presence of residual urine acting as a culture medium and the damage associated with back pressure. Apart from these situations, UTI in the absence of pyelonephritis is probably benign.

The presentation of UTI is variable but with increasing age the symptoms are similar to those in the adult (Table 15.1). In nearly 50 per cent of children there is a history suggestive of urinary symptoms in the first year of life with dysuria, frequency and haematuria becoming common presenting features from the age of 2. Loin pain is uncommon in the very young even when renal parenchymal infection exists. Some children present with acute abdominal pain and vomiting, and appendicitis may be suspected.

The male and female ratio in the newborn is 2.5 to 1, whereas, in older children UTI is 20 times more common in girls than boys. This female preponderance is usually attributed to the short urethra in the female. Bacterial invasion of the bladder is facilitated by periurethral colonisation with faecal oragnisms, local irritation from threadworms and from chemicals such as chlorine in

Table 15.1 Presentation of urinary tract infections in infancy and childhood (adapted from Smellie 1979)

Symptoms	Age				
	0–1 month	1 month to 2 years	2–5 years	5–12 years	Total
	N = 45	N = 45	N = 44	N = 66	N = 200
Failure to thrive					
Feeding problem	24	16	3		43
Screaming attacks					
Irritability					
Diarrhoea					
Vomiting	16	30		2	48
Fever	5	17	25	33	80
Convulsions	1	3	4	3	11
Haematuria		3	7	4	14
Frequency and dysuria		2			44
Abdominal or loin pain			10	37	47

swimming baths and surface tension lowering agents such as bubble bath. Recent surveys, in normal school girls, have shown that 1–2 per cent have a urinary infection at any one time and that around one-half of these children have abnormalities on radiological examination. Up to 20 per cent of girls with UTI will have scarred kidneys by the age of 5 but the incidence of scarring does not seem to increase much thereafter.

Diagnosis

The key to the diagnosis of UTI is the microscopic and bacteriological examination of the urine. The concept of significant bacteriuria continues to be frequently misunderstood; provided the urine is properly collected, bacteria colonising the urinary tract will tend to be present in numbers of more that 10^5 organisms/ml whereas contaminants entering the urine during voiding will rarely exceed 10^3 organisms/ml. Urine microscopy is useful for early diagnosis of bacteriuria with one bacterium per high power field corresponding to 5×10^4–10^5 bacteria/ml when uncentrifuged urine is examined.

obtained midstream urine specimens in hospital has made an enormous contribution to the management of UTI in children. The method can be used at all ages, remembering that the preputial folds of non-circumcised boys contain large numbers of bacteria, especially Proteus species, even after cleaning and must be irrigated before a urine culture is taken. Clean catch urine samples can be collected from small babies, and avoid the need for unreliable bag specimens. The mother should be taught how to collect the specimen into a sterile dish, usually about one hour after the feed whilst the nappy is still dry, and to inoculate both sides of the dip slide immediately (Fig. 15.1). In older children the dip slide may be held in an established stream of urine in order to wet it sufficiently. False-positive cultures and unnecessary investigation are therefore avoided. Bladder catheterisation and suprapubic urine aspiration need only be undertaken in an emergency or when equivocal results have been obtained on dip-slide culture.

Bacterial multiplication starts rapidly in vitro and after 24 hours at room temperature urines have similar bacterial numbers irrespective of the

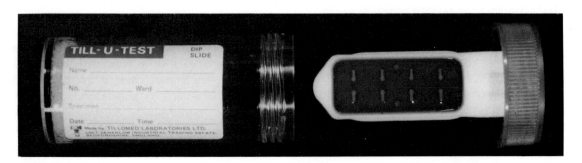

Fig. 15.1 The dip slide

The examination of the urine for pus cells alone is of little value in the diagnosis; 90 per cent of patients with symptomless UTI show an increased number of pus cells in the urine, but only around one-third to one-half of patients with overt infection have an increased whiet cell excretion.

Accurate diagnosis requires careful attention to the method of collection and storage of urine and whether or not antibiotic treatment has been commenced at the time of sampling. The demonstration that dip-slide cultures, inoculated during voiding in the home, are as reliable as carefully

number present at voiding. It is essential, therefore, if midstream samples are to be stored before transportation that they should be dept cold from the moment of voiding. At 0–4°C the bacterial count remains unchanged for at least 48 hours.

Management

The management of UTI is based on the confirmation of infection in at least one urine sample, unless the child is clinically ill. Antibiotics are given, usually for 2 weeks, after which an intravenous urogram (IVU) should be arranged. If this is completely normal with no evidence or ureteric dilation the child should be followed for 2 years with regular measurements of blood pressure and examination of urine samples. As a preliminary investigation, ultrasound of the renal tract is useful and may provide helpful infoemation if undertaken at intervals as part of a follow-up programe. If further infections occur a micturating cystourethrogram (MCUG) is necessary. If reflux is present, usually grade I or II, prophylactic antibiotics, low-dose co-trimaxazole (Septrin) or nitrofurantoin (Furadantin), are prescribed and follow-up is continued for a further 2 years. This regimen is associated with a reduced emergence of resistant strains of bacteria. At the end of this period, a limited IVU and MCUG should be repeated and, if normal, the child discharged. Recurrent infections during prophylaxis suggest the need to assess renal growth frequently and to consider surgical reimplantation of the ureter if the infection cannot be controlled and scarring develops. If the initial IVU is abnormal, a MCUG is carried out immediately. Grade III reflux in a child under one year, and grade III or IV in older children, are indications for surgery (Fig. 15.2).

The natural history of UTI is poorly understood but there is evidence to suggest that in the absence of any structural abnormality the effect of treatment is negligible. Diligent management can, however, prevent the development of renal scarring in children with vesicoureteric reflux and recurrent infections.

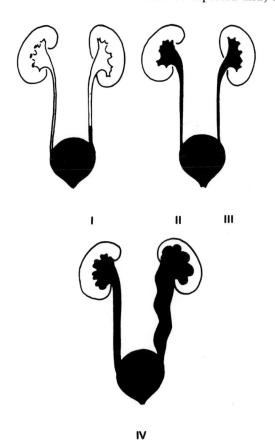

Fig. 15.2 Grades of reflux: grade I — reflux into lower end of ureter without dilatation; grade II — reflux entering up to kidney on micturition only; grade III — reflux entering up to kidney both during bladder filling and during voiding; grade IV — reflux with dilatation of ureter or renal pelvis

ENURESIS
(See also Chapter 11)

Pathogenesis

Children acquire full bladder control at different ages and most children with a continence problem are enuretic rather than incontinent. The majority of children are dry during the daytime by the age of 3 years and dry at night by 4. Ten per cent of 5-year olds wet the bed, as do 5 per cent of 10-year olds. Nocturnal enuresis is more common than diurnal enuresis and occurs in any phase of sleep, except rapid eye movement sleep. Enuresis is classified as primary when the child has never been dry at night, but is usually dry during the day. Secondary enuresis is less common and occurs after a period of nocturnal continence and is frequently associated with emotional disturbances. Children with enuresis are probably all psychiatrically normal although emotional problems may well develop in severe, long-standing cases. Stress is more likely to influence enuresis in the 3 and 4-year olds and emotional or behavioural disturbance is more common in girls and children with diurnal enuresis. There is a strong familial association in nocturnal enuresis, if a parent was enuretic there is a 40 per cent chance of the child being enuretic, and if a sibling is enuretic the child has a 25 per cent chance of having the same problem. Enuresis is more frequently encountered in social classes IV and V. Decreased functional, rather than structural bladder capacity is associated with enuresis, and when the child becomes continent this is associated with an increase in functional capacity.

Management

The basis for successful management requires knowledge of the family and social history development milestones, and details of toilet training. Physical examination must include palpation of the abdomen which may reveal abnormalities of the kidneys or bladder, or evidence of constipation. Examination of the spine for evidence of spina bifida occulta or diastematomyelia, neurological examination to include gait and reflexes, and examination to exclude muscle wasting are also essential. The blood pressure should be recorded and urinalysis undertaken to exclude infection, as up to 10 per cent of children with a continence problem have UTI. When neurological and urinary tract disease have been excluded, a plan of treatment should be embarked upon, having explained carefully to the parents that the child is normal and that the problem is one of an inappropriate physiological reflex. Parental support is essential and a positive rather than a punitive attitude is required. Simple practical measures such as cutting down evening fluids, and encouraging voiding when awakened, can be effective particularly when combined with a reward system such as the star charts. Around one-third of children will become dry with these measures, however, the problem must be regularly reviewed and if there is no improvement after 3 months an enuresis alarm can be tried. If used properly the bell or buzzer alarm can l be used to cure up to 80 per cent of children, and with relapsers dryness is achieved faster. Success will be more rapidly achieved if the principle of the alarm is carefully explained to the child and parents and should only be used if the child has his own bed. The child must get up after the alarm has rung and empty his bladder even if he has wet the bed. The alarm should be used until there has been a run of dry nights for one month.

The tricyclic antedepressant, imipramine, can be used and has been found to be more effective than placebo. A dose of 25 mg is used initially and any benefit should be noticed within 3–4 weeks although increments in dosage may be necessary in individual cases. If there is no improvement after 2 months the drug should be discontinued. The parents must be warned to keep the drug locked away because overdose can be fatal for a young child.

Diurnal enuresis, usually associated with nocturnal enuresis is less common and more difficult to manage than nocturnal enuresis alone. The functional bladder capacity is even smaller, so frequency and urgency are commonly encountered. On urodynamic investigations many of these children are found to have unstable bladder contractions. Treatment is as for nocturnal enuresis with more emphasis on interval bladder training. The use of anticholinergic drugs is indicated in certain cases and may decrease the frequency of unstable contractions and increase bladder capacity.

Incontinence

Incontinence is the inappropriate voiding of urine as a result of neurological or urinary tract disease. It is important to diagnose surgically correctable abnormalities such as posterior urethral valves, ectopic ureters and meatal stenosis. A micturition history should suggest such an abnormality and the appropriate radiological investigation undertaken. Mental subnormality is associated with incontinence, the pattern of bladder activity being appropriate to the child's mental age. Neuropathic bladder, such as that associated with spina bifida, is a rare condition in childhood but, because of the serious implications, the diagnosis must be made early and the long-term problems and surveillance of these children managed jointly between hospital and general practitioner.

HAEMATURIA

With the introduction of the dip stick test the detection of blood in the urine has become very easy; although it needs to be confirmed microscopically. Establishing the cause of haematuria and its clinical significance is not so easy; Table 15.2 lists some causes of haematuria in children. How does the clinician approach the diagnostic

Table 15.2 Classification of haematuria in infants and children

Glomerular causes
Acute glomerulonephritis
Other types of glomerulonephritis
(membranous, membranoproliferative)
Henoch-Schönlein nephritis
Systemic lupus erythematosus
Haemolytic uraemic syndrome
Recurrent haematuria syndromes
(Alport's syndrome, IgA (Berger's) disease)

Non-glomerular causes
Infections of the urinary tract
(acute pyelonephritis, tuberculosis)
Renal trauma
   direct
   indirect (shock or hypoxaemia, especially in the neonate)
Renal stones
Foreign bodies (urethral) and penile excoriation such as a meatal ulcer after circumcision
Urological malformations (obstructive uropathy)
Cysts and tumours (polycystic disease, Wilms' tumour, leukaemia)
Haematological disorders (haemophilia, sickle cell disease)
Drugs

---

problem of the child with blood in his urine? Inquiry may elicit a history of previous macroscopic haematuria, suggesting recovering acute nephritis, a pedigree of a familial nephritis or whether the haematuria is associated with other symptoms. Physical examination must include the genitalia and abdomen and a search for oedema. Urine microscopy is needed to confirm erythrocyturia and the finding of casts suggests a renal cause. Bacteriuria and pyuria indicate infection and the need for urine culture. Proteinuria (1+ or more by dip stick) should be quantified by timed collection and renal function estimated from the serum creatinine. If these tests are normal the child and his parents should be reassured and an annual urine check and measurement of blood pressure are all that is required. If macroscopic haematuria or proteinuria develop this will demand further assessment. Urography should be undertaken sparingly and mainly in children with symptoms in addition to haematuria. Ultrasound is an invaluable and non-invasive first-line investigation. There is hardly ever an indication for cystoscopy.

The child with glomerular disease is likely to present with an acute nephritic syndrome, nephrotic syndrome, haematuria and/or proteinuria, or acute or chronic renal failure. Unfortu-

nately, the mode of presentation does not enable renal pathology to be predicted and the prognosis appears to be more closely related to the histological classification than to the clinical syndrome.

The ability to study glomerular disease whilst it is still evolving and the rationalisation of treatment have been simplified by undertaking a renal biopsy. Careful selection of cases, and undertaking the procedure under controlled conditions has made the technique relatively safe and it causes only minor discomfort.

ACUTE POST-STREPTOCOCCAL GLOMERULONEPHRITIS

In epidemic years acute post-streptococcal glomerulonephritis is the most common cause of haematuria in children, and is probably the most common cause of haematuria resulting from immunological injury. It is a disease with a characteristic clinical pattern, although it may present with varying degrees of clinical severity. It is generally thought to be a benign disease in children in contrast to other types of glomerulonephritis.

The disease usually follows 7–14 days after group A, beta-haemolytic streptococcal infection. In most cases the preceding infection is localised to the upper respiratory tract, but in some cases it may follow a streptococcal skin infection. Acute glomerulonephritis occurs most commonly between the ages of 3 and 7 years and is considered rare in children under the age of 2 years. The typical syndrome comprises sudden onset of oliguria, haematuria, proteinuria, reduced glomerular filtration rate, oedema and hypertension. The disease, however, may be mild and be manifest by the presence of haematuria only. A positive throat culture for the organism is found in only 15 per cent of cases. The anti-streptolysin O titre which rises within the first 3 weeks of the disease can be detected in more than 80 per cent of patients, similarly the third component of serum complement (C3) is markedly reduced in up to 90 per cent of cases. These markers usually return to normal within 3 months, however, the haematuria may persist for more than one year.

When the only manifestation is haematuria, all other possible causes must be excluded. A 10-day course of a suitable antibiotic, usually penicillin, is given to eradicate streptococcal infection. If there is evidence of fluid overload, oliguria, or a raised blood pressure, the child should be admitted to hospital. The salt and water retention are responsible for the hypertension which can be life threatening and associated with pulmonary oedema, hypertensive encephalopathy and cerebral haemorrhage. Long-term bed rest is not useful and does not affect the eventual outcome. Some exacerbation of haematuria after exercise or during an upper respiratory tract infection is sometimes seen during the healing phase and can be disregarded as long as it is not associated with a deterioration of renal function.

HENOCH-SCHONLEIN NEPHRITIS

Approximately 30 per cent of children with Henoch-Schonlein purpura develop a nephritis. The clinical picture may vary from haematuria with proteinuria to renal failure. Typically the rash is present to make the diagnosis. Only a small proportion of affected children (20 per cent) develop chronic glomerulonephritis and perhaps 5 per cent of these may reach terminal renal failure within one or 2 years after the onset of the disease. In the remainder, the haematuria and proteinuria slowly disappear though this may take several years and exacerbations of haematuria during intermittent infections are common and need not cause concern. The overall prognosis is uncertain, but a 10-year survival of around 95 per cent is likely. The follow-up should continue until all renal abnormalities have disappeared. Those children with persistent manifestations appear to be particularly at risk and the prognosis is worse for those with acute nephritis or nephrotic syndrome than with haematruia or proteinuria alone.

NEPHROTIC SYNDROME

Physiology

The nephrotic syndrome consists of a disturbance of glomerular permeability resulting in albuminuria, hypoalbuminaemia and oedema. Hypoalbuminaemia reduces the plasma colloid osmotic pressure resulting in a seepage of fluid from the intravascular to the intestitial compartment resulting in oedema. The critical plasma albumin concentration is 25 g/l. The loss of fluid from the intravascular compartment results in hypovolaemia and, as it is the plasma volume that is depleted, there is a rise in haemoglobin concentration and packed cell volume. The fall in blood volume leads to poor renal perfusion, and hypovolaemia, if prolonged, may progress to peripheral circulatory collapse, renal failure and death.

In childhood the majority of cases respond to corticosteroid therapy and have only minimal histological changes in the glomeruli evident on light microscopy. The term 'minimal change nephrotic syndrome' has gained popular usage although the expression 'steroid responsive nephrotic syndrome' has the merit of focussing on the most important objective. The condition occurs with a frequency of about one case per 100 000 total population per annum and is more common in boys than girls. The peak age is 3 years and it rarely presents under the age of 3 months but can occur throughout adult life. About 15 per cent of children with nephrotic syndrome will have a more serious lesion such as focal sclerosis or membranoproliferative disease. A number of clinical and laboratory characteristics may be associated with minimal changes nephrotic syndrome and are therefore viewed as favourable prognostic signs (Table 15.3). Relapses are often precipitated by upper respiratory tract infections.

Table 15.3 Features of 'minimal change nephrotic syndrome'

Age at presentation (between 1–14 years)
No haematuria
Normal blood pressure and renal function
Highly selective heavy proteinuria (i.e. albumin)
Early response to corticosteroid therapy
Normal serum complement (C3) concentration

Management

Hypovolaemia

A hypovolaemic crisis is characterised by vomiting, abdominal pain, faintness and signs of peripheral circulatory failure, and may occur early in relapse even before much oedema is clinically evident. It is a medical emergency and the child should be hospitalised and given a rapid intravenous infusion of plasma.

Diet

An adequate protein intake is necessary to compensate for urinary losses of albumin. The protein intake of a child on an ordinary western diet is probably adequate. Rigorous dietary sodium restriction is usually impractical and unnecessary in children, although excess dietary salt and high sodium-containing foods should be avoided.

Infection

The nephrotic child is prone to infection and, historically, the major reduction in mortality in the syndrome followed the introduction of penicillin rather than corticosteroids. Septicaemia due to Gram-negative or gram-positive organisms and primary peritonitis due to *Streptococcus pneumoniae* should be suspected in every sick nephrotic, and there is much to be said for penicillin prophylaxis against pneumoccal infection in the oedematous child.

Corticosteroids

Prednisolone is the corticosteroid of choice and, for the induction of remission, a high dose of 2 mg/kg body weight every 24 hours should be given until response, i.e. freedom from proteinuria (Albustix 0 or trace) for 2 days, followed by stepwise withdrawal over a 6-week period. The same regimen should be used for the treatment of relapse. Common errors in corticosteroid therapy are to use too low a dose, to start reducing dosage before remission has been achieved and to interpret response in terms of control of oedema rather than elimination of proteinuria.

Most steroid responsive nephrotics will go into remission within 2 weeks of therapy. Two-thirds of the responders will relapse and for the first two or three relapses the objective should be to tail off corticosteroids completely. The frequent relapser, three within 12 months, is considered steroid dependent and can be satisfactorily maintained on alternate day prednisolone therapy. Up to 0.5 mg/kg body weight on alternate days as a single morning dose can be used without much toxicity, and even higher doses are possible in younger children. This regimen should be continued for at least 6 months and, if the child has been relapse-free, the dosage reduced to see if it is still necessary. Careful growth records must be maintained so that if further maintainance therapy is required the risks can be accurately assessed. The side effects of corticosteroid therapy are well known (Table 15.4) but can be minimised with careful supervision.

Table 15.4 Side-effects of corticosteroid therapy

Growth retardation (less with alternate day therapy)
Susceptibility to infection
Hypertension and oedema
Cushingoid features (obseity and striae)
Osteoporosis
Increased protein catabolism (associated with increased appetite)
Diabetes mellitus
Gastrointestinal complications
   perforation
   haematemesis
   pancreatitis
Intracranial hypertension (during steroid withdrawal)
Addisonian crisis

Immunosupressive drugs such as cyclophosphamide, have been established as valuable therapy in the frequently relapsing nephrotic child who has become steroid dependent and in some cases steroid resistant. However, the potential toxity of these agents is always worrying and it is generally agreed that if a nephrotic can be maintained in remission on a corticosteroid regimen that does not cause significant side effects, then cyclophosphamide therapy is not warranted. In the long run most children stop relapsing, though a few persist beyond adolescence, and the prognosis of the steroid responsive nephrotic child is fundamentally good.

HYPERTENSION

There has been an increasing interest in, and awareness of, systemic hypertension as a problem of childhood and adolescence. Too frequently blood pressure is measured in a hasty, casual

Table 15.5 Blood pressure measurements in normal children

Age (years)	Mean (mmHg)		95th percentile (mmHg)	
	Systolic	Diastolic	Systolic	Diastolic
0–0.5	80	45	110	60
0.5–3	95	55	115	80
4–7	100	65	120	85
8–10	105	70	130	90
11–15	115	70	140	90

fashion without attention to detail, the greatest errors occuring in young infants and obese children. Blood pressure should be determined with the child lying or sitting on the mother's lap and relaxed. It is of little value if the child is crying. As a rule of thumb, a cuff containing a bladder that will cover two-thirds of the upper arm without impinging on the antecubital fossa should be used. The bladder should encircle as close to the full circumference of the arm as possible. Normal ranges for blood pressure are shown in (Table 15.5) and it remains controversial at what level hypertension should be diagnosed. It is clear, however, that a single hypertensive should be rechecked and a pattern is consistently above the normal range the child should be investigated to exclude treatable causes. Elevated blood pressures are uncommon in childhood. A careful family history for evidence of hypertension or cardiovas-

cular disease should be taken, particularly in those who are asymptomatic. Hypertension may also be secondary and it is important to exclude other disorders such as renal disease (Table 15.6).

The most frequent symptoms include headaches, nausea, vomiting and anorexia, heart failure, convulsions and other central nervous system signs such as facial palsy or hemiplegia. Renal parenchymal disease accounts for nearly 80 per cent of sustained hypertension in children, and approximately 10 per cent of this group will have a renovascular basis. Appropriate urography, ultrasound and isotope scanning, and arteriography may reveal the pathology, but the majority of children with chronic hypertension will not have a surgically correctable cause. This group are therefore committed to long-term drug therapy with the associated problems of compliance adherence to dietary restrictions and regular clinic attendance for evaluation. Traditionally, the management of mild hypertension consists of using a diuretic, thiazide or frusemide, adding a beta-blocking agent such as propranolol, and a peripheral vasodilator such as hydrallazine or monoxidil in the refractory or more severe cases. Children who present with a hypertensive emergency may not only demonstrate a severe elevation of blood pressure, but also acute complications such as pulmonary oedema, hypertensive encephalopathy and renal failure. These patients require immediate control and maintenance of blood pressure to normal levels and in addition therapy for each complication.

Table 15.6 Aetiology of hypertension

Renovascular	Renal artery stenosis
Parenchymal renal disease	Nephritis, reflux nephropathy, obstructive uropathy, tumours, cystic disease, dysplasia, chronic renal failure
Cardiovascular	Coarctation of the aorta
Endocrine	Adrenal cortex; congenital adrenal hyperplasia, Cushing's syndrome Adrenal medulla; phaeochromocytoma, neuroblastoma Hyperthyroidism
Metabolic	Heavy metal poisoning, hypercalcaemia salt and water overload
CNS	Raised intracranial pressure, Guillin-Barré syndrome
Essential	

ACUTE RENAL FAILURE

Acute renal failure (ARF) is a syndrome characterised by sudden disruption of glomerular and tubular function. It may be transient, prolonged, reversible or irreversible. The kidneys are unable to regulate urine flow and composition as manifested by disturbances of fluid, electrolyte and acid-base balance, together with failure of elimination of the products of nitrogen metabolism. Essential for normal renal function are an adequate blood supply of healthy kidneys and a patent functioning non-obstructed urine collection and excretion system. Oliguria exists when the daily urinary output is less than 300 ml/m^2 surface area. Classically ARF is divided into prerenal, renal and postrenal causes, aetiological factors in each of these areas being womewhat dependent on the age of the child (Table 15.7), ARF is recognised by a rising blood urea and creatinine concentration.

Table 15.7 Causes of acute renal failure in infancy and childhood

Prerenal
Hypovolaemia
   acute gastroenteritis
   nephrotic syndrome
   post surgery
   burns
   salt wasting disease (renal and adrenal)

Hypotension
   septicaemia
   hypothermia

Renal
Acute glomerulonephritis
Renal venous thrombosis
Haemolytic uraemic syndrome
Congenital glomerular and tubular disease
Nephrotoxins

Postrenal
Congenital obstructive uropathy

The history and physical examination will frequently indicate the diagnosis. A history of vomiting and diarrhoea suggest salt and water depletion, and hypernatraemic dehydration is common in infants with gastroenteritis who have received high solute feeds. A poor urine stream in young infants suggests urethral valves and obstructive uropathy. A palpable bladder and enlarged kidneys indicate intravesical obstruction. Bilateral gross enlargement of the kidneys is suggestive of polycystic disease and, in acute onset of renal failure, haematuria and enlarged hard kidneys may be caused by renal venous thrombosis. The history and clinical features may be helpful in the diagnosis of nephritis, nephrotic syndrome or haemolytic uraemic syndrome. Short stature, anaemia and evidence of renal osteodystrophy are suggestive of chronic renal disease.

The management of ARF in the child, especially the infant, is different from that in the adult. Treatment and diagnosis proceed concurrently. Detailed knowledge of fluid and electrolyte balance, and the nutritional requirements of the infant are necessary, as is access to the complex technology for specific investigation. The specific and frequently life-threatening problems of hyperkalaemia, hypoglycaemia, hypocalcaemia, acidosis and hypertension each require individual assessment and treatment.

CHRONIC RENAL FAILURE

Chronic renal failure is the outcome of many disease processes but, in children, it is predominantly secondary to chronic glomerulonephritis or pyelonephritis (reflux nephropathy). Therapy for chronic renal failure may basically be divided into medical management, and dialysis and transplantation. Careful management of the uraemic child (Table 15.8) before dialysis or transplantation not only improves survival and prevents acute deterioration which can cause further renal failure damage, but also can ensure that affected children lead relatively normal lives. Frequent outpatient monitoring is essential and careful attention must be directed at each of the items shown in Table 15.8. It is essential to maintain close liaison with personnel such as paediatric dietician and pathologist so that appropriate action can be taken in the

Table 15.8 Potential problems in chronic renal failure

Biochemical disturbances
Sodium, potassium, calcium, phospate and acidaemia
Nutrition
Plasma proteins and urea production
Infection
Urinary tract and non-renal infections
Renal osteodystrophy
Hypertension
Anaemia
Growth and skeletal maturation
Social development
Schooling and family relationships
Emotional development

management of individual problems as they occur. It is therefore understandable that the management of children with end-stage kidney disease should be carried out in specialist paediatric nephrology units. The results of dialysis and transplantation to date, undoubtedly justify considering treatment for all children. Each case must be assessed carefully by a paediatrician and the paediatric nephrology team, not forgetting the considerable stress and discipline that will face the patient and family.

FURTHER READING

Chantler C 1979 The kidney. In: Godfrey S & Baum D Ch. 10 (eds) Clinical paediatric physiology
Edleman C M (ed) 1978 Paediatric kidney disease
Smellie J M 1979 In: Black & Jones (eds) Renal disease, 4th edn. Blackwell Scientific Publishers, Oxford

16

Gynaecological disorders

The gynaecological diseases which affect children reflect the endocrine background of the particular age-period. In utero a girl's genital organs are stimulated by hormones which have passed across the placenta from the mother and the appearance of the genitalia reflect this in a newborn baby. After this, disorders characteristic of oestrogen deficiency occur, until the changes of puberty appear and a girl begins to produce her own oestrogens. The special disorders of the adolescent are mainly abnormalities of menstruation. Tumours, fortunately rare in childhood, may occur at any time.

NORMAL SIGNS IN THE NEWBORN

During the first few weeks of life the passive hormone stimulation which the baby has from the mother gives rise to several physiological manifestations. Breast swelling is seen in many babies, male and female, born at term; left alone, as it should be, this swelling usually regresses quickly and only rarely does it persist for more than one month. Baby girls often show congestion and swelling of the vulva and there is sometimes a prominent hymen and a white discharge which can be plentiful (Fig. 16.1); rarely the discharge may be streaked with blood from breaking down endometrium which has also responded to maternal hormones. These changes, too, disappear quickly and call for no treatment. Hymenal tags are very common and disappear spontaneously (Fig 16.2).

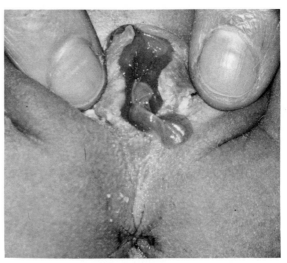

Fig. 16.2 Pronounced hymenal tag in a newborn child. This shrank and disappeared spontaneously (by permission of Marcel Dekker, New York)

VAGINAL CYSTS

Small cysts of the hymen or paraurethral glands are sometimes seen. They rarely need treatment

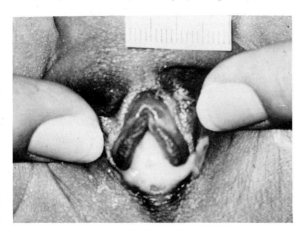

Fig. 16.1 Newborn child showing congestion and oedema of the vulva and profuse vaginal discharge (by permission of Marcel Dekker, New York)

and usually disappear spontaneously. However, one condition, hydrocolpos, is more important since it calls for early and correct treatment. It must be differentiated from a cyst.

Hydrocolpos

Hydrocolpos is an abnormality in which there is an imperforate membrane at the lower part of the vagina behind which a quantity of milky fluid collects as a result of the hormone stimulation mentioned above. The child may be fretful due to the collection of fluid and may be unable to pass urine since the bladder neck is blocked by the large swelling. Physical signs include a lower abdominal cystic swelling — the bladder perched on top of a pelvis full of fluid — and an imperforate membrane visible when the vulva is inspected (Fig.16.3). A rectal examination, made with a little finger, will indicate the cystic swelling anteriorly.

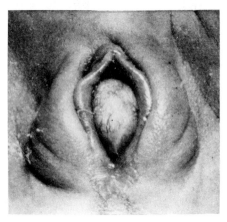

Fig. 16.3 Bulging membrane in a newborn child with hydrocolpos

If the diagnosis is correctly made, treatment is simple; the membrane is incised and the fluid released. It must be emphasised that the diagnosis is often made incorrectly and the abdomen may be opened with serious results.

INTERSEX

Doubt about the sex of the infant, although rare, is usually evident at birth and is discussed in Chapter 20.

VULVOVAGINITIS

After the first month or so of life the child's genital organs receive very little sex hormone stimulation and the disorders seen reflect this oestrogen lack. The most common condition is vulvovaginitis (Fig. 16.4). This arises because the vagina of the child has no protective acid secretion such as it has during the first few weeks of life and during the reproductive period.

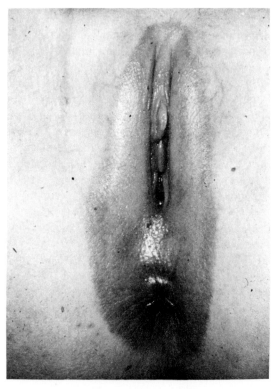

Fig. 16.4 Vulvovaginitis in a child (by permission of Marcel Dekker, New York)

Bacterial organisms which are easily introduced into the child's vagina may establish themselves and cause an infection. These are usually non-specific organisms of low virulence, but may be pyogenic perhaps affecting the child elsewhere such as the tonsils or the middle ear; gonococcal infection is seen occasionally. Swabs from just within the introitus can be obtained, without disturbing the child, and should be placed in appropriate transport medium and sent at once for bacteriological study. This may reveal a specific organism in which case the child may respond to an antibiotic to which that organism is susceptible. In many instances, however, there will be no specific bacteriological findings and treatment may be carried out by the application of a little oestrogen cream to the child's vulva each night for 1–2 weeks. This improves the acidity of the vagina and allows the infection to be overcome. Treatment should not be continued for more than 2 weeks or there may be too great an oestrogen absorption and general effects. An important part of management is to ensure that the vulva is not irritated by substances applied to it. Strong antiseptic materials must be avoided, nothing should be put in the bath water, the vulva should be carefully dried with a soft towel and perhaps a little bland cream applied. Daily bathing is essential. Other possible causes of vulvovaginitis include threadworm infestations, and these should always be looked for, or rarely, a foreign body in the vagina. In the latter instance, the discharge is usually blood-stained and foul smelling which should always call for careful investigation.

Not all children with vulvitis have a vaginal discharge as the cause. Some have a local skin disorder which may also be affecting other parts of the body. One lesion sometimes seen is lichen sclerosis, a vulval dystrophy in which whitish patches appear on the vulva skin and there is soreness and irritation which leads to scratching (Fig. 16.5). The condition can usually be kept under control by the hygienic measures described above or, if there is secondary infection following scratching, an antibiotic cream may be used. There is a strong tendency to improvement at puberty.

LABIAL ADHESIONS

This is also common in childhood. The labia minora adhere together in the midline leaving a tiny opening through which urine is passed. If the vulva is carefully inspected it will be seen to be flat and featureless and there is usually a vertical translucent area in the midline where the labia are joined (Fig. 16.6). This condition is often

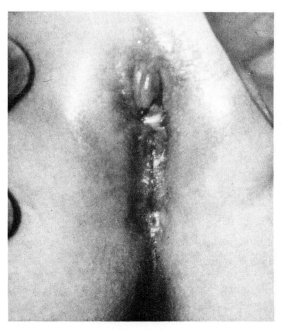

Fig. 16.6 Labial adhesions in a little girl

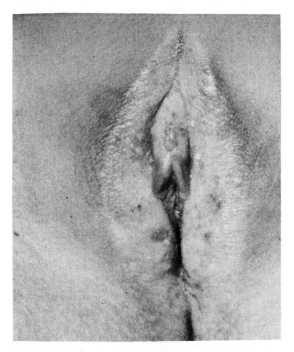

Fig. 16.5 Lichen sclerosis of the vulva in a little girl

mistaken for congenital absence of the vagina; it does not resemble this since here the vulva looks otherwise normal apart from the absence of the vaginal introitus. Once it is certain that the diagnosis is labial adhesions they often separate spontaneously if a little oestrogen cream is applied nightly to the vulva for 1–2 weeks. Alternatively, the adhesions may be broken down with a blunt probe, but this can cause discomfort. Referral for advice is wise.

VAGINAL BLEEDING

This may be serious and should never be ignored. Its causes include:
1. A vaginal foreign body
2. A malignant vaginal or cervical tumour
3. Precocious puberty (see Chapter 20)
4. A local vulval lesion such as a prolapsed urethra or scratching of lichen sclerosis.

In any of these conditions referral for investigation is indicated.

Around the time of puberty, girls may present with irregular or heavy menstrual periods, infrequent periods or dysmenorrhoea. Irregularity is common during early menstrual life and alone calls for no treatment. Given time, the periods nearly always become more regular as the condition has a very strong tendency to spontaneous cure. Hormones must be withheld and reassurance given; iron may be helpful to treat anaemia. If there is no significant improvement in 3–6 months referral to a special unit is indicated. Infrequent periods are relatively common at this time of life and the intervals between the periods diminish as time goes by. Should this not happen referral for further advice would again be indicated.

Painful periods

Dysmenorrhoea is often a difficult symptom to treat and it may reflect anxiety in the child's mother as much as anything else. It is usually wise to attempt to educate mother and daughter in the physiology of menstruation and to prescribe simple analgesics in the first instance; strong analgesia should be avoided if at all possible. If simple measures of this kind are not successful, the advice of a gynaecologist should be sought.

Amenorrhoea

Failure to menstruate is is not an uncommon cause

of concern and consultation. This symptom should never be considered in isolation, but always in association with the occurrence of the other signs of secondary sexual development. A normal girl in the UK may menstruate for the first time any time between the ages of 10 and 16. If a girl aged 15 is seen who has not menstruated, it may therefore be tempting to think that this is not abnormal; provided the other signs of secondary sexual development are progressing normally this is likely to be so, but if there are no signs of secondary sexual development then this requires further investigation. A clue to the likely cause of failure to menstruate may be obtained by considering the other signs of secondary sexual development. Thus, if secondary development other than menstruation is good it is likely that there is an anatomical cause such as congenital absence of the vagina or an imperforate vagina; if secondary sexual development is absent or very poor, it is likely that there is a hormonal cause for this and either the ovaries are incapable of function or the hypothalamus and pituitary are not stimulating them. If there are any heterosexual changes this is a serious situation demanding urgent investigation. The other conditions, with one exception, are not urgent, but referral for gynaecological advice would usually be wise. However, haematocolpos may present as an acute emergency.

This condition resembles hydrocolpos, except that the fluid accumulating in the vagina and pelvis is retained menstrual blood. The patient, who is likely to be about 15 or 16, will have good secondary sexual development, but will not have menstruated although she may well have experienced intermitted pelvic pain as the blood collects. When there is enough blood to fill the pelvis she may develop acute retention of urine. The physical signs will then show a lower abdominal cystic swelling, as in hydrocolpos, a tense bluish bulging membrane of the introitus and a cystic swelling felt anteriorly on rectal examination. The patient should be sent into hospital quickly so that the membrane may be incised and the fluid released.

FURTHER READING

Dewhurst J 1980 Practical pediatric and adolescent gynecology. Marcel Dekker, New York

17

Respiratory diseases

RESPIRATORY DISEASES

PULMONARY FUNCTION TESTS IN CHILDREN

It is possible to perform simple lung function tests in children from the age of 5 years. The tests, which require cooperation, consist primarily of lung volume measurements such as vital capacity, forced expiratory volume in one second, and peak expiratory flow rate (Fig. 17.1, Table 17.1). Flow-volume curves are useful in assessing small airway obstruction (Fig. 17.1). Pulmonary function testing in babies requires special complicated apparatus, usually only available in research departments.

The new technique of ventilation-perfusion lung scan is very useful in evaluating lung function at all ages of childhood. Radioactive Krypton (half-life 13 sec.) is inhaled and its lung distribution measured using a gamma camera; technitium-labelled microspheres are injected (half-life 6 hours) and become trapped in the pulmonary capillaries, thus outlining pulmonary perfusion. This technique can be used to assess outcome by serial measurement of lung ventilation-perfusion ratios after significant lung disease.

Arterial blood gases reflect the final pathway of

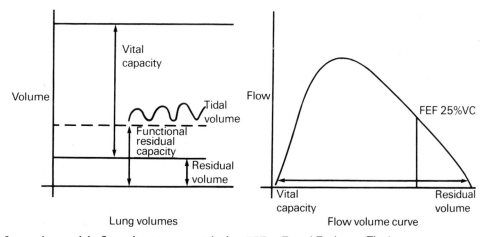

Fig. 17.1 Lung volume and the flow-volume curve on expiration (FEF = Forced Expiratory Flow)

Table 17.1 Respiratory function in children

Age	5 years	10 years	15 years
Vital capacity (ml)	1200	2200	3500
FEV$_1$ (ml)	1000	2000	3300
PEFR (l/min)	140	280	400

gas-exchange and can be measured at any age. Inspired oxygen concentration at the time of sampling must be noted. The most common sampling site is the radial artery, but the brachial and posterior tibial vessels can also be used. The femoral arteries should be avoided if at all possible. Capillary blood gas sampling gives reliable measurements for acid-base and carbon dioxide concentrations but not for oxygen. Transcutaneous oxygen sensors, properly calibrated, offer a useful means of serial assessment.

INFECTIONS

Respiratory tract infection in infants and children is extremely common; it is the most frequent reason for seeking medical advice in this age group. The majority of infections affect the upper respiratory tract; approximately 20 per cent cause significant symptoms in the lower tract. Pulmonary alveolar growth continues until the age of 8 years and severe infection before this age carries the potential for permanent disruption of lung development and later sequelae.

The epidemiology of respiratory tract infection in childhood is dependent on several factors including the virulence and dose of the organism, and host resistance. The host's resistance is related to age, degree of immunological development, previous experience of infection and stage of lung growth. These factors influence the environment in which the invading organism finds itself and thus its potential for causing disease. Certain physical factors are also important in determining the severity of infection; these include low birth weight, male sex, obesity, younger age groups, previous significant respiratory difficulties and the presence of congenital malformations. External environmental factors such as atmospheric pollution, parental smoking exposure to active infection and seasonal variation of disease incidence are also important. The clinical pattern of disease is related to the part of the respiratory tract most affected.

Upper Respiratory tract infection

Coryza (common cold)

This infection is relatively mild and is characterised by a mucoid nasal obstruction, sore throat and often cervical adenopathy. Fever may be present. Many different viruses are implicated in the aetiology, but the most common include rhinovirus, respiratory syncytial virus, influenza, parainfluenza and coxsackie virus. Management is symptomatic. Antibiotics are not indicated except where there is clear evidence of a secondary bacterial infection or a more serious underlying disease such as bronchiectasis or cystic fibrosis is present.

Acute infection of tonsils, adenoids and pharynx

Infection of the tonsils, adenoids and pharynx is common and occurs principally in the 3–8-year age group. It is characterised by fever, sore throat, malaise and occasionally vomiting. Examination of the throat reveals infection of the pharynx, peritonsillar area and the tonsils themselves. There is usually an associated enlargement of cervical lymph nodes. The tonsils are enlarged and inflamed with tiny haemorrhages and exudate. The surrounding inflammation of pharynx and adenoids frequently leads to cough and nasal obstruction.

A virus is the aetiological agent in approximately 90 per cent of cases; the most frequent isolates include respiratory syncytial virus, influenza, parainfluenza, coxsackie, echo and adenovirus. The most prominent bacterial pathogen is the group A beta-haemolytic streptococcus. Infectious mononucleosis may also present with florid tonsillitis while Corynebacterium diphtheriae, although rare, should not be forgotten, particularly if there is a prominent exudate.

Tonsillitis may occasionally be epidemic, particularly in closed communities with outbreaks of streptococcal infection or pharyngo-conjunctival fever due to adenovirus.

Treatment consists of an adequate fluid intake and symptomatic measures such as the control of fever and sore throat. Penicillin should be given 6-hourly, for 10 days, when a streptococcal infection is suspected. If the patient is vomiting or otherwise unlikely to take the drug, intramuscular long-acting penicillin is useful. Erythromycin is a suitable alternative to penicillin if there is a history of penicillin allergy.

Complications of bacterial infection are fortunately rare, largely because of the widespread use of antibiotics. Immediate problems include peritonsillar or pharyngeal abscess and acute cervical adenitis. In peritonsillar or pharyngeal abscess there may be marked dysphagia and obvious displacement of tissues on examination. A retro-pharyngeal abscess may be seen on a lateral neck X-ray. The neck may be held extended in order to facilitate breathing through the partially-obstructed airway. Cervical adenitis may occur in association with acute tonsillitis and occasionally leads to abscess formation. Treatment of these problems includes the appropriate antibiotic in large doses, and occasionally surgical drainage.

Late complications of streptococcal infections include rheumatic fever and acute glomerulonephritis. The liberal use of penicillin has probably resulted in a significant reduction of these diseases.

Chronic or recurrent infection of tonsils and adenoids

Recurrent and frequent infection of the tonsils and adenoids is common in young children. A significant increase in incidence is seen on starting play-school or nursery, followed then by a natural decrease to the adult frequency at the age of 7–8 years. With this pattern of illness in mind relatively few children should require adenotonsillectomy in their early years, and the current decrease in the popularity of this operation should continue (see Table 17.2). It is probable that less than one child in 25 in the general population needs

Table 17.2 Indications for and against tonsillectomy and adenoidectomy

For
Adenoidectomy
  Persistent nasal obstruction due to large adenoids
  Recurrent otitis media if large adenoids are thought to block the lower end of the Eustachian tube
Adenotonsillectomy
  Sleep apnoea syndrome
Tonsillectomy
  Recurrent cervical adenitits or peritonsillar abscess because the tonsils are an ineffective barrier against repeated
  Pharyngeal infection
  Recurrent tonsillitis, significantly affecting growth and weight gain
  Suspected tonsillar tumour
Against
Parental pressure on doctor
Large tonsils which cause no symptoms. Large tonsils are frequently wrongly assumed to be unhealthy. Parents should be reassured that lymphoid atrophy frequently reduces the size of the tonsils after about the eighth year
Short palate. Any child with a submucous or frankly cleft palate or bifid uvula should not have his adenoids removed because of the the risk of aggravating nasal speech due to pharyngopalatal incompetence

removal of tonsils and adenoids by the age of 8 years.

In a number of children removal of tonsils and adenoids is, however, of significant benefit; these include those who have frequent severe attacks, three to four a year, which cause significant systemic symptoms, general ill health and interfere with normal growth. In the younger age group, 1–3-years old, a small number of children have severe mechanical airway obstruction due to adeno-tonsillar hypertrophy; these children are chronic mouth breathers with persistent nasal obstruction and nasal discharge, they usually snore at night and may have difficulty sleeping due to recurrent obstruction with short periods of sleep apnoea. In some cases, cor pulmonale will develop due to pulmonary hypertension and right heart failure. Chronic infection may also contribute to recurrent middle ear problems and hearing difficulties. Adenotonsillectomy, in this group may produce a dramatic improvement in the child's general health, appetite and growth.

Otitis media

Otitis media or middle ear infection occurs as a result of an infecting organism travelling up the Eustachian tube, helped by forceful nose blowing or coughing. The commonest bacterial organisms include *Streptococcus pneumoniae*, *Haemophilus influenzae* and *Straphylococcus aureus*; viruses may also cause the disease.

Once an infection has been established, the mucosal lining of the middle ear produces an inflammatory exudate. If the Eustachian tube is blocked by the exudate or oedema, the exudate increases in volume, may become frankly purulent and may lead to pressure necrosis and perforation of the tympanic membrane, resulting in a discharge from the ear and subsequent relief of earache. With treatment, the exudate resorbs or drains through a patent Eustachian tube, so normal middle ear function is restored. If the exudate does not resolve, and becomes thick and gelatinous, a chronic secretory otitis, or glue ear, supervenes and there is interference with sound conduction (conductive deafness). Conditions which interfere with middle ear ventilation through the Eustachian tube, such as enlarged adenoids or vasomotor rhinitis may predispose to recurrent otitis.

Most children will have suffered an attack of otitis media by the age of 6 years. Older children may accurately describe symptoms of pain and deafness. Babies may present with fever and deafness, or non-specific symptoms such as, diarrhoea, vomiting, persistent crying or irritability. The ears of all fretful and febrile babies should always be examined. In early otitis, the edge of the drum may be reddened and there are commonly dilated vessels on the handle of the malleus. This effect can also be produced, to a lesser extent, by crying. The drum in addition is dull and loses its lustre. Later the drum becomes very red and the normal anatomical landmarks are no longer visible. The drum may subsequently bulge and perforate, in which case the external auditory canal will be full of debris and pus.

The management of acute otitis media:
1. Relief of pain with aspirin or paracetamol. These drugs will also reduce an associated fever.
2. All children with red tympanic membranes should receive a course of an appropriate antibiotic. *Haemophilus influenzae* is common in children under 5 years; ampicillin or amoxicillin is appropriate but if the child is allergic to penicillin, erythromycin or co-trimoxazole are also effective. In order children, penicillin is a better choice of drug because *Streptococcus pneumoniae* and *Strept. pyogenes* are the common pathogens. If the membrane has perforated a swab should be taken of the discharge and the antibiotic treatment changed according to the results of culture. Treatment should be continued for at least one week. Ear drops have no place in the treatment of acute otitis media.
3. The use of a decongestant given orally may help to restore Eustachian tube patency and function, and facilitate drainage.
4. Follow-up must continue until the doctor is satisfied that the infection has settled, that any drum perforation has healed and that hearing has returned to normal.

Complications of otitis media:
1. Glue ear with hearing loss
2. Chronic suppurative otitis media
3. Mastoiditis
4. Meningitis
5. Intracranial abscess
6. Lateral venous sinus thrombosis.

The occurence of complications other than glue ear are now much less common, largely due to the widespread use of effective antibiotics.

Glue ear

Glue ear is not uncommon and is due to the persistence of a gelatinous exudate in the middle ear. This condition is often undetected with important consequences to hearing and learning. It is characterised by a dull bluish discoloration of the tympanic membrane, which is often retracted and immobile. A fluid level may be seen behind the ear drum.

Evidence of transient hearing loss may occur in up to 30 per cent of children following acute otitis media. In the older child, a tuning fork may be used to determine whether bone conduction is greater than air conduction (Rinne's test), demonstrating a conductive hearing loss in the affected ear. Simple audiometry may be used to show a loss of hearing at various frequencies and below certain levels of intensity. The testing of hearing in younger children may need to be done by the use of the Stycar miniature toy method. (See chapter 3)

Treatment:
1. If a hearing loss is found, the administration of a decongestant may restore Eustachian tube function and result in medical drainage of the middle ear.
2. If after 6 months, hearing is still abnormal or gets worse despite treatment, then a myringotomy may be needed. The surgeon incises the tympanic membrane under direct magnification and sucks out the gelatinous glue from the middle ear.
3. Adenoidectomy may be done at the same time if it is thought that enlarged adenoids are causing obstruction to the lower end of the Eustachian tube.
4. The insertion of grommets into the myringotomy incision leaves a ventilation tube in situ which will allow re-aeration of the middle ear. The grommets extrude themselves after a few months and may sometimes be found lying in the external auditory meatus. While a child has grommets in place it is necessary that a close fitting protective

hat or earplugs are used if the child goes swimming. Diving should be prohibited as water may enter the middle ear.

Sinusitis

Acute infection of the sinuses is only seen in the older child as the maxillary and ethmoid sinuses remain relatively small and the frontal sinuses do not develop until the early school years. The sphenoidal sinus appears even later. Acute sinusitis is usually viral in origin and causes fever, pain, headache and nasal discharge; bacteria include *Streptococcus pneumoniae* and the group A beta-haemolytic streptococcus. Treatment is with penicillin for 10 days, but erythromycin is a useful alternative. Decongestants may also be useful. Chronically infected sinuses may need surgical drainage; the possibility of other diagnoses such as IgA deficiency, allergic rhinitis or cystic fibrosis should be considered.

Lower respiratory tract infection

Laryngotracheobronchitis (croup)

Larygotracheobronchitis, or croup, is due to an acute inflammation of the upper portion of the lower respiratory tract. Acute inflammation of the epiglottis is considered separately (see below). Laryngotracheobronchitis is most commonly viral and is frequently due to parainfluenza viruses; respiratory syncytial virus and rhinoviruses are also prominent pathogens.

Croup occurs mainly in late infancy and early childhood with a peak incidence between the ages of 6 months and 4 years. It presents with initial upper respiratory tract symptoms followed by the development of hoarseness and a barking croupy cough. Stridor commonly occurs and, if airway obstruction increases, indrawing of respiratory muscles is seen on inspiration. The rate of clinical progression is much more gradual, and the patient less toxic, than with epilottitis. Signs of significant airway obstruction require hospitalisation for close observation, and respiratory support including oxygen, and occasionally endo- or naso-tracheal intubation to bypass the obstruction may be needed. General care involves minimal handling, adequate fluid intake, added humidity and oxygen if necessary. Antibiotics are not specifically indicated unless additional bacterial pathology is suspected.

Epiglottitis

Acute epiglottitis is an extremely dangerous condition; it is seen in the age range 6 months to 6 years with a peak incidence in the second year of life. Infection with *Haemophilus influenzae* type B is the commonest cause; β-haemolytic streptococci cause only a few cases.

The patent presents with a rapid onset of toxicity, fever and sore throat; within a few hours there is respiratory obstruction, drooling of secretions at the mouth, and neck extension to ease the passage of air through the obstructed airway. Clinically, there is inspiratory stridor with indrawing of respiratory muscles and, as hypoxaemia and hypercapnia worsen, restlessness and cyanosis appear. Acute airway obstruction and respiratory arrest may occur at any time.

If epiglottitis is suspected no attempt should be made to visualise the throat and no instruments should be put into the mouth because of the risk of acute complete obstruction. The child should be taken immediately to hospital; visualisation of the epiglottis is then undertaken *only by an experienced person* who can intubate immediately or, if this fails, perform a tracheostomy to relieve obstruction. A lateral neck X–ray is not to be recommended unless the diagnosis is seriously in doubt, as the additional handling can precipitate total obstruction. In an acute emergency, the passage of a large-bore needle into the trachea below the cricoid cartilage may be life-saving. Supportive therapy includes the use of intravenous antibiotics (ampicillin or chloramphenicol for ampicillin-resistant Haemophilus organisms), fluid therapy and antipyretics. Once the obstruction is bypassed, oxygen is rarely needed.

Pertussis (whooping cough)

This is a potentially serious disease in infants and young children. Pertussis epidemics have now recurred because of the recent increase in unimmunised children in the community and it has been estimated that nearly three-quarters of those who are not protected are likely to contract the illness, with varying severity, before school age. Classical pertussis is due to infection with *Bordetella pertussis* although other organisisms such as adenovirus, *Bordetella parapertussis* and *Bordetella bronchiseptica* have been implicated in pertusis-like syndromes.

The incubation period is 10–14 days. The illness begins with a mild cough and mucoid nasal discharge which is followed by a spasmodic paroxysmal cough in the second week, this can result in cyanosis, vomiting and the production of small quantities of tenacious mucus. The cough typically lasts for several weeks and has been called the 100 day cough — its name in Chinese. It may recur again during a subsequent respiratory infection although generally in a milder form. Young infants tend to have a more severe course and may contract the illness before they are due to be immunised.

Complications include sub-conjunctival haemorrhage, bronchopneumonia and lobar or segmental lung collapse which can lead to respiratory failure in severe cases. A small but important mortality occurs in the order of 0.5–1 per 1000 cases.

Management is symptomatic. There is no efficient medication to stop the paroxysms. Erythromycin given to family contacts is effective in preventing spread of classical pertussis and reduces the length of time the patient is infectious, but does not otherwise modify the course of the illness.

Bronchiolitis

Bronchiolitis is an acute infection caused principally by respiratory syncytial virus, other viruses implicated include parainfluenza, influenza and adenovirus. It occurs commonly during the first 6 months of life but is seen throughout the first year. Seasonal epidemics occur with peak incidence in winter and early spring.

At the bronchiolar level there is a marked inflammatory response which leads to small airway obstruction with wheezing and hyperinflation. In more severe cases, there may be pneumonia with areas of lung collapse or consolidation. On examination the infant is tachypnoeic with coryzal signs, there is a low grade fever and obvious chest hyperinflation with inspiratory indrawing and expiratory wheeze. Widespread expiratory rhonchi are heard on auscultation and patchy crepitations are heard on inspiration. The liver is usually palpable below the costal margin secondary to hyperinflation, associated cardiac failure is rare. In severe cases, respiratory failure may supervene with cyanosis due to hypoxaemia and an elevated arterial carbon dioxide tension ($PaCO_2$) on blood gas analysis.

Management is supportive with humidified oxygen given if necessary. Humidity itself may be of symptomatic value but does not modify the course of the illenss. Adequate fluid intake is important but should not exceed daily requirements. Antibiotics are not indicated. Severe cases may require artificial ventilation.

Underlying conditions such as cystic fibrosis, recurrent aspiration and immunodeficiency should be considered in children with unusually severe bronchiolitis.

There remains considerable debate about the relationship of acute bronchiolitis to asthma. Up to 50 per cent of children with acute bronchiolitis may go on to have recurrent wheezing episodes typical of asthma. This is much more likely if there is a family history of atopic disease.

Pneumonia

Pneumonia is common at all ages but, particularly so, in infants and young children. The commonest pathogens in the younger age group are viral, such as respiratory syncytial virus, although the other respiratory viruses can also cause severe infection, especially adenovirus. In older children, viruses continue to be important but bacterial infection becomes increasingly common; *Streptococcus pneumoniae* is the predominant pathogen, although the incidence of *Mycoplasma pneumoniae* infection increases towards adolescence. Infection with other bacteria is rare but can be severe; these organisms include *Staphylococcus aureus*, β-*haemolytic streptococci* and *Haemophilus influenzae*. Gram-negative organisms such as *E. coli, Klebsiella* and *Pseudomonas aeruginosa* are only seen in debilitated children or those with underlying disorders such as immune deficiency or cystic fibrosis. *Pneumocystis carinii*, adenovirus, cytomegalovirus and measles can produce serious interstitial pneumonia in immunosuppressed children.

In the young child, the infection is bronchopneumonic with signs of fever, tachypnoea, dry cough and increased work of breathing. Auscultation of the chest may reveal areas of diminished air entry and creptitations over the affected lung. X-ray confirms widespread areas of patchy consolidation usually bilaterally.

In the older child, the infection is more lobar in type. Air entry is diminished over the affected area and crepitations are heard. Dullness to percussion and bronchial breathing occur when more complete consolidation is present. In severe cases, respiratory failure occurs and ultimately circulatory failure due to cor pulmonale with associated hypoxaemia and acidosis.

Management is supportive; skilled nursing care is important, in hospital if necessary. Daily fluid intake should be limited to 75 per cent of normal as inappropriate antidiuretic-hormone secretion can occur leading to cerebral oedema and even convulsions. Humidified oxygen is given via head box, oxygen tent or face mask. Arterial blood gases should be monitored.

Antibiotics are indicated whenever bacterial infection is suspected. Trap-sputum specimens or blood culture may help to identify the organism. Penicillin is the usual drug of choice with erythromycin as an alternative for the penicillin-sensitive patient. If there is a likelihood of staphylococcal infection, cloxacillin and possibly gentamicin may be required. Erythromycin is the treatment of choice for infections by mycoplasma. Antibiotics which are active against Gram-negative organisms may be particularly appropriate for the child who has already been in hospital or those with other disorders. The choice of antibiotics should be confirmed by the results of bacteriological cultures. Physiotherapy is helpful in facilitating clearance of secretions and re-expansion of consolidated lobes of lung.

Empyema is a rare complication and is usually due to *Staphylococcus aureus* although anaerobic organisms also occur. Adequate antibiotic therapy and drainage are vital for proper resolution.

Tuberculosis

Tuberculosis in children is fortunately much less common now; however, it is still encountered in clinical practice and remains an important cause of morbidity and mortality.

The illness is caused by the organism *Mycobacterium tuberculosis*, although, rarely, infection due to atypical mycobacteria, particularly affecting the cervical lymph glands, is seen. The bacilli are usually acquired by airbone transmission from an infected person; the organ most frequently involved in primary infection is the lung. The organism multiplies and causes a primary focus to appear, this undergoes slow fibrosis over a period of many months and may eventually either calcify or disappear. Simultaneously, there is multiplication of the organism and tissue reaction within the regional (hilar) lymph nodes. The size of this reaction depends upon the age and nutritional state of the host. Resistance is less vigorous in the young or malnourished child.

Six weeks after infection the patient becomes sensitised to tuberculoprotein and the diagnostic delayed hypersensitivity reaction in skin becomes positive. This is the basis of the Mantoux test in which 0.1 ml (10 tuberculin units) of 1: 1000 dilution of PPD (protein purified derivitive) is injected intradermally. An indurated area of 5 mm diameter or greater is produced within 48 hours in those who are sensitive. If significant disease is suspected 0.1 ml of 1: 10 000 solution should be used to avoid a severe or painful skin reaction. The Mantoux test is the most reliable test for diagnostic purposes. It may be falsely negative in those with severe infections and is inhibited by steroid therapy.

Screening of larger populations may be carried out using the multiple puncture Heaf test. A spring-loaded gun produces a circle of six epidermal punctures through a tuberculin PPD solution placed on the skin surface. Positive reactions produce induration at the puncture sites, in those with vigorous reactions they may coalesce. The tuberculin n test uses a device with four points or tines, which have been coated with tuberculin; they are pressed against the skin for 5 seconds. The Mantoux test is probably the most efficient.

Systemic symptoms may occur in association with the primary infection and include fever, lethargy, anorexia, weight loss, hepatosplenomegaly and rarely erythema nodosum and phlyctenular conjunctivitis. The vast majority of children with primary tuberculosis will, however, show no significant systemic upset and are only detected by routine testing for tuberculoprotein sensitivity in school screening programmes.

The late complications affect a number of organs. Progressive primary lung infection including collapse, consolidation, bronchiectasis, pleural effusion and, rarely, empyema may occur. The central nervous system may be involved by tuberculous meningitis, usually within 6–12 months of the primary infection. This complication still carries a high morbidity and mortality. There may be involvement of bones and joints on 1–3 years after initial infection and renal tuberculosis may occur several years later. The most serious complication is miliary tuberculosis with generalised haematogenous spread throughout the body.

Children who are shown to have had primary infection either by the presence of physical signs or by tuberculin conversion from negative to positive reaction, should be given antituberculous chemoprophylaxis in order to prevent late complications (principally tuberculous meningitis and miliary tuberculosis). The most suitable drugs in childhood are para-aminosalicylic acid (PAS), isoniazid (INH), streptomycin and rifampicin. PAS and INH are given to those who show Mantoux conversion in the absence of other signs. Where there is clinical infection triple therapy is used with parenteral streptomycin with PAS and INH in combination. Rifampicin is a useful alternative but should be used with caution, especially if INH is also given, because of the risk of hepatotoxicity in children. Drugs should be continued for at least 14 months.

Management should also be directed towards improving the patient's general wellbeing and nutritional status in addition to chemotherapy specifically directed against the organism.

Protection may be achieved by the use of BCG vaccine. This is an attenuated bovine strain (Bacille-Calmette-Guèrin) which is given intradermally. It is currently offered to tuberculin-negative schoolchildren in late childhood (11–13 years of age) but may be given in the neonatal period to those at high risk of exposure, such as children of certain immigrant groups in the UK or those who are likely to travel abroad to countries with a high prevalence rate of tuberculosis.

STRIDOR

Stridor is noisy breathing heard on inspiration or expiration due to obstruction of airflow in large airways including the larynx and trachea. The amount of stridor will vary with the rate of breathing and the degree of obstruction present; it may be absent during quiet breathing or when obstruction is severe. Inspiration stridor is usually associated with laryngeal or vocal cord problems, although it may also occur in significant upper tracheal lesion. Bidirectional stridor is more typical or tracheal narrowing below the vocal cords.

Aetiology

The causes of stridor are listed in Table 17.3. By far the most common is laryngomalacia, which is a benign self-limiting condition in which inspiratory stridor occurs during the first few months of life. This varies with the baby's activity, crying and position, and is less prominent when the

Table 17.3 Causes of stridor

Laryngomalacia
Laryngotracheobronchitis (croup)
Diptheria
Acute epiglottitis
Allergic oedema
Vocal cord paralysis
Vocal cord cysts
Cleft larynx
Laryngeal web
Sub-glottic haemangioma
Sub-glottic stenosis
Cystic hygroma
Foreign body
Tracheal stenosis
Vascular ring

infant is prone. It is due to indrawing of the laryngeal tissues during inspiration in the presence of a small larynx and elongated epiglottis. The prognosis is excellent and most children will outgrow this problem by late infancy.

Stridor due to acute infections such as epiglottitis and laryngotracheobronchitis, should be treated with appropriate antibiotics and intubation to bypass the obstruction if necessary (see Chapter 26).

Investigation to establish the aetiology of stridor includes a chest X–ray, including a lateral film, lateral neck X–ray and barium swallow to exclude lesions pressing on the trachea such as cysts or a vascular ring. More detailed investigations involve laryngoscopy to assess vocal cord movement and to exclude supraglottic lesions and bronchoscopy to exclude tracheal pathology, such as tracheal stenosis, bronchomalacia and haemangioma.

Clinical features and management

Stridor varies in severity according to the degree of obstruction and may be absent at rest or when lying prone depending on its aetiology. In supraglottic or vocal cord lesions it is usually inspiratory but, within the trachea, narrowing of this type usually produces bidirectional stridor. Wheezing is normally absent as this originates in smaller airways, although it can occur with significant tracheal obstruction causing retention of secretions.

Treatment is dependent on the lesion found but may include surgical correction for vascular ring, or laryngotracheoplasty to enlarge the trachea where significant permanent narrowing has occurred as in subglottic stenosis. In a number of cases, the airway obstruction cannot be relieved immediately and elective tracheostomy has to be performed until sufficient tracheal growth or resolution of the primary problem has occurred. Infants and children with a tracheostomy may be managed successfully at home. After operation the parents are instructed in the technique of tracheal toilet and suction; they are provided with a supply of catheters and a suction pump for use at home. In these cases, weekly hospital visits occur in order to change the tube. As improvement occurs a silver, valved tube may be inserted which allows expiration to occur normally through the glottis and stimulates speech development.

INHALATION OF FOREIGN BODY

Inhalation of foreign bodies is not uncommon in infants and young children. A peanut or other food stuff are the commonest cause but many other objects such as small plastic toys, beads and occasionally seeds or pine needles may be inhaled. Frequently, there is an acute episode of cough, choking or wheeze at the time of inhalation or symptoms may develop gradually over the next few hours or days. In some cases, however, the diagnosis is delayed and the child may present with chronic cough and sputum production or recurrent pneumonia. It is in this situation that the risk of permanent lung damage, including the development of chronic bronchiectasis is greatest. Most objects lodge in the mainstream bronchi, more often on the right side than the left.

Diagnosis is based on an accurate history and careful physical examination which reveals diminished air entry on the affected side and hyperinflation if there is significant air trapping behind the foreign body. Alternatively there may be collapse-consolidation and bronchial breathing.

X-ray of the chest may show typical hyperinflation on the affected side especially on an expiratory film. Chest screening may also reveal hyperinflation with air trapping and diminished respiratory movement on inspiration. Areas of pneumonic consolidation or complete collapse may also be found depending on the duration of the condition.

Bronchoscopy is essential if foreign body inhalation is suspected. Removal of the object should be followed by adequate physiotherapy and antibiotics to clear the lung of retained secretions and aid the resolution of any secondary bacterial infection. In cases where the diagnosis is delayed, careful follow-up should be undertaken to assess lung function on the affected side. This may be permanently compromised by the presence of bronchiectasis or chronic peripheral pulmonary vascular disease.

CYSTIC FIBROSIS

Cystic fibrosis is a serious, life-long disorder affecting exocrine glandular secretions throughout the body. The incidence in Caucasians is about 1 in 2000 live births; it is less common in other racial groups. The inheritance is autosomal recessive with a gene carrier rate estimated at one in 25 of the adult population. Adult carriers are quite normal and cannot be distinguished biochemically from the normal population. No antenatal diagnosis yet exists to detect babies before birth.

The illness may present in a number of ways. Ten to 15 per cent present with intestinal obstruction due to meconium ileus in the neonatal period. Most other children with cystic fibrosis present in infancy or pre-school years with recurrent lower respiratory tract infection, frequent pale bulky stools and failure to thrive. Increasing numbers are now being detected at birth by screening tests such as immunoreactive trypsin measurement on blood spot taken with the Guthrie test.

Clinical features

The major clinical features affect the respiratory tree and the digestive tract. The abnormal secretions in the respiratory tract, although initially of normal viscosity, become abnormally viscid in the presence of infection. This tends to occur from an early age and causes increasing damage to the small airways leading to obstruction, sputum retention and overinflation. Chronic bronchial wall thickening occurs as infection worsens and eventually there is microabscess formation with irreversible pulmonary damage and bronchiectasis. Upper respiratory tract symptoms with chronic sinusitis and recurrent nasal polyposis are common problems in the older child.

Major digestive difficulties are seen in most cases. These are due primarily to pancreatic insufficiency with decreased trypsin, lipase and bicarbonate concentrations in duodenal juice. There may be meconium ileus in the neonatal period (see Chapter 23), or recurrent abdominal pain with partial or complete bowel obstruction in later life. The latter is typically due to impacted faecal material in the ileo-caecal region and can be relieved by gastrografin enema. Frequently, there is also a history of poor weight gain, abdominal distension, and offensive stools which contain fat globules on microscopy. The children have an excellent appetite, unlike those with small bowel malabsorption, unless an acute respiratory infection complicates their chronic pulmonary dysfunction. In toddlers, the bulky stools can cause rectal prolapse.

A number of other clinical features may also develop including biliary cirrhosis, portal hypertension and oesophageal varices, gastric hyperacidity and diabetes mellitus due to pancreatic fibrosis. Heat exhaustion due to excess salt loss can occur in hot climates. In adult life, males are always infertile due to fibrosis of the vas deferens while females have reduced fertility and tend to have exacerbation of their chest symptoms during pregnancy. Their breast milk has a high sodium content. It is important to note that intellectual function is not affected.

The diagnosis is confirmed by measurement of sodium or chloride content in sweat collected by iontophoresis. A concentration of 70 mmol/1 on a sample weighing more than 100 mg is diagnostic. Analysis of duodenal juice bicarbonate, trypsin and lipase concentrations following pancreatic stimulation may be helpful in difficult cases.

Management

1. Pulmonary

Treatment must be carried out every day. The most important aspect is care of the chest and this must be kept as clear of sputum as possible by encouraging postural drainage and physiotherapy three times daily from the time of diagnosis. Antibiotics should be used in high dosage for 2–3 week courses during intercurrent respiratory tract infections to prevent lower respiratory tract consolidation with pathogenic organisms such as *Staphylococcus aureus*, *Pseudomonas aeruginosa* and *Haemophilus influenzae*. Continuous antibiotics may occasionally be indicated for prolonged periods if there is established infection. A significant number of cystic children also develop wheeze; if this is due to reversible airway disease, as tested by peak flow measurement, then bronchodilators such as salbutamol, terbutaline or theophylline may be useful. There is some evidence that these agents may also promote mucociliary clearance. If allergy is thought to have a prominent part in symptoms then Intal may be beneficial. Mucolytic agents such as acetylcysteine are not generally recommended but do have a role in individuals with particularly viscid sputum which is difficult to clear.

2. Nutritional

Nine out of 10 patients with cystic fibrosis have nutritional problems primarily related to pancreatic insufficency. Management is aimed at providing a high calorie, high protein, high carbohydrate and low fat diet. Oral pancreatic enzyme replacement is given with meals using compounds such as Pancrex, Cotazym or Nutrizym. The dosage has to be tailored to the individual and will vary depending on the fat intake and level of pancreatic insufficiency at that time. Vitamin supplements are added to replace vitamins A, B, C, D and E. Vitamin K is given if there is hepatic dysfunction. A good salt intake is also essential and salt tablets may be indicated in hot climates where excess salt loss in sweat and heat exhaustion can occur.

3 Social and family

Cystic fibrosis is a life-long condition with a variable prognosis; life expectancy can be from a few months or years at one extreme to the middle-forties at the other. The majority now survive to adult life. The overall management of the child and the family must include adequate counselling and support for the parents and the patient throughout childhood, adolescence and adult life. This involves the physician, physiotherapists, nurses and social workers. Most children can lead a reasonably normal life and attend normal school if given appropriate support. In adult life they can take jobs which do not require heavy physical effort or involve exposure to smoke or dust. Many now marry and it is important to counsel about the management of the illness in adult life. Males with cystic fibrosis are sterile. Cystic fibrosis management is essentially hospital based; the Cystic Fibrosis Research Trust provides funding for research and also meetings and literature for affected families.

BRONCHIECTASIS

Bronchiectasis is a chronic lung condition caused by bronchial dilatation in the presence of infection and is characterised by chronic cough and purulent sputum production. It is the pathological end-result of a number of disease processes listed in Table 17.4. The affected child may present with

Table 17.4 Causes of bronchiectasis

Cystic fibrosis
Lower respiratory tract infection
Immunodeficiency
Foreign body inhalation
Abnormal lung development
Recurrent aspiration

dyspnoea, cough, sputum production, finger clubbing, hyperinflated chest and with diminished air entry and coarse crepitations heard over the affected area.

A number of organisms, which can infect the lung, may produce these changes including *Staphylococcus aureus*, *Streptococcus pneumoniae*, *Haemophilus influenzae*, *Klebsiella aerogenes*, *Pseudomonas aeruginosa*, *Bordetella pertussis* and adenovirus. Investigation of the child with bronchiectasis should include full blood count, immunoglobulins, Mantoux test, sweat test and X–rays possibly including a radioisotope lung scan. Bronchography is only rarely required nowadays, although bronchoscopy is essential if initial investigation fails to reveal a cause or if a foreign body is suspected.

Treatment is similar to that in cystic fibrosis. This will include regular physiotherapy and intermittent or continuous antibiotics depending on the pathogen isolated from regular sputum cultures. The aim is to keep the lung free of infection so that recovery and resolution may occur and further deterioration is prevented. Surgery may be indicated to deal with the primary cause, for example, removal of a foreign body or cyst. There is considerable postoperative morbidity following chest surgery in these patients and therefore lobar removal is rarely indicated as more than one lobe is frequently affected and good results can be obtained with conservative management.

18

Heart disease

CONGENITAL HEART DISEASE

Major advances in the precise diagnosis of congenital heart disease have been made in the last decade. Angled angiographic views and real-time ultrasound now allow precise anatomical detail to be available before surgery. Parallel with these diagnostic advances, a new descriptive nomenclature allows a better understanding of complex lesions. The use of deep hypothermia and cardioplegic solutions have, over the same period, revolutionised surgery of infants and small children with congenital heart disease.

Medical treatment of infants and children with congenital heart disease has not altered significantly. It is well described in major texts and will not be dealt with in this chapter. One major addition to medical management is the pharmacological control of the patency of the ductus arteriosus. Indomethacin is used to close and prostaglandin to maintain patency in duct-dependent lesions such as pulmonary atresia.

Readers interested in individual lesions should refer to one of several comprehensive monographs. This chapter is intended to give a broad overview of the subject. Indications for invasive or non-invasive investigations, medical treatment and surgery are presented along with classical features on X–ray, electrocardiogram and echocardiogram.

Acyanotic lesions with left to right shunt
Atrial septal defect (ASD)

This represents 10 per cent of congenital heart lesions; 70 per cent are of the secundum variety.

1. Secundum atrial septal defect

A defect in the atrial septum in and around the area of the foramen ovale; it is occasionally multiple.

Presentation: Usually asymptomatic in childhood, the lesion being found by chance at school or welfare clinic examination or during an incidental illness. Development of pulmonary hypertension, pulmonary vascular disease and atrial arrhythmias will occur after the third or fourth decade.

Clinical findings: Pulmonary ejection systolic murmur and mid-diastolic tricuspid murmur. Both murmurs are due to increased pulmonary flow. Second sound is fixed and widely split.

ECG: Right axis deviation, RSR pattern in V4R and VI, terminal S in left chest leads.

Chest X-ray Cardiomegaly, prominence of right atrium, right ventricle and main pulmonary artery, plethoric lung fields.

Echocardiography Paradoxical septal movement with right ventricular cavity enlargement. Sector scan invariably visualises the defect and localises it to septum secundum.

Management Surgical closure of the defect is entirely safe with minimal mortality, and should be performed before school entrance.

2. Primum atrial septal defect

The defect is low in the atrial septum close to the atrioventricular junction. Usually associated with cleft septal leaflet of the mitral valve which is abnormally anterior and rightward in position. It represents the simplest type of atrioventricular defect, previously called endocardial cushion defect.

Presentation: Often symptomatic in childhood (compare with secundum ASD) depending on degree of mitral regurgitation. Rarely presents in cardiac failure in infancy. Many children present as incidental finding at medical examination.

Clinical findings: Pulmonary systolic and tricuspid diastolic flow murmurs with fixed split of the second heart sound (as in secundum ASD). Associated apical pansystolic mitral murmur in the presence of mitral regurgitation through the cleft mitral valve.

ECG: Left axis deviation with partial incomplete right bundle branch block. Left ventricular volume overload pattern with mitral regurgitation.

Chest X-ray: Cardiomegaly, plethoric lung fields, right and left ventricles may be enlarged.

Echocardiogram: Paradoxical septal movement with right ventricular cavity enlargement, anterior mitral leaflet touches septum during diastole, left ventricle and left atrium may be enlarged. Sector scanning usually shows a defect low in the interatrial septum and can differentiate it from secundum ASD. Both atrioventricular valves insert onto interventricular septum at same level, while normally septal tricuspid leaflet inserts more apically than mitral septal leaflet.

Management: Surgical closure is the treatment of choice with slightly higher risk than for secundum ASD. Mitral valve cleft usually requires repair or even replacement.

3. Complete atrioventricular defects

These lesions represent the more complex end of the atrioventricular defect spectrum. Usually (but not always) associated with ostium primum ASD, and perimembranous inlet ventricular septal defect. Atrioventricular valve rings are formed medially and two bridging leaflets, formed by both atrioventricular valves, span the combined defect. It was previously known as common atrioventricular canal and is commonly associated with Downs syndrome. It may also occur in association with tetralogy of Fallot or double outlet right ventricle.

Presentation High pulmonary blood flow and pulmonary hypertension result in failure to thrive and heart failure in infancy. Murmurs may be restricted to systole at left sternal edge with accentuated pulmonary component of second heart sound. However, if pulmonary hypertension is not too severe then the murmurs of mitral regurgitation, VSD and ASD may be heard. Cyanosis is rare. Increased anteroposterior chest diameter.

ECG Left axis deviation, biventricular hypertrophy.

Chest X-ray Cardiomegaly with maybe four chamber enlargement. Main pulmonary artery enlarged; pulmonary plethora.

Echocardiogram Both M-Mode and 2-D scanning demonstrate bridging leaflets crossing the atrioventricular defect. 2-D can further demonstrate both atrial and ventricular defects and may indicate site of insertion of anterior bridging leaflet into septum or right ventricle. Echo features of pulmonary hypertension may be present.

Management and treatment In view of complexity of anomaly and risk of surgery in infancy, heart failure is treated medically at first. Failure to thrive thereafter, indicates the need for surgical intervention. Pulmonary artery banding to diminish pulmonary blood flow and pressure is probably the safest procedure in infancy. Thereafter, despite mortality between 10 per cent and 20 per cent total correction is treatment of choice. The atrioventricular defect is patched and the mitral valve reconstituted or replaced.

Persistent ductus arteriosus (PDA)

This is the commonest congenital cardiac lesion (12 per cent) and is twice as common in girls as boys. It is frequently associated with prematurity, maternal rubella and shows increased incidence in populations living at high altitude.

Presentation The timing and type of presentation is determined by size of duct. Large ducts cause cardiac failure, failure to thrive, feeding difficulties in early infancy. Smaller shunts may be asymptomatic and found at routine medical examination, presenting only as a murmur.

Clinical findings Continuous machinery murmur in the second left intercostal space. It may be confused with venous hum which is a normal finding and goes away with compression of the neck, rotation of the head or laying the child flat. In infancy the classical continuous murmur may not be heard, (the diastolic component may be missing). Large ducts will have mid-diastolic mitral flow murmurs and accentuated pulmonary component of the second heart sound. Peripheral pulses and pulse pressure are large volume indicating a leak from the aortia into the pulmonary artery.

ECG Left ventricular hypertrophy, sometimes biventricular hypertrophy, left ventricular volume overload. Small ducts may have normal ECGs.

Chest X-ray Large ducts have pulmonary plethora, prominence of the main pulmonary artery, and enlargement of left ventricle and left atrium. Small ducts may have normal chest X-rays.

Echocardiogram: Left ventricular and left atrial enlargement are recognised with volume overload pattern of contraction in the left ventricle. M-Mode echocardiography was the method of choice but the newest high frequency cross-sectional transducers now give easy and accurate pictures of the ductus in small infants from the suprasternal and high parasternal approaches.

Management and treatment: Large ductuses in small infants require digoxin, diuretics and fluid restriction to control their heart failure. Although a percentage will close spontaneously, surgical treatment is usually indicated. The ducts in pre-term infants between 28 and 32 weeks gestation may close with indomethacin, a prostaglandin synthetase antagonist. Success rate is, however, much less than surgery and there are side-effects, including gastric erosion and disturbance of renal function.

In general, all persistent ducts should be closed regardless of size or age of the child. Surgery, even in the pre-term neonate, has a low mortality.

Ventricular septal defect (VSD)

Incidence In childhood, this is one of the commonest congenital cardiac anomalies. Between 60 per cent and 70 per cent of all defects close spontaneously.

Presentation Symptomatology and clinical findings vary with size of defect and therefore size of shunt. Small defects present in asymptomatic children as incidentally discovered murmurs. Large defects customarily present during the first 2 months of life with heart failure, difficulty in feeding, dyspnoea and chest infections. Heart failure depends on the size of the left-to-right shunt, which appears after the customary fall in pulmonary artery pressure and resistance after birth. A small number of children have ventricular septal defects and pulmonary vascular resistance which never falls; pulmonary vascular disease then occurs with reversal of the shunt and cyanosis.

There is an increased antero-posterior diameter of the chest with Harrison's sulcus, and a pansystolic murmur in the fourth and fifth intercostal space left sternal edge, with or without a thrill. Mitral diastolic flow murmurs present in shunts where pulmonary flow is more than twice systemic. The presence of pulmonary hypertension is suggested by increase in loudness of pulmonary component of the second heart sound, and right ventricular parasternal heave.

Chest X-ray This is normal in small defects. Cardiomegaly, left ventricular, left atrial enlargement and pulmonary plethora occur with large defects. Pulmonary hypertension is associated with prominence of the main pulmonary artery.

ECG. This shows sinus rhythm with normal QRS axis. Biventricular hypertrophy is common in bit shunts, and as pulmonary vascular resistance increases right ventricular hypertrophy becomes dominant. Deep Q waves in the left chest lead are common with large shunts, left ventricular volume overload pattern. Recent studies suggest that defects in certain areas of the septum (trabecular and perimembranous) have a higher likelihood of spontaneous closure.

Echocardiogram Enlargement of left ventricle and left atrium is seen with left ventricular volume overload pattern. Abnormal pulmonary valve echoes may strongly suggest pulmonary hypertension. Two-dimensional echocardiography can now reliably diagnose ventricular septal defects and locate the area of the defect in the interventricular septum.

Management and treatment Since 60 per cent of all defects close spontaneously, most small defects will require no medical treatment, apart from penicillin cover for dental extractions. Followup is continued until the defect is considered closed.

Small infants with large defects in heart failure are treated with digoxin and diuretics. Catheterisation is undertaken in these infants at least once during the first year of life to assess the degree of pulmonary hypertension, size of shunt and eliminate other associated lesions, e.g. PDA. If the pulmonary artery pressure is low, regardless of the size of shunt, conservative management is indicated as some of these defects will still close.

When the pulmonary artery pressure is raised, repeat catheterisation between 6 and 18 months is indicated, as some will get smaller but others will develop pulmonary hypertension. Primary closure is recommended in these children after 18 months, but many with large shunts and high pulmonary vascular resistance will require primary closure in the first year of life. Mortality from surgical correction after the age of two is very low (less than 2 per cent). In the first year of life it may be twice as high.

Obstructive lesions of the right heart

Pulmonary stenosis (PS):

Incidence: Pulmonary valve stenosis represents 10 per cent of all congenital heart disease and may be mild, moderate or severe. The common lesion is at valvar level, but more rarely subvalve or supravalve stenosis, or branch artery stenosis may be found.

1. Severe pulmonary valve stenosis

Presentation: Age and mode of presentation depend on severity of stenosis. Virtual pulmonary atresia may present in the immediate neonatal period with cyanosis, heart failure, tricuspid regurgitation. More commonly severe stenosis presents with a loud ejection systolic murmur in a well-nourished infant who is not in heart failure. The second heart sound is single and there is usually no ejection click (compare this with mild pulmonary stenosis). Cyanosis may be present if an ASD coexists but this is rare.

Chest X-ray This shows normal pulmonary vascularity. The pulmonary artery appears prominent due to post-stenotic dilatation. There is a hypoplastic appearance to the peripheral pulmonary arteries. Right ventricle and right atrium are frequently enlarged.

Echocardiogram: Right ventricular hypertrophy and the site of obstruction are readily seen using the cross-sectional technique. Doming and thickening of the pulmonary valve are frequently visualised.

Management and treatment Pulmonary valvotomy is method of choice; the stenosed valve is split along its commissures on cardio-pulmonary bypass or profound hypothermia. Outside the neonatal period, surgery has a low mortality. Infants with very severe pulmonary stenosis have poorer outlook depending on the size and function of the right ventricle. A very small right ventricular cavity with virtual pulmonary atresia may be better served by aorto-Pulmonary shunting. Post-valvotomy residual pulmonary ejection murmurs are the rule and, frequently, early diastolic murmurs due to pulmonary regurgitation occur. Successful pulmonary valvotomy using a balloon angioplasty catheter is now possible, even in quite severe cases; mortality is comparable to surgery.

2. Mild pulmonary valve stenosis

Presentation Usually discovered at a routine medical examination in middle childhood. The child is asymptomatic. Pulmonary ejection murmur with a wide split of the second heart sound and an ejection click. The presence of ejection click confirms that the stenosis is not severe.

ECG This may be normal or show mild right ventricular hypertrophy.

Chest X–ray: Again, this may be normal or show slight post-stenotic dilatation.

Echocardiogram: Usually shows normal limits.

Management and treatment: Catheterisation is necessary to confirm the severity of stenosis. If the systolic pressure difference across pulmonary valve is greater than 60–70 mmHg, the lesion is considered severe and valvotomy is indicated. Under 30 mmHg systolic pressure difference, the condition is considered mild and although follow up is indicated, progression of severity is almost unknown. The intermediate group sometimes progress to become more severe and require surgery at a later stage.

3. Fallot's tetralogy

Incidence. This is the most common form of cyanotic congenital heart disease — 10 per cent of all cardiac anomalies. Four features make up the tetralogy, ventricular septal defect, aortic over-riding, pulmonary infundibular stenosis and right ventricular hypertrophy. Deviation of the infun-dibular septum produces pulmonary infundibular obstruction associated with infundibular hyper-trophy. Right ventricular hypertrophy results from pressure overload of the right ventricle. Deviation of the infundibular septum leads to the aortic override. Underlying haemodynamics are that blood in the right ventricle is prevented from wholly entering the pulmonary artery because of the stenosis, flows across the ventricular septal defect into the aorta, thus providing partly oxygen-ated blood in the systemic arterial circulation.

Presentation and clinical findings The degree of pulmonary outflow tract obstruction determines the type of presentation and the age at presen-tation. If obstruction is very severe, the presen-tation may be in early infancy with cyanosis. However, the classical presentation is with a murmur in an asymptomatic child whose cyanosis develops during the first 6–12 months. Probably, increasing infundibular stenosis is the cause in this group.

Dyspnoea, especially when feeding in infants, increases with age. Squatting is characteristic of older children; after exertion they squat on their haunches. Hypercyanotic spells are common when the pulmonary anatomy is severely hypoplastic. Infundibular spasm, perhaps related to increased circulating catecholamines, further narrows down the outflow tract and reduces pulmonary blood flow. Increasing right-to-left shunting occurs and unconsciousness may ensue. These spells are an indication for early treatment.

Ejection systolic murmur at the pulmonary area, single second heart sound or greatly reduced pulmonary component of the second heart sound are features; the more severe the narrowing, the shorter the murmur. During a hypercyanotic spell, the murmur may shorten dramatically. Cyanosis and finger clubbing are common, and right ventricular hypertrophy is present clinically. Other congenital abnormalities, particularly of the gastrointestinal or genito-urinary tracts are common.

Chest X–ray: Right ventricular enlargement, with uptilting of the apex (coeur en sabot). A small main pulmonary artery and branch is evidence of a right-sided aorta in 25 per cent of cases. There is a concave pulmonary artery segment.

ECG: This indicates right ventricular hyper-trophy, right axis deviation, seldom right atrial enlargement.

Echocardiogram: Override of interventricular septum by the aorta is well recognised by either ultrasonic technique. The pulmonary artery is seldom seen. VSD and right ventricular outflow tract narrowing can be recognised using 2-D echo.

Management: In infancy profound cyanosis and cyanotic spells are best treated surgically by aorto-pulmonary shunting. The Waterston shunt (ascending aorta to right pulmonary artery) has fallen from favour because it produces unilateral increase in pulmonary blood flow and deformity of the right pulmonary artery. A Blalock Taussig shunt (subclavian to right or left pulmonary artery) remains a better and more physiological shunt, but it is often technically difficult or impossible in tiny infants. Modified Blalock Taussig shunts, in which Goretex or similar tubing is anastomosed to the side of the subclavian artery and the corres-ponding pulmonary artery, now is the method of choice. The patency rate of these is higher in in-fants than the Blalock Taussig shunt. Hypercyano-tic attacks may be treated acutely with oxygen administration, correction of acidaemia and a beta-blocker, such as propranolol. Over 5 kg body weight, if the anatomy is not severe, total correc-tion is the method of choice. Total correction con-sists of closure of the VSD, resection of the outflow tract and, if necessary, placement of either a gusset or a conduit in the outflow tract.

The most severe form of Fallot's tetralogy is pulmonary atresia with VSD. Clinical presentation differs in that a pulmonary ejection murmur is usually absent. The presentation is usually in infancy and the child may depend entirely on a PDA for pulmonary blood flow. Under these circumstances, prostaglandin may be infused to maintain patency of the duct until palliation by aortopulmonary shunting is achieved. Recently, long-term oral prostaglandins have been shown to be successful, but they must be given frequently, every 1–2 hours, and the child must, remain in hospital during treatment. Long-term correction of pulmonary atresia depends on the size of the pulmonary arteries and includes closure of the VSD and insertion of a valved conduit from the right ventricle to the pulmonary artery.

Obstructive lesions of the left heart
Aortic stenosis

Incidence This represents 7 per cent of congenital heart disease, but 1 per cent of normal population has a bicuspid aortic valve. Stenosis may be at valvar, subvalvar or supravalvar level, 83 per cent of lesions are at valvar level and 9 per cent at subvalvar level. Subvalve aortic stenosis may be due to a thin discrete membrane in the left ventricular outflow tract, or a fibro-muscular narrowing. Supravalvar aortic stenosis is commonly associated with hypercalcaemia, mental retardation and the typical facies. Biscuspid aortic valve need not cause clinical problems in childhood, but frequently results in calcific aortic stenosis in middle-age.

Presentation Aortic stenosis only rarely causes heart failure in infancy. Most children grow and develop normally and are asymptomatic. Referral is usually because of an incidentally discovered murmur. Severe aortic stenosis in older children may cause dyspnoea, syncope or even angina. In infancy, severe stenosis may be associated with heart failure, an enlarged heart and extreme dyspnoea.

Auscultatory findings The ejection systolic murmur in the aortic area is conducted to the suprasternal notch and carotids. The aortic component of the second heart sound is frequently reduced. Ejection click at the left sternal edge suggests a lesion at valve level. The intensity of the murmur usually predicts the severity of stenosis and size of aortic valve gradient. Left ventricular apex is not displaced but heaving in character. A small volume, slow rise peripheral pulse is common. Subvalve aortic stenosis has a systolic murmur heard further down left sternal edge and the differential diagnosis is from ventricular septal defect. Supravalve aortic stenosis frequently shows higher pulse pressure in the right arm, as preferential flow of blood occurs down right subclavian artery.

ECG ECG shows normal axis, left ventricular hypertrophy varying with intensity of stenosis. Left ventricular strain pattern with ST depression and T wave inversion in left chest leads is common in severe lesions. ECG is unreliable in assessing severity.

Chest X-ray This may be normal. Left ventricular and left atrial enlargement, and dilatation of ascending aorta associated with severe valvar stenosis. Subvalve aortic stenosis is less likely to have a post-stenotic dilatation.

Echocardiogram M-Mode echo is the most accurate way of assessing left ventricular hypertrophy. The more severe the stenosis the greater the LVH. 2-D echo reliably identifies biscuspid aortic valve and categorically identifies sub- or supravalve aortic stenosis.

Management and treatment: In view of the unreliability of the ECG, the assessment of severity of aortic valve stenosis is best accomplished by measurement of peak systolic pressure difference across the aortic valve at cardiac catheterisation. Usually, aortic stenosis in childhood does not produce symptoms; a systolic pressure difference across the obstruction of 70 mmHg or more is considered severe, and of less than 30 mmHg as mild. Prediction of severity from clinical findings is notoriously unreliable in the intermediate group. If stenosis is mild, no restriction of activity is indicated but antibiotic prophylaxis for dental extractions or surgical procedures is obligatory. The risk of bacterial endocarditis is high. More severe aortic stenotics may die suddenly with exertion and competitive exercise should be banned; syncope is a bad prognostic sign. In severe aortic stenosis, valvotomy is the treatment of choice either in infants or older children. Mortality for valvotomy in later childhood is under 5 per cent, but in infants may be over 20 per cent. Subvalve aortic stenosis if severe also necessitates surgery. Results in discrete membranous lesions are very good, but abolition of stenosis is difficult in long fibromuscular obstructions and mortality is higher. Supravalve aortic stenosis if severe is treated by widening of the aortic root.

After valvotomy, many children have aortic regurgitation and almost certainly most will require aortic valve replacement after they have achieved their full growth.

Coarctation of the aorta

Incidence This accounts for 5 per cent of all cardiac lesions. It is the commonest cause of heart failure in acyanotic newborn babies. It is commonly associated with other cardiac lesions including bicuspid aortic valve (50 per cent of cases), ventricular septal defect, persistent ductus arteriosus.

Juxta-ductal coarctation
(often called the adult type)

A localised constriction, often diaphragm-like, with abrupt reduction in aortic size and post-stenotic dilatation. It may present in infancy with heart failure, but is usually an incidental finding later in childhood. If untreated, it will in adult life, lead to aortic rupture, intracranial haemorrhage and heart failure. Collateral circulation usually develops from the subclavian artery and its branches to below the coarctation. Flow murmurs through these collaterals are easily heard over the back of the chest. An ejection systolic murmur over the base of the heart usually means the presence of a biscupid aortic valve. An isolated coarctation without aortic valve anomaly may have very little anterior murmur. Systemic upper limb hypertension is present with impalpable or barely palpable and delayed femoral pulses.

ECG The ECG is normal in mild cases. Left ventricular hypertrophy, sometimes with strain pattern in severe coarctation.

Chest X-ray Cardiomegaly with increase in size of left ventricle is seen in severe cases; rib-notching appears when there are arterial collaterals. Visible indentation at the site of the coarctation may be seen.

Echocardiogram Evidence of bicuspid aortic valve on the echocardiogram is invaluable. Left ventricular hypertrophy will indicate the severity of coarctation. 2-D echocardiography from suprasternal notch can recognise the degree and site of coarctation.

Management and treatment Surgical resection is the treatment of choice. Operative mortality in later childhood is virtually zero, so surgery should be undertaken before puberty. Thereafter, an increasing number of patients will have persistent systemic hypertension despite resection.

Tubular hypoplasia: (Infantile type)

Coarctation of tubular form involving the aortic isthmus probably results from reduced aortic blood flow in the fetus. Several intracardiac lesions, such as VSD, persistent ductus arteriosus, or aortic stenosis are associated with this type of coarctation. In addition to diffuse tubular hypoplasia, a localised constricttion is frequently found at the site of the ductus. The clinical features are protean and depend on underlying associated cardiac lesions as well as the coarctation. Hypertension in the upper limbs is often present. The femoral pulses may vary depending on patency of persistent ductus arteriosus. Heart failure in the neonatal period is very common.

ECG Right ventricular hypertrophy more than left with diffuse ST–T wave changes is common. Dominant left ventricular hypertrophy is rare at this age.

Chest X-ray Cardiomegaly, plethoric lung fields, pulmonary venous congestion are all frequent. Findings depend again largely on associated lesions.

Echocardiogram It is occasionally possible to demonstrate narrowing of isthmus suprasternally using 2-D echo, but most frequently the ultrasound is used to demonstrate the associated cardiac lesions.

Management and treatment Initially, anticongestive therapy and oxygen are indicated. Prostaglandins may be used to keep the duct open temporarily, as these children deteriorate rapidly when the duct closes. Surgery is the treatment of choice. The duct is usually ligated at the same time and if a large left-to-right ventricular shunt is present, pulmonary artery banding may also be undertaken. Mortality varies with associated lesions, severity of aortic hypoplasia and age at presentation. Gussets of prosthetic material or pericardium may be used to enlarge the coarcted area, or a flap of subclavian artery may be brought down and included in the anastomosis.

Abnormalities of cardiac connections
Univentricular heart

This heading covers a clinically disparate group of conditions, including lesions known in the past as single ventricle, tricuspid atresia and mitral atresia. The common factor in all is the presence in the myocardial mass of one functional ventricle. A ventricle by definition has three parts; an inflow portion including an atrioventricular valve, a trabecular and an outflow portion. If only one chamber within the myocardial mass fulfils these criteria the heart is univentricular and any other chamber is described as rudimentary. Univentricular hearts may be of double inlet type where both AV valves drain into the single ventricular cavity, or there may be absence of the right or left atrioventricular connection (tricuspid or mitral atresia). Almost any variety of ventriculoarterial connections is possible, including pulmonary atresia, transposition of the great arteries and truncus arteriosus. Coarctation, persistent ductus arteriosus and pulmonary stenosis are frequently found in association with univentricular heart. Coarctation and ductus may be haemodynamically embarrassing and , on the other hand, pulmonary stenosis may be of benefit by preventing the lungs from receiving the full force of systemic pressure and flow when pulmonary artery is connected to the main ventricle.

Presentation and clinical features Most present early in infancy and fall into two group:
1. Those with pulmonary oligaemia due to pulmonary stenosis or pulmonary atresia will have clinical problems similar to the tetralogy of Fallot
2. Those with pulmonary plethora and high pulmonary artery pressure, will present in failure and have similar clinical features to large ventricular septal defects.

ECG Superior or leftward axis is common, particularly in absent right atrioventricular connection. Chest leads are very variable but may fail to show evidence of activity from more than one ventricle.

Chest X-ray Chest X–ray varies according to pulmonary blood flow; high pulmonary blood flow with pulmonary plethora or low pulmonary blood flow with oligaemia. Children in heart failure with high pulmonary blood flow have large hearts.

Echocardiogram Both M -Mode and 2-D echocardiography can make the diagnosis correctly and reliably. Both techniques will show the failure of development of the posterior inlet septum, which is the prime feature. 2-D echocardiography is the method of choice for assessing presence or absence of atrioventricular connections and mode of connections, and can usually demonstrate rudimentary chambers.

Management: Medical therapy is indicated for children in heart failure. In infancy, surgery is always palliative; removal of coarctation, ligation of duct and banding of the pulmonary artery is frequently necessary, and severe obstruction to pulmonary blood flow necessitates an aortopulmonary shunt. Long-term total correction is much more experimental.

Total anomalous pulmonary venous drainage

This represents approximately 1 per cent of congenital heart disease. The pulmonary venous blood drains not to the left atrium but to a systemic vein with supradiaphragmatic or infradiaphragmatic drainage. In the supradiaphragmatic type, a common channel forms from confluence of the pulmonary vein and drains into the right or left superior vena cava, innominate vein, coronary sinus or right atrium direct. Infradiaphragmatic drainage is usually to the portal vein via a common descending channel through the diaphragm, but may also be to the inferior vena cava. Mixed drainage may also occur.

Presentation Most cases present in the first year of life especially if there is obstruction to pulmonary flow. Presentation is usually in the first year of life. This and mode of presentation vary with the site of drainage and the degree of obstruction. The more severe the obstruction (as in drainage to the portal system) the earlier the presentation and the sicker the child. Resultant right heart failure with cyanosis in the neonatal period usually is seen with obstruction and is most likely due to portal vein drainage. Pulmonary hypertension is present at or above systemic level and the outlook is bad without urgent surgery. Anticongestive therapy helps only briefly. If obstruction is absent and there is a high flow situation, survival is possible for months or even a year with mild cyanosis, failure to thrive, signs of a large left-to-right atrial shunt and variable evidence of pulmonary hypertension. Auscultatory findings are then those of right ventricular volume overload with pulmonary systolic ejection and tricuspid diastolic flow murmur.

ECG Right ventricular and right atrial enlargement, with often very little left ventricular activity is the rule.

Chest X–ray: Obstructed cases show intense reticular mottling of the lung fields due to pulmonary venous congestion with a small heart. Non-obstructive cases show pulmonary plethora, with enlargement of the right ventricle and right atrium. The anomalous ascending vein is large and dilated, but in infancy frequently not obvious on the straight X–ray of the chest. The classic snowman appearance due to supracardiac anomalous veins is seldom present in infants.

Echocardiogram Echocardiography is essential to make the diagnosis. Right ventricular enlargement, right atrial enlargement, signs of pulmonary hypertension with a small left atrium and left ventricle are invariable. 2-D echocardiography can allow recognition of posterior confluence of the pulmonary vein and may demonstrate the site of drainage. Cardiac catheterisation is indicated immediately the diagnosis is suspected.

Management and treatment Surgical correction is indicated in every case to anastomose the confluence of pulmonary veins to the left atrium. The surgical mortality in infancy and in the obstructed cases is very high (up to 50 per cent for obstructed and up to 25 per cent for non-obstructed cases).

Transposition of the great arteries (TGA)

Definition and incidence By definition the aorta arises from the morphological right ventricle and the pulmonary artery from the morphological left. TGA constitutes 7 per cent of all cases of congenital heart disease; 20 per cent of cases have an associated VSD, and 5 per cent have VSD with pulmonary stenosis. Transportation haemodynamics are found frequently in univentricular heart and double-outlet right ventricle.

Presentation The presentation is usually in the first few days of life with severe cyanosis and often congestive failure. In the presence of a VSD, presentation may be delayed for a month or more, and children are relatively less cyanosed. The differential diagnosis is from lung disease or the persistent fetal circulation syndrome.

Clinical findings It is usually found in large full-term infants. There is deep central cyanosis single loud heart sounds, and frequently no murmurs are audible. If VSD, PDA or PS are present, then the murmurs of these lesions may be heard. Cardiac failure and severe acidaemia are common.

ECG Right ventricular hypertrophy is usually marked with right axis deviation. Left ventricular activitiy only increased when there is PDA or VSD.

Chest X-ray This shows prominence of right ventricle and right atrium. If great arteries lie one behind the other, then narrow upper mediastinal shadow gives classic egg on its side appearance; Although this is classical it is not typical. In presence of PDA or VSD, pulmonary plethora is seen.

Echocardiogram 2-Dechocardiography demonstrates very accurately the ventriculoarterial connections. Note that transposition of the great arteries is not an abnormal relationship of the great arteries, but an abnormality of connections. Contrast echocardiography viewed from the suprasternal approach demonstrates the diagnosis very accurately as the aorta fills with contrast from the systemic venous system preferentially.

Management: Confirmation of diagnosis is urgent. In absence of major intracardiac defect, effective pulmonary blood flow is minimal and condition is incompatible with life for more than a few hours or days. Cardiac catheterisation is performed as soon as diagnosis is suspected, because delay will lead to increasing hypoxaemia, acidaemia and death. At the diagnostic catheterisation, balloon atrial septostomy is performed by passing a catheter with deflated balloon across the foramen ovale to the left atrium. After inflation the balloon is pulled back to rupture the flap of the foramen ovale. An ASD is created with bidirectional shunting at atrial level, allowing improvement in effective pulmonary blood flow, and survival of the child for up to a year. Definitive correction is usually by Mustard's procedure. The existing atrial septum is excised and baffle, usually of pericardium, is used to redirect blood from the venae cavae to the mitral valve and from the pulmonary veins to the tricuspid valve.

The risk of death from balloon atrial septostomy is minimal. The mortality associated with Mustard's operation is between 5 per cent and 15 per cent. Some children do not have good mixing of oxygenated and deoxygenated blood after atrial septosomy and require a Blalock-Hanlon surgical atrial septectomy as a closed procedure during the first few months of life. Recently, attempts to switch the great arteries have gained favour, but mortality is still greater than 50 per cent. At present, therefore, use of this procedure in uncomplicated TGA is contraindicated.

Patients who also have VSD and PS have severe central cyanosis, pulmonary oligaemia and require a shunt procedure, as described for tetralogy of Fallot. In later childhood this condition is treated by the Rastelli procedure; a patch is inserted from the left ventricle through the VSD to the aortic root. Pulmonary valve and artery are closed and a valve conduit from right ventricle to pulmonary artery inserted.

ARRHYTHMIAS AND CONDUCTION DEFECTS IN CHILDHOOD

Incidence and aetiology

Clinically significant arrhythmias are much less common in paediatric cardiology compared with adult medicine. However, ambulatory tape monitoring has shown that unsuspected ectopic rhythms such as ventricular or atrial ectopics, or transient bradycardias or tachycardias, are remarkably common in the normal infant and young child. The correlation between these disturbances and sudden infant cot death is as yet unconfirmed.

Association of arrhythmias with major forms of congenital heart diesease is fortunately rare.

Lesions associated with rhythm and conduction abnormalities

1. Ebstein's anomaly of the tricuspid valve: frequently Woolf-Parkinson-White syndrome and paroxysmal atrial tachycardia
2. Anatomically corrected transposition of the great arteries: atrioventricular block, paroxysmal atrial tachycardia, atrial fibrillation or flutter
3. Dilated cardiomyopathy and hypertrophic obstructive cardiomyopathy: supraventricular tachycardia, atrioventricular block.

Investigation of arrhythmias in childhood involves the use of 24-hour ambulatory tape monitoring, exercise testing when arrhythmias are precipitated by exertion and sometimes invasive intracardiac electrography.

Paroxysmal supraventricular tachycardia

This is the commonest form of arrhythmia in childhood, and presents as rapid regular tachycardia between 150 and 300 beats per minute, depending on age. The condition shows characteristically intermittent attacks which start and stop suddenly, and last from a few beats to several days. Prolonged attacks lead to cardiac failure. There is frequent association with an abnormal conduction pathway across the atrioventricular junction, as in Woolf-Parkinson-White syndrome (10 per cent of children with paroxysmal atrial tachycardia). Between attacks in this condition the ECG is characterised by short PR interval (less than 0.12 of a second) with slurring of the up-stroke of the R wave.

Infants under one year developing paroxysmal atrial tachycardia may present as failure to thrive, colic of respiratory distress. Even at very fast rates, short attacks leave the baby relatively untroubled. Listlessness and irritability accompany attacks of longer duration and heart failure may ensue with hepatomegaly, cardiac enlargement on X–ray and even pulmonary oedema. Precipitating factors may include respiratory and other infections. Identification of paroxysmal tachycardia during an attack is easy by electrocardiogram, rate of 180–300 per minute without variation in RR interval and absent P waves.

Management and prognosis

Prognosis is generally good. Some remit spontaneously during early childhood but some will persist into adolescence. Woolf-Parkinson-White anomaly usually means a persistent tendency throughout life. In infancy the acute paroxysm is stopped with DC shock with or without digoxin. Digoxin is frequently satisfactory for continuing control, but the newer anti-arrhythmics such as disopyramide, verapamil and amiodarone may be necessary in resistant cases. Practolol was highly effective but has been withdrawn from general use, the other beta lockers are not so efficacious.

Other arrhythmias in childhood

Atrial fibrillation and atrial flutter are rarely seen, except in association with cardiomyopathy or after surgery. Ventricular premature beats are common in normal children, but ventricular tachycardias are virtually unknown except with cardiomyopathy after surgery.

Atrioventricular block

Prolongation of the time taken for the depolarising impulse to travel from the sino-atrial node into the ventricular mass via the bundle of His is due to atrioventricular block. First-degree block is found in otherwise normal children, with atrial septal defect, and in Ebstein's anomaly. It is also associated with myocarditis or digoxin therapy. The PR interval is longer than the expected value for the patient's age and heart rate. Second and third degree block are frequently associated with congenital heart disease and myocarditis. In second degree, occasional P waves are not conducted to the ventricles, sometimes as a random phenomenon or as part of the Wenckeback phenomenon where the PR interval lengthens progressively until a complete QRS is dropped.

Third degree or complete heart block is almost always congenital in origin, except following surgical correction, often after correction of tetralogy of Fallot. Sometimes the diagnosis may be made prenatally. Many children are asymptomatic. Heart rate under one year of age may be as high as 60–70 beats per minute, but thereafter slows to rates of under 40 per minute as the child nears adult life. It is not the benign condition as was previously thought. Patients are either asymptomatic and lead normal lives or require pacemaker insertion because of Stokes-Adams attack and syncope. Improved pacemaker design now allows cases which are symptomatic in early childhood to be treated satisfactorily. Insertion of such units in neonatal period, while rare, is not unknown and can be carried out successfully. There is little place for medical therapy.

Benign systolic murmurs

The majority of murmurs referred by the general practitioner, paediatrician or school health doctor will be benign systolic murmurs. Reliable identification of a murmur as benign can be difficult as there is no characteristic auscultatory feature. Most are quiet, although venous hums in the upper chest and back can be quite loud. These hums result from flow of blood through the great veins of the neck and alter with neck movement; they will usually disappear when the child is examined lying flat.

Although benign murmurs are usually quiet, short and soft, such murmurs may also be found in congenital heart disease.

To make the diagnosis of a benign systolic murmur, the following features should be present:
1. The child must be free of cardiac symptoms
2. A normal single first heart sound must be heard with a normal physiological splitting of the second heart sound
3. No added clicks or diastolic murmurs are hear
4. The murmur usually becomes loudest in the supine position and decreases in intensity when assuming the upright posture:
5. Cardiac rhythm and blood pressure must be normal
6. The ECG, chest X–ray and echocardiogram should all be within normal limits

CARDIAC FAILURE IN INFANCY

This may be a surprisingly difficult diagnosis to make. Dyspnoea, respiratory distress, hepatomegaly, oedema, tachycardia and cardiomegaly are all important signs. Apart from the last, all these findings may result from non-cardiac illnesses.

1. Dyspnoea

This results in slowness or inability to feed in the neonate, and it frequently occurs with other problems, e.g. upper respiratory tract infection, simple nasal obstruction, pneumonia or bronchiolitis. Other features include laboured respiration and use of accessory respiratory muscles, including flaring of the alae nasi. Increased antero-posterior chest diameter, the "blown chest", also occurs in both cardiac and severe respiratory diseases.

2. Hepatomegaly

A sensitive indicator of severity of heart failure, but it may also be due to metabolic disorders or intrinsic liver disease. Over-inflation of the lungs with bronchiolitis may result in the liver being pushed down so that it is easily palpable. Percussion of the upper edge of the liver will differentiate this from true hepatomegaly.

3. Peripheral oedema

Commonly seen also in renal disease and it may be confused with lymphoedema, as in Turner's syndrome.

4. Tachycardia

It is also associated with infection or metabolic imbalance.

5. Cardiomegaly on chest X–ray

Clinical assessment of cardiomegaly can be difficult in infancy. The chest X–ray is more reliable and echocardiography can diagnose cardiac chamber enlargement.

Thus the diagnosis of heart failure should not be made in the absence of radiological cardiomegaly.

In the older child the signs are those of tachycardia, dyspnoea, hepatomegaly, raised jugular venous pressure and peripheral oedema, as in the adult. Again a large heart is seen on chest X–ray.

BACTERIAL ENDOCARDITIS
Incidence and aetiology

A chronic disease which is rarely found before the age of three. Low-grade intermittent fever, rigors, anaemia, petechiae, splinter haemorrhages under the nails and generalised wasting with splenomegaly are common findings. Sudden acute haemodynamic abnormalities follow bacterial destruction of semi-lunar or atrioventricular valves. Vegetations are usually found on congenitally abnormal structures or following rheumatic damage. Persistent

ductus arteriosus, ventricular septal defect, coarctation of the aorta and aortic stenosis are lesions most commonly affected. Atrial septal defects and pulmonary stenosis are less frequently involved.

The infecting organism varies according to age. The most common organism in childhood is still *Streptococcus viridans* following dental extraction. After cardiac surgery, staphylococcus is the most common organism.

Dental extractions, scaling and other forms of surgery should be covered in known cases of congenital heart disease by an appropriate antibiotic. Penicillin is the drug of choice for dental work or ear, nose and throat operations, but erythromycin is the alternative when there is penicillin allergy. Following cardiac surgery staphylococcal infection is well prevented by flucloxacillin. Therapy is proven blood culture-positive bacterial endocarditis should be for a minimum of one month, initially given intravenously until the temperature is normal. The assessment of efficacy of treatment is by clinical evaluation, temperature recording and back titration against the organism.

Regimen for guidance of dentists and family doctors

1. When penicillin is *not* contra-indicated: by intramuscular injection *half an hour* before the operation. Benzylpenicillin injection (crystalline penicillin) 300–600 mg and 6 hours later the oral administration of phenoxymethyl penicillin (Penicillin V) 125–250 mg 6 times daily (or equivalent) for 3 days or as long as infection persists.
Or: Triplopen (benetranine procaine and benzyl penicillins) *half an hour* before operation, 1 ml up to 6 years of age, 2 ml 6 years and over, and 24 hours later the oral administration of phenoxymethyl penicillin (Penicillin V) as above.
2. When the patient is hypersensitive to penicillin: by oral administration *2 hours* before operation. Erythromycin estolates 250–500 mg and then 6 hours later 125–250 mg four times daily for 3 days or as long as infection persists.
3. When penicillin is contra-indicated other than because of hypersensitivity, e.g. when the child has received small doses of prophylactic penicil-

lin therapy within previous 8 weeks: by intra-muscular injection *half an hour* before operation. Cephaloridine 250–500 mg and 6 hours later the oral administration of erythromycin estolate 125–250 mg four times daily for 3 days or for as long as infection persists.

RHEUMATIC FEVER

The incidence of this disease has drastically declined in the Western world and it is now rare in the UK. Aetiologically there is a relationship to previous infection with group A streptococcus. There is probably a cross reaction with heart muscle when heart antigens resemble those of the streptococcus, causing an autoimmune reaction.

Clinical findings and presentation

It is rare before 3 years, but more common between 5 and 15 years of age; a preceding strep-tococcal infection (usually sore throat) is almost invariable. There is general malaise with insidious onset and joint pain affecting the large joints and flitting from joint to joint. Pallor, sweating an pyrexia are usual. Rashes of the erythema margi-netum or nodosum type are found, and a small percentage will have rheumatic nodules on the extensor surfaces of the upper limbs.

The sedimentation rate is raised, a leucocytosis is present and the anti-streptolysin O titre is high and rises as the disease process continues. C-reac-tive protein in the patient's serum indicates ongoing rheumatic activity.

Rheumatic Carditis

Occurs in approximately 15 per cent of cases and is indicated by the following findings:
1. Development of cardiac murmurs, sytolic or diastolic, and indicative of cardiac dilatation and mitral incompetence
2. Pericardial friction rub
3. Increasing cardiac size on chest X-ray
4. Frank cardiac failure with peripheral oedema and other standard signs.

Treatment

1. Penicillin to eradicate any residual streptococcal infection
2. Bed rest but not total immobility
3. Salicylates in large doses for the arthritic symptoms.

If carditis is considered to be present, then digoxin and diuretics are prescribed when cardiac failure is recognised. Evidence has been put forward for treating a patient with carditis with corticosteroids. This evidence is not firm, although it is believed that the recovery rate in significant cardiac involvement is improved.

Prognosis

Recovery of joints is complete and the major risks for these patients are:
1. Further relapses, (either of rheumatic fever or Sydenham's chorea, which is commoner in girls). Prophylactic penicillin should therefore be continued orally indefinitely
2. Development of a chronic rheumatic valve disease. Mitral valve is affected three times more commonly than the aortic valve, and thus any patient with proven rheumatic fever merits long-term followup after recovery.

19

Haematology

NORMAL RANGES OF HAEMATOLOGICAL VALUES

When interpreting haematological results in children, especially in the newborn, it is important to know the normal range for the age. The main changes in haemoglobin, red cells and leucocytes are shown in Figure 19.1. One should also note that:

1. Haemoglobin values are lower in the preterm infant than in the term baby. The highest haemoglobin concentrations are in cord blood or a few hours later (normal range 17–22 g/dl). Concentrations below this indicate a high risk of anaemia in subsequent weeks. The haemoglobin drops to its lowest level at around 9 weeks of age and this is sometimes called physiological anaemia; values as low as 9.8 g/dl are then within normal limits

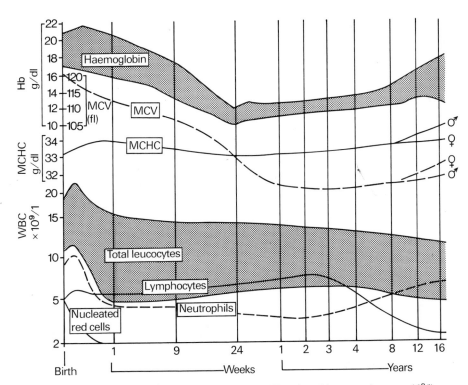

Fig. 19.1 Normal range of blood counts from birth to adult life. Hb (g/dl) and total leucocyte (count × 10⁹/l) ranges are shaded. Means values are given for mean corpuscular volume (MCV fl) and mean corpuscular haemoglobin concentration (MCHC g/dl). Cell counts are expressed as count × 10⁹/l and mean values are given for lymphocytes, neutrophils and nucleated red cells. (Data derived from tables of normal ranges given by Willoughby 1977, and Dacie & Lewis 1975)

2. The mean corpuscular volume (MCV) is high in preterm babies and at birth. After 9 weeks the MCV falls to adult values

3. It is normal to find nucleated red cells in the blood in the first few days of life

4. Leucocyte counts in the preterm infant are low. In all infants the count rises to a maximum 12 hours after birth mainly due to a short-lived neutrophil leucocytosis. Thereafter, lymphocytes are commoner than neutrophils until the age of 4–6 years when the lymphocyte count falls to adult values.

5. Coagulation times in the newborn infant are slightly prolonged, and platelet counts are marginally lower

6. Fetal haemoglobin persists above adult levels until 6 months of age; this must be remembered when investigating haemoglobinopathies in young infants.

HAEMATINICS AND VITAMINS

Iron

The commonest cause of anaemia in children is iron deficiency. Infants are particularly susceptible to iron deficiency for the following reasons:

1. Over 75 per cent of the body iron at birth is in the circulating red cells, bleeding can thus cause severe iron depletion

2. Human milk contains low amounts of iron (1.5 mg/l) and iron intake does not increase until a mixed diet is achieved. Up to 1 mg of iron must be absorbed daily to avoid deficiency. The circumstances shown in Table 19.1 predispose to iron deficiency anaemia.

Table 19.1 Conditions with predisposition to anaemia

Low birth weight and prematurity

Feeding with cow's milk (which contains only 0.5 mg iron/l)

Blood loss: placenta praevia, blood exchange between twins at birth, haemorrhage and venepuncture

Problems associated with the non-industrialised world: Hookworm anaemia and inadequate dietary iron

Coeliac disease and other malabsorption syndromes

Folic acid

Folic acid occurs in the form of polyglutamates in green vegetables. It is present in adequate amounts in human and dried cow's milk but not goat's milk. The daily requirement for infants is between 20–50 µg a day. Older children require up to 2 mg daily. Deficiency of folic acid is uncommon. Factors associated with folate depletion are shown in Table 19.2.

Table 19.2 Factors associated with folate depletion

Overheating milk and vegetable foods

Prematurity and low birth weight (infants less than 2 kg)

Infection

Malabsorption syndromes

Haemolysis

As a side effect of anticonvulsant therapy

Maternal folate depletion

Vitamin B12

Vitamin B12 is required as a co-factor in DNA synthesis and for metabolism of certain one-carbon molecules. There is a hepatic store at birth and it is present in adequate amounts in milk, eggs, meat and fish. Vitamin B12 dietary deficiency is rare, but does occur in vegetarian Gujarati Indians. B12 deficiency anaemia in childhood has several aetiologies (Table 19.3).

Table 19.3 Aetiologies of B12 deficiency anaemia

True juvenile pernicious anaemia: an autoimmune disease with antibodies to gastric parietal cells and intrinsic factor

Transcobalamin II deficiency: a defect in B12 transport (recessive inheritance)

Imersuland's syndrome: a defect of ileal receptors for vitamin B12 (recessive inheritance)

Maternal pernicious anaemia

Vitamin E

This vitamin is an antioxidant essential for normal red cell membrane function. Preterm infants are susceptible to Vitamin E deficiency and may develop haemolytic anaemia. Some neonatal units give routine supplements of the vitamin to extremely preterm infants.

Vitamin K

Deficiency of vitamin K leads to failure by the

liver to synthesise coagulation factors II, VII, IX, X giving a bleeding tendency with a prolonged prothrombin time. At birth, stores of vitamin K are derived from the mother and are rather variable; subsequently gut bacteria supply sufficient amounts. About one in 500 normal neonates has low levels of vitamin K and develops haemorrhage disease of the newborn. This is preventable by the routine intramuscular administration at birth of 1.0 mg synthetic vitamin K.

DISORDERS DUE TO MATERNOFETAL EXCHANGE

Maternal antibodies (IgG), drugs administered to the mother, and maternal infection can all cause haematological problems in the fetus and neonate (Table 19.4).

Table 19.4 Haematological disorders associated with materno-fetal exchange

Transfer of maternal antibody
Haemolytic anaemias
   Rh haemolytic disease
   ABO haemolytic disease
   haemolytic disease due to less common antigen differences (Kell, Lewis, Duffy)
   maternal autoimmune haemolytic anaemia

Megaloblastic anaemia
   maternal antibody to intrinsic factor
   transfer of LE (lupus erythematosus) factor

Neutropenia
   immunoneutropenia

Maternal drug ingestion
Haemolytic anaemia
   associated with infant G6PD deficiency e.g. sulphonamides, dapsone, quinine

Bleeding tendency
   warfarin, barbiturates, salicylates

Thrombocytopenia
   quinine, sulphonamides, thiazide diuretics (these drugs act in combination with a maternal antibody)

Haemolytic disease of the newborn

Rhesus disease

The rhesus (Rh) system consists of several red cell membrane antigens C, c, D, E, e, controlled by three gene pairs. Individuals lacking the D antigen (termed Rh negative) will make antibodies to red cells from Rh-positive individuals. Haemolytic disease of the newborn occurs when a sensitised Rh-negative mother gives birth to a Rh-positive infant. Sensitisation occurs in two ways:

1. Fetomaternal blood leak in the previous pregnancy usually at delivery
2. Prior transfusions of mother with Rh-positive blood.

The disease typically affects the second or subsequent pregnancies. IgG anti-D passes across the placenta and causes a haemolytic aneamia in the infant. Severe haemolysis causes cardiac failure (hydrops fetalis) and intrauterine death. Less severe haemolysis results in the birth of an anaemic and jaundiced infant at risk from brain damage from unconjugated bilirubin (kernicterus) and phototherapy or exchange transfusion is often indicated. Mild haemolysis without anaemia or clinical jaundice does not require treatment. The condition is now uncommon because of successful prevention and treatment of established haemolytic disease of the newborn in the following ways:

1. Blood group of all mothers checked at first antenatal visit
2. Rh-negative mothers at risk (Rh-positive father) are tested regularly in pregnancy for anti-D antibodies
3. No antibodies detected or antibodies in low titre not rising: give anti-D to mothers within 72 hours of delivery if infant is Rh positive
4. Rising antibody titres:
   a. before 28–32 weeks: amniocentesis and bilirubin estimation, fetal transfusion for high or rising bilirubin indicating a severe anaemia
   b. after 32 weeks: amniocentesis shows rising bilirubin, consider premature delivery by Caesarian section.

ABO haemolytic disease

ABO haemolytic disease is less common because maternal anti-A and anti-B antibodies are usually large IgM molecules and cannot cross the placenta. The disease usually affects Group A infants of a group O mother. Typically the disease is mild to moderate in severity. First-born infants can be affected. The direct Coombs' test is negative, and the blood film shows spherocytes. Phototherapy may be necessary.

ANTENATAL DIAGNOSIS OF HAEMOLYTIC DISORDERS

Parents of affected children seek advice about the risk of having further infants affected by lethal disorders or conditions which grossly impair normal life. Genetic counselling is necessary as a first step. The nature of the disease and the risks of future pregnancies are discussed with the parents. Specific investigation may be indicated, especially for haemophilia and β-thalassaemia.

Amniotic fluid sampling

The amniotic fluid can be used to measure abnormal fetal metabolites (markers for disease) or to obtain amnion cells for cellular and chromosome analysis (which therefore indicates the baby's sex). Male fetuses are sometimes aborted when the mother is a carrier of haemophilia.

Fetal blood sampling

This is done by fetoscopy and used in the diagnosis of haemophilia (assessment of factor VIII antigen and its coagulation antigen by immunoassay) and thalassaemia major where rates of β-haemoglobin chain synthesis (defective in thalassaemia) can be measured in the circulating fetal normoblasts.

THE PRETERM INFANT

Preterm infants are particularly susceptible to bacterial infection which can prove fatal unless diagnosed and treated early. Infection should be suspected when toxic granulation, vacuolation or a left shift of neutrophils is seen (appearance in the blood of non-segmented juvenile cells). The neutrophil count is not helpful since although it may rise initially it falls in life-threatening infections. Serious bacterial infection in neonates and

particularly in preterm infants frequently triggers off disseminated intravascular coagulation with bleeding due to microangiopathic haemolytic anaemia. The haematological management of perterm infants is shown in Table 19.5.

Table 19.5 Haematological management of preterm infants

1. *Maintain a high index of suspicion for bacterial infection:* request careful evaluation of the blood film; treat early with broad spectrum antibiotics

2. *Investigate bleeding tendencies:* give vitamin K if prothrombin time is prolonged and correct disseminated intravascular coagulation with appropriate factors, fresh frozen plasma, cryoprecipitate or platelets

3. *Preterm infants develop an exaggerated physiological anaemia:* this can be minimised by giving routine supplements of iron (30 mg daily) folic acid (1 mg daily) and vitamin E (25 iu daily). Blood transfusion is required if the haemoglobin at birth is less than 13 g/dl. Remember venesection for investigations can cause significant blood loss

ANAEMIA IN CHILDHOOD

Thalassaemia syndromes (See also Chapter 25)

Adult haemoglobin (HbA) is formed from two α globin chains and two β, γ, δ or ε chains. Thalassaemia is a defect of the genes organising globin synthesis. HbA is made in reduced amounts in the heterozygous state (thalassaemia minor) and in negligible amounts in the homozygous state (thalassaemia major). Fetal haemoglobin ($\alpha 2 \gamma 2$) and haemoglobin A2 ($\alpha 2 \delta$) synthesis is not impaired. The thalassaemia defect causes a severe disorder of red cell maturation associated with massive destruction of defective cells in the bone marrow, and chronic haemolysis (Table 19.6). The gene occurs commonly in people of Mediterranean and Oriental origin.

Clinical features and management

Thalassaemia minor. A lifelong mild asymptomatic anaemia which requires no treatment. Iron therapy should not be given.

Thalassaemia major. Due to chronic haemolysis: failure to thrive, bony abnormalities including skull bossing and mongoloid face, hepatospleno-

Table 19.6 Typical laboratory profile for β-thalassaemia

	Thalassaemia minor	Thalassaemia major
Haemoglobin	10.4 g/dl	5.1 g/dl
MCV	67 fl	58 fl
Red cell count	4.8×10^{12}/l	4.9×10^{12}/l
Film comment	Iron deficiency appearance	Leptocytes, poikilocytes, hypochromia, target cells, 10% nucleated red cells/100 WBC
Serum iron	30μmol/l	42 μmol/l
saturation	94%	98%
Serum ferritin	350 μg/l	780 μg/l (normal upper limit 340 μg/l
HbA2	3.1%	2.8%
HbF	1.1%	97%

megaly. Due to chronic anaemia: haemosiderosis, bronzing of skin, cardiac failure. Treatment involves blood transfusion, iron chelation with desferrioxamine (home use of subcutaenous infusion pump) and splenectomy.

Sickle cell anaemia

A haemoglobinopathy caused by synthesis of an *abnormal* globin chain (compare this with thalassaemia), where there is a defect in the formation of normal haemoglobin. A single substitution of valine for glutamine on the β globin chain leads to a haemoglobin molecule abnormally susceptible to precipitation when the blood oxygen tension falls. The crystallisation of the molecule deforms the red cell to a sickle shape, which is rigid and blocks capillaries, leading to hypoxia and further sickling in the sickle crisis (homozygotes only) (Table 19.7). The disorder is common in West Africans.

Clinical features

Heterozygotes. None.

Homozygotes. Tall thin build, chronic anaemia with frequent painful crises of haemolysis and sickling, often precipitated by infection, dehydration, or acidosis. Chronic haemolysis leads to gallstones, bony changes, leg ulcers and dactylitis. There is an increased incidence of Salmonella arthritis.

Mangement

Painful crises require treatment of the precipitating cause, and support with fluids, bicarbonate, and adequate analgesia. Before major operations red-cell exchange is necessary.

Glucose-6-phosphate-dehydrogenase (G6PD) deficiency

A group of red cell enzymer defects. The defect

Table 19.7 Typical laboratory profile for sickle cell disease

	Sickle cell trait (heterozygote)	Sickle cell disease (homozygote)
Haemoglobin	Normal	10.0 g/dl
Film	Normal	Target cells Occasional sickle cells Howell-Jolly bodies
'Sickledex' screen	Positive	Positive
Hb electrphoresis	Two bands: A and S	One band in the S region

Table 19.8 Typical laboratory profile for G6PD deficiency

	During attack	Between attacks
Haemoglobin	5.2 g/dl	12.4 g/dl
Reticulocytes	13%	1.2%
White count	$18.0 \times 10^9/l$	$6.4 \times 10^9/l$
Film	Crescent cells and spherocytes seen	Normal
Heinz bodies	Numerous	None seen
Urine	Methaemoglobin	Normal
Brilliant cresyl blue decolouration screen and G6PD assay	May be normal because reticulocytes contain the enzyme	Abnormal

causes haemoglobin to be unusually susceptible to damage by oxidation. It precipitates in the red cell as Heinz bodies, and causes acute intravascular haemolysis. Inheritance is sex-linked, female carriers having intermediate enzyme levels between normal and affected individuals. There are several varieties: African (primaquine sensitive), European (including favism), and Oriental (Table 19.8).

Clinical features

Acute attacks of haemolysis with prostration, pallor, rigors, loin pain and methaemoglobinuria; precipitated by ingestion of oxidants or occasionally by non-specific factors including infection.

Management

Prevent haemolytic episodes by identifying and avoiding precipitating causes. Treat acute attack symptomatically with analgesia and fluids. Occasionally methylene blue and vitamin C (antioxidants) may be required.

Hereditary spherocytosis

A chronic haemolytic anaemia of varying severity due to defective red-cell membrane sodium transport. Red cells accumulate fluid and become spheres with increased osmotic fragility (Table 19.9). Inheritance is autosomal dominant.

Table 19.9 Typical laboratory profile for spherocytosis

Haemoglobin	10.5 g/dl
MCV	78 fl
Reticulocytes	12%
Film comment	Numerous spherocytes
Direct Coombs' test	Negative
	Increased fragility
Immediate and 24-hour incubated osmotic fragility	

Clinical features

Chronic haemolysis, mild jaundice, pallor, spenomegaly, gallstones and occasionally leg ulcers and bony changes. Aplastic crises following viral infections and haemolytic crises can occur.

Management

Splenectomy is indicated if the disorder is severe.

Autoimmune haemolytic anaemia

In childhood this is usually an acute haemolytic episode often following viral infections, presenting with pallor, jaundice and occasionally purpura (Table 19.10).

Management

Steroid therapy and blood transfusion may be necessary. The condition is usually self limiting.

Table 19.10 Typical laboratory features of autoimmune haemolytic anaemia

Haemoglobin	6.1 g/dl
MCV	108 fl
Reticulocytes	28%
Nucleated red cells	12/100 leucocytes
White count	$14 \times 10^9/1$
Film comment	Spherocytes and polychromasia, toxic granulation
Direct Coombs' test	Positive

Aplastic anaemia

Bone marrow stem cell failure leads to grossly reduced production of red cells, granulocytes and platelets. Fanconi type aplasia is a congenital bone marrow hypoplasia often with other mesodermal abnormalities. Aplasia may follow viral infection such as hepatitis A or as an idiosyncratic response to drugs and toxins such as chloramphenicol, pesticides and model aeroplane glue. However, in 50 per cent of cases no antecedent cause can be determined. These cases are termed idiopathic aplastic anaemia (Table 19.11).

Table 19.11 Typical laboratory features of severe aplastic anaemia

Haemoglobin	6.0 g/dl
Reticulocytes	0.2% ($12 \times 10^9/1$)
White count	$2.4 \times 10^9/1$ (2% neutrophils, 98% lymphocytes)
Platelets	$15 \times 10^9/1$
Bone marrow aspirate	Hypocellular particles with reduced haematopoiesis in all lines
Bone marrow trephine	Hypocellular fatty marrow with occasional foci of lymphocytes. Haematopoietic cells are severely reduced

Clinical features

Presentation with pallor, bruising and infection. Absence of splenomegaly and bone pain helps to distinguish this condition from acute leukaemia and thrombocytopenic purpura. Fanconi patients have a characteristic facial appearance, café-au-lait spots and a tendency to short stature, microcephaly, hypoplastic or horsehoe kidneys, cardiac defects and bony abnormalities of thumb and radius.

Management

Mild cases and patients with Fanconi-type aplasia respond to androgens such as oxymethalone. Severe cases, patients with life-threatening bleeding requiring transfusions should be considered for bone marrow transplantation, if a donor can be found. Around one-third of the patients may respond to immunosuppressive treatment with antilymphocyte 10 globin or large doses of methyl-prednisolone.

HAEMORRHAGIC DISORDERS

A scheme for investigation and diagnosis of bleeding disorders is shown in Table 19.12. Some of the commoner coagulation disorders are described.

Haemophilia syndromes

These include factor VIII deficiency (haemophilia A), factor IX deficiency (haemophilia B) and von Willebrand's disease (VIII deficiency with a platelet disorder). The incidence of severe inherited bleeding disorders in the UK is in the order of 150 per million. One-half of these patients have classic haemophilia (factor VIII deficiency) (Table 19.13).

Clinical features.

Haemophilia is characterised by recurrent haemarthrosis which can lead to crippling deformities due to joint destruction and pressure damage on adjacent nerves and blood vessels. Trauma can lead to relentless bleeding into confined spaces such as muscle sheaths and the retroperitoneal area causing dangerous pressure damage to adjacent structures. Presentation is often in the first year of life but less severe cases may present later in childhood. In von Willebrand's disease, nosebleeds and

Table 19.12 Investigating haemorrhagic disorders (Screen: platelet count, prothrombin time (PT), kaolin cephalin coagulation time (KCCT), blood film)

Finding	Indicates	Further investigations
Two or more abnormalities + red cell fragmentation	Disseminated intravascular coagulation with microangiopathic haemolytic anaemia	Fibrinogen titre or thrombin time Fibrin degradation products (FDPs) Identify cause of DIC
Prolonged PT	Liver defects Vitamin K deficiency Hereditary defect of factor VII (rare)	Give vitamin K and test again Factor VII assay
Prolonged KCCT	Haemophilia von Willebrand's disease Other hereditary defects	Factor VIII assay and Factor VIII antigen estimation Platelet aggregation tests Other factor assays
Prolonged PT and KCCT	Hereditary factor X, II or I deficiency Dysfibrinogenaemias (rare)	Fibrinogen titre Thrombin time Factor assays Plasma electrophosis, search for cryofibrins
No abnormality detected	Platelet function defect Vascular purpuras von Willebrand's disease in 'good phase'	Platelet aggregation Bleeding time Examination of patient for telangiectasia Retest at a later date

Table 19.13 Typical coagulation results of haemophilia syndromes

	Haemophilia (VIII deficiency	von Willebrand's disease
Prothrombin time	14 s	14 s (control 14 s)
Kaolin cephalin coagulation time	170 s	58 (control 35 s)
Factor VIII coagulation assay	4%	50%
Factor VIII antigen	105%	48%
Bleeding time	Normal	Prolonged
Platelet aggregation with ristocetin	Normal	Impaired

gastrointestinal haemorrhage are characteristic and haemarthroses are less common.

Management

The care of these disease is specialised and should be carried out in conjunction with a haemophilia centre. Home treatment with intravenous freeze-dried factor VIII has done much to improve the quality of life of children with severe haemophilia. They should be encouraged to attend normal schools.

Disseminated intravascular coagulation (DIC)

A variety of triggers to the coagulation process can provoke DIC. Three pathological processes are involved in the syndrome:
1. Consumption of coagulation protein and platelets with a consequent tendency to bleed
2. Small vessel fibrin deposition with damage to susceptible organs such as kidney, brain and lungs, and damage to red cells by intravascular fibrin strands causing red-cell fragmentation and haemolysis

3. Activated fibrinolysis causes breakdown of fibrin producing circulating fibrin degradation products, a useful laboratory marker of DIC.

Two clinical entities are recognised: consumption coagulopathy and microangiopathic haemolytic anaemia, which represent the two ends of the spectrum of clinical presentations.

Consumption coagulopathy

Acute bleeding tendency is the major problem e.g. Waterhouse-Friedrichson syndrome (Table 19.14).

Clinical features. (e.g. meningococcal septicaemia) Presentation is with severe toxaemia and meningitis, bleeding from venepuncture sites, purpura and nosebleeds. Rapid improvement with intravenous antibiotic therapy and transfusion with frozen plasma and platelets.

Table 19.14 Typical laboratory features of consumption coagulopathy

Haemoglobin	12.4 g/dl
WBC	16 × 10α/l
Film comment	Left shift, toxic granulation and Döhle bodies
Platelets	26 ×10⁹/l
Prothrombin time 18 s,	18 s, control 12 s
Kaolin cephalin coagulation time	64 s, control 5 s
Fibrinogen titre	< 1 in 16
Fibrinogen degradation products	40 units per ml

Microangiopathic haemolytic anaemia

Organ damage is the major problem. The coagulation protein consumption is chronic and partially

Table 19.15 Typical features of microangiopathic haemolytic anaemia

Haemoglobin	8.2 g/dl
WBC	7.2 × 10⁹/l
Film comment	Fragments, schistocytes and burr cells, polychromasia
Platelet count	90 × 10⁹/l
Fibrin degradation products	40 units per ml
Prothrombin time	14 s, control 12 s
Kaolin cephalin coagulation time	38 s, control 35 s

compensated, e.g. haemolytic uraemic syndrome (Table 19.15).

Clinical features. Presentation is with uraemia, mild jaundice and renal failure.

Management. Treat acute renal failure and replace coagulation factors and platelets if there is a serious bleeding tendency. Heparin can prevent further fibrin deposition but its use is disputed.

Thrombocytopenia

A low platelet count may be due either to decreased production of platelets by megakaryocytes or increased consumption. Table 19.16 lists the causes of thrombocytopenia.

Idiopathic thrombocytopenic purpura (ITP)

This condition is usually an acute self-limiting disorder in childhood and frequently follows viral infection.

Clinical features

Abrupt onset with bruising, bleeding and epistaxes

Table 19.16 Causes of thrombocytopenia

Due to decreased megakaryocyte production
Drug induced, aplastic anaemia, acute leukaemia, congenital amegakaryocytic thrombocytopenia (TAR syndrome), Wiskott-Adrich syndrome

Due to increased platelet consumption
Maternal anti-platelet antibodies, maternal idopathic thrombocytopenia (ITP), drug-induced autoantibodies, ITP, consumption coagulopthy and microangiopathic haemolytic anaemia (e.g giant haemangiomas)

Congenital infections
Rubella, syphilis, toxoplasmosis

about 2–6 weeks after a viral infection. The bleeding tendency is often less severe than the bleeding count would suggest. The laboratory features are given in Table 19.17

Table 19.17 Typical laboratory features of ITP

Haemoglobin	12.8 g/dl
WBC	8.4 g 10⁹/l
Platelets	10 × 10⁹/l
Bleeding time	15 minutes (normal range 7–11 minutes)
Prothrombin time and kaolin cephalin coagulation time	Normal
Bone marrow aspirate	Cellular with increased megakaryocyte numbers many of which are rounded, small and darkly staining. No increase on blasts is seen

Management

Treatment is not always necessary. Steroids are indicated if bleeding is severe or life-threatening.

Splenectomy is effective if the disease becomes chronic.

DISEASES ASSOCIATED WITH AN INCREASED TENDENCY TO INFECTION

A scheme for investigating a suspected immune deficiency is outlined in Table 19.18.

Neutropenia

Reduction in circulating granulocyte numbers associated with an increased risk of bacterial and fungal infection may be due to:

1. Defective stem cells: cyclic neutropenia, aplastic anaemia, drug-induced e.g. anti-cancer chemotherapy (predictable), chloramphenicol idiosyncrasy
2. Defective neutrophil maturation: Kostmann type, Schwachmann type
3. Excessive consumption: immune neutropenia (transfer of maternal antibody); drug-induced autoantibody e.g. quinidine and amidopyrine idiopathic autoantibody

Table 19.18 Investigating a suspected immune defect (Screening test: full blood count including differential leucocyte count, immunoglobulins)

Finding	Possibilities	Further investigation
Neutropenia	Transient — associated with infection Drug induced Congenital (including cyclic neutropenia)	Repeat neutrophil counts History of drug ingestion Bone marrow aspirate, trephine Cell cultures (CFU-C assay)
	Hypersplenism	Test maternal serum for antibodies to neutrophils
Neutropenia with pancytopenia	Aplastic anaemia Acute leukaemia secondary to chronic infection, disseminated malignancy	Family studies Bone marrow aspirate and trephine CFU-C assays Microbiological culture
Lymphopenia with or without hypogammaglobulinaemia	Transient — associated with infection congenital immune deficiency disease: severe combined immune deficiency, di George syndrome, ataxia telangectasia Common variable immune deficiency, Bruton-type hypogammaglobulinaemia	Repeat blood counts X-ray for thymic shadow T and B lymphocyte numbers PHA and mixed lymphocyte culture, lymphocyte response
Normal or raised blood count	Granulocyte function defects: Chronic granulomatous disease, myeloperoxidase deficiency, Chediak-Higashi syndrome, chemotactic defects — lazy leucocyte syndrome, specific defect to staphylococcus (Job's syndrome)	NBT (nitro blue tetrazolium) test Candida and staphylococcal killing test Chemotaxis, and granulocyte kinetic studies

4. Defective mobilisation from bone marrow:
lazy leucotye syndrome.

Clinical and laboratory features

Fungal infections classically affecting the mouth
and throat, skin, perianal region lungs and bones.
Immunoglobulins are often increased due to
chronic infection and splenomegaly is common. In
cyclic neutropenia there is a clear history of short-
lived episodes of infection occurring at 3-weekly
intervals. The severity varies according to the
condition and aetiology. Neutrophil counts greater
than $0.2 \times 10^9/1$, compensatory monocytosis and
eosinophilia are good prognostic features. Death
in infancy is likely in Kostmamann's type neutropenia, but others are compatible with prolonged
life and the disorder due to maternal antibody is
self limiting.

Management

This depends on the aetiology. Supportive care
may include the use of oral, non-absorbable antibiotics to reduce the risk of infection from body
flora; early use of intravenous antibiotics if
systemic infection occurs; and long-term antibiotic
cover for pulmonary infections. In life-threatening
conditions, bone marrow transplantation is indicated.

Defective granulocyte function

A number of rare conditions present with bacterial
and fungal infections, and failure to thrive associated with normal granulocyte numbers but
defective function. These conditions include

chronic granulomatous disease (CGD), a defect of
intracellular neutrophil killing; myeloperoxidase
deficiency; lazy leucocyte syndrome, a defect of
neutrophil chemotaxis; Chediak-Higashi syndrome,
defective lysozymal vacuoles; and Job's syndrome, a particular susceptibility to staphylococcal
infection.

Many of these conditions are compatible with
prolonged survival, but bone marrow transplantation is being increasingly used with success in
CGD.

Laboratory features

In these conditions the neutrophil count is normal
or raised and the diagnosis can only be made by
tests of granulocyte function (see Table 19.4).

**Impaired lymphocyte function and antibody
synthesis:**

There is a large group of conditions where an
increased tendency to overwhelming infection
form bacteria, fungi and viruses are due to defective lymphocyte function (see Chapter 13).

FURTHER READING

Barrett A J 1980 Bone marrow transplantation. Archives of
    Disease of Childhood 55: 750–752
Dacie & Lewis 1975 Practical haematology. Churchill
    Livingstone, Edinburgh, p 12
Glader B E (ed) 1978 Perinatal haematology. In: Clinics in
    Haematology, Sanders, London
Voke J, Madgwick C, Normandy K 1980 Haemophilia centre
    handbook, Immuno Ltd,
Willoughby M L (ed) 1977 Paediatric haematology. Churchill
    Livingstone, Edinburgh

20

Endocrine and metabolic disease

DIABETES MELLITUS

Juvenile-onset diabetes mellitus affects approximately one in every 1500 children under 15 years of age and is almost invariably insulin dependent. Onset can occur at any age from birth to adolescence with a peak incidence between 5–12 years of age. The aetiology remains unknown although there is a seasonal variation in incidence and onset often follows a viral infection. There is no definite pattern of inheritance but diabetic children have a higher number of first degree relatives with diabetes than non-diabetic children suggesting genetic predisposition or an autoimmune basis for the disease. Environment may also play a large part in the development of the condition.

Diabetes mellitus presents more acutely in childhood than in the adult, the onset being marked by tiredness, polyuria, polydypsia and weight loss. These symptoms may have been present for 4–6 weeks or only noticeable for a few days. Other warning signs of developing diabetes include secondary nocturnal enuresis, monilial or staphylococcal skin infections and blurring of vision. When the diagnosis is suspected the child should be referred immediately to avoid progression to diabetic keto-acidosis.

Most children are not seriously ill when first seen and the diagnosis is usually made before the stage of dehydration and coma is reached. The diagnosis is confirmed by finding glycosuria on urine testing plus an elevated blood glucose level; a glucose tolerance test is seldom required in children.

Management

The management of diabetes aims to achieve blood glucose levels as near normal as possible by obtaining a balance between calorie intake, insulin requirements and energy expenditure. At the same time the child must be helped to lead a full and active life. Many factors such as exercise, illness and anxiety may disturb the diabetic balance but insulin dosage and dietary intake are the two factors which can be manipulated to improve blood glucose control.

1. Insulin

In the majority of children presenting with mild symptoms, treatment is commenced with a single daily injection of a long-acting insulin such as Rapitard insulin given before breakfast. Intermittent doses of short-acting insulin before main meals over the initial 24-hour period will give some indication of daily insulin requirement. Whatever the selected dosage of insulin, alterations will be necessary during the first few days, and an appropriate regimen may not be achieved until the child is in the home environment. In the early months following diagnosis, there is often a honeymoon period when insulin requirements decrease markedly for a variable length of time. This is due to the child's pancreas producing small amounts of endogenous insulin and the daily insulin dosage must be reduced accordingly.

If good diabetic control is not achieved on a single daily injection of long-acting insulin, this regimen may have to be modified by adding some short-acting insulin or by giving insulin twice a day. Many adolescent patients find their diabetic control much improved on twice daily insulin and their lifestyle more flexible. Insulin is now available as standard 100 unit/ml insulin and a special small disposable syringe is available for children. The new purified mono-component insulins are less antigenic, effective in smaller dosage than the standard insulins and are increasingly used for newly diagnosed diabetics. Changing from standard to mono-component insulin may lead to a reduction in total dosage and an alteration in duration of action which can precipitate hypoglycaemia. Injection sites should be checked at intervals as some children prefer to inject repeatedly into the same area which is less painful but may adversely affect absorption if local hypertrophy occurs. Lipoatrophy may develop at injection sites but can be avoided by changing to mono-component insulin.

2. Diet

Diets for diabetic children should provide adequate daily calories for growth and energy requirements, food being offered at regular intervals during the day to complement insulin action. Usually this means three main meals of breakfast, lunch and evening meal with snacks mid-morning, mid-afternoon and at bedtime. The carbohydrate content of the diet is calculated as 100 g per day for a child aged one year and an additional 10 g for each subsequent year of age. Protein and fats are not usually restricted. Portions of carbohydrate are divided between meals, providing approximately 25 per cent of each main meal and 5–10 per cent of each snack. This is only a rough guide and food intake must be adjusted to the appetite and energy requirements of the individual. Initially food is weighed but with experience food allowances can be gauged accurately without weighing. Concentrated sweet foods should be avoided as the glucose is absorbed too rapidly for the available insulin.

3. Control

Assessment of blood glucose control is based on the presence or absence of symptoms of hyperglycaemia or hypoglycaemia, and on routine urine testing for glycosuria using the Clinitest two drop method. This provides an indirect and retrospective assessment of blood glucose; ideally the bladder should be emptied twice in succession and

the second specimen tested. Urinalysis is performed four times a day at first, before main meals and at bedtime but, when the diabetes is stable, twice daily testing is adequate. Testing before breakfast and the evening meal gives an indication of the duration and strength of action of the long-acting insulin. Blood glucose monitoring is now possible at home and some adolescents manage their diabetes using the finger prick blood test in preference to urine tests. Serial values are needed to assess control over a 24-hour period.

Diabetic keto-acidosis

The child presenting with severe dehydration and keto-acidosis is dangerously ill and requires emergency treatment. Symptoms include recent weight loss, vomiting, abdominal pain and hyperventilation. The patient is clinically dehydrated and drowsy with marked Kussmaul respiration. In severe cases there is peripheral circulatory collapse, oliguria and coma. Pneumonia and salicylate poisoning should be considered in the differential diagnosis. When severe abdominal pain is present there may be tenderness and guarding and exclusion of an acute abdominal condition is very difficult. Correction of the dehydration and acidosis will gradually relieve the pain if it is secondary to the keto-acidosis.

The three main principles of treatment are rehydration, correction of hyperglycaemia with insulin, and correction of the metabolic acidosis.

1. Correction of dehydration is the first priority and an intravenous infusion of 0.9 per cent saline should be commenced immediately to run at 10–20 ml per kg body weight over the first hour. At the same time blood is taken for estimation of blood glucose, urea and serum electrolytes, pH and bicarbonate and for blood culture. If the patient is shocked, plasma may be given initially followed by 0.9 per cent saline. The patient should be weighed if possible and the degree of dehydration estimated clinically. Fluid replacement is then calculated as the approximate percentage of body weight lost, e.g. 5 or 10 per cent dehydration, plus maintenance fluid requirements for 24 hours. One-half of this total fluid requirement should be given in the first 8 hours and the remainder over the following 16 hours. The amount of fluid required

may have to be readjusted according to urine output as an osmotic diuresis may persist if the blood glucose level is slow to fall. After the first 2 hours the intravenous (i.v.) fluid should be changed to 0.45 per cent saline to avoid sodium overload, and 4.2 per cent dextrose/0.18 per cent saline introduced when the blood glucose falls below 14 mmol/l.

Strict measurement of fluid intake and output is essential to indicate when the patient is in positive fluid balance. A specimen of urine should be obtained as soon as possible and tested for glucose and ketones. Bladder catheterisation is rarely necessary except in the comatose, severely dehydrated patient. Oral fluids should not be given and, if vomiting persists or the patient is unconcious, the stomach should be emptied via a naso-gastric tube. In the concious patient small amounts of ice may be sucked to relieve intense thirst.

Potassium should be added to the i.v. fluid as there is a deficit in total body potassium in keto-acidosis, and 26 mmol/l of fluid is adequate. Ideally, the potassium should only be added after insulin has been given, after the patient has passed urine, and when the initial serum potassium is known.

2. Soluble or short-acting insulin is always used in emergency treatment and may be given as inter-mittent intramuscular i.m. doses or as a continuous i.v. infusion. Using the i.m. route the initial dose is 0.5 units/kg body weight up to a maximum of 10 units, followed by 0.1 units/kg 2-hourly accord-ing to blood glucose levels. Subcutaneous insulin is poorly absorbed in the dehydrated patient and the i.m. route is preferred.

Constant i.v. infusion of insulin produces excel-lent blood glucose control but requires extremely close patient observation and facilities for hourly blood glucose estimations with promptly available results. The initial dosage is 0.1 units/kg over the first hour up to a maximum dose of 10 units, the insulin being administered by a syringe pump connected to the i.v. infusion. Insulin must not be added to the main i.v. infusion fluid as accurate control of dosage is difficult. The subsequent hourly insulin dose is adjusted according to the rate of fall of blood glucose.

3. Correction of acidosis using i.v. sodium bicar-bonate may be necessary if the arterial pH is less than 7.1. Above this level rehydration and insulin alone may lead to spontaneous correction of the acidosis. If sodium bicarbonate is used the amount required is that needed to half correct the base deficit and should be diluted in the main infusion fluid. The amount can be calculated from the formula:

$$\text{mmol bicarbonate} = 1/10 \text{ (base excess} \times \text{body weight in kg)}$$

Use of bicarbonate increases the risk of cerebral oedema because of the extra sodium load, and may induce hypokalaemia due to the more rapid shift of potassium into the cells.

Frequent clinical re-assessment is essential in managing diabetic keto-acidosis and the basic guide-lines for treatment must be modified according to the patient's response. Blood samples for glucose, electrolytes, pH and bicarbonate should be repeated at 2–4 hourly intervals until the metabolic imbalance is corrected. Flow sheets are invaluable for monitoring fluid balance and biochemical changes.

Once rehydration is achieved and the clinical condition improved the child may be established on a 4-hourly sliding scale of soluble insulin given according to urine and blood glucose measure-ments. When a regular diet is tolerated long-acting insulin is introduced and the diabetes stabilised as in the non-emergency presentation.

Hypoglycaemia

In achieving blood glucose levels as near normal as possible there is a risk of episodic hypogly-caemia. Excess insulin, delayed meals, omitting a snack or unexpected vigorous exercise can all precipitate hypoglycaemia. Most children learn to anticipate a mild attack of hypoglycaemia by recognising the symptoms of headache, hunger and faintness and take preventive action by eating glucose. All children should carry glucose tablets or sweets with them wherever they are, especially at school or on the playing field. Irritability is a common sign of hypoglycaemia which parents may notice. Severe nocturnal hypoglycaemia may cause loss of conciousness and convulsions which are extremely frightening for both parents and child, and carry the risk of neurological damage.

Treatment of the unconcious patient consists of

an i.m. injection of glucagon 1 mg which will improve concious level sufficiently for the patient to take oral glucose. Parents should know how to inject glucagon and keep an ampoule at home. An intravenous infusion of dextrose may be required if the child is vomiting, if the hypoglycaemia has been prolonged or has resulted from excess long-acting insulin.

Long-term management

Most diabetic children enjoy active and healthy lives and rarely require hospital admission. Successful long-term management is based on education of the child and his family at the time of diagnosis, providing them with a full understanding of the disease and its treatment. During the initial hospital admission the family are taught to test urine, inject insulin and regulate the diet. Many families are grateful for an initial period of hospitalisation as a breathing space during which they can adjust to the diagnosis. Much of the information provided is not absorbed at this time and understanding of the management of diabetes comes gradually once the child is at home. Teaching can be done at home by a community nurse experienced in diabetes and many problems such as hypoglycaemia resolved as they arise in the home environment.

Opportunities must be available for the family to ask questions and contact with other families who have a diabetic child may be helpful. A telephone number of a doctor or nurse experienced in diabetes should be available to families 24 hours of the day to provide guidance in the event of an emergency. Periodic visits either to the general practitioner or hospital clinic, usually 3-monthly when stable, provide an opportunity to monitor growth and maturation and resolve any fresh problems.

Various factors affect long-term diabetic control, particularly in children who are growing and changing physically and emotionally. Frequent episodes of keto-acidosis are not uncommon in adolescent girls, and often precede menstruation. Emotional disturbances may produce hyperglycaemia and ketosis, and poor diabetic control may be a reflection of unhappiness or family instability. Other forms of stress such as school examinations, have a similar effect. During adolescence there is often a natural rebellion against the discipline of routine and diet but this usually resolves with family support. Re-education of a teenage patient may be helpful, especially if the diagnosis was made very early in life, as this may encourage self-confidence and independence from parents. The transition from paediatric to adult diabetic clinic can be a difficult step, and fears of long-term complications such as blindness often resurface at this time.

Illness may temporarily increase insulin requirements and patients are advised to test their urine more frequently if they feel unwell. If a child is vomiting or anorexic the normal dose of insulin should be given, and calorie equivalents to the diet taken in fluid form. To avoid major crises a doctor should be contacted if a diabetic child has vomited more than twice in succession, if heavy glycosuria is persisting despite increase in insulin dosage, If ketonuria is present or if the child feels unwell.

GROWTH

Growth and development are two of the main parameters for assessing health and well-being in children, and measurement of height, weight and head circumference should be an integral part of paediatric examination. Normal growth depends on thyroxine, growth hormone and androgens which produce the pubertal growth spurt.

Short stature

Initial assessment of the short child is based on a careful history and physical examination including details of pregnancy, birth history and time of onset of growth retardation. Measurement of height and weight must be accurate and values plotted on a standard growth chart (see Chapter 3). All measurements must be evaluated in the context of family size and the heights of parents, grandparents and siblings should be recorded. A height below that expected for the family is likely to be significant. If the child's height is below the third percentile for his age it is important to ascertain whether he has always been among the smallest in his class. History of changes in size of clothes or shoes suggests recent growth. Physical examination will reveal signs of systemic disease, malnutrition or genetic abnormalities, e.g. unusual facies, webbing of the neck or abnormal palmar creases.

Investigation of a child whose height is below the third percentile should include routine urinalysis and estimation of skeletal maturation by measuring the radiological bone age. An X-ray of the left wrist (knee in infants under one year) can be compared with standards provided by Greulich and Pyle. If the bone age is significantly delayed, serum T4 (thyroxine) and TSH levels should be performed to exclude hypothyroidism. A skull X-ray may show evidence of a pituitary tumour such as a craniopharyngioma. When there is a history of progressive growth retardation then measurement of growth velocity is essential. Two height recordings taken 6 months apart are adequate to demonstrate the rate of growth. A normal height velocity excludes both hypothyroidism and growth hormone deficiency. If there has been a definite fall off in height then growth hormone levels should be measured. Random values are difficult to interpret and specific stimulation tests are required which also evaluate other aspects of pituitary function.

Table 20.1 Causes of growth retardation in childhood

Intrauterine growth retardation
Malnutrition
Chronic systemic disease
Genetic defects
Psychosocial deprivation
Endocrine disorders
Hypothyroidism, hypopituitarism, excess glucocorticoids
Russell-Silver dwarfism
Cystic fibrosis, renal failure, coeliac disease, cardiac defects
Turner's syndrome, achondroplasia, osteogenesis imperfecta

Table 20.1 lists the main causes of short stature in childhood. Hypothyroidism and hypopituitarism are the most important endocrine causes, Hypopituitarism or isolated growth hormone deficiency may both be congenital or acquired, the acquired form occurring in children who have received cranial irradiation for CNS leukaemia or tumour. Growth hormone is secreted by the anterior pituitary and acts via somatomedin which directly increases the growth rate of epiphyseal cartilage.

Children with growth hormone deficiency may grow well for the first 2 years of life before becoming noticeably short. They may suffer episodes of neonatal hypoglycaemia. In appearance they are small and slightly obese with round, doll-like faces. Intelligence is normal. Those patients proven to be growth hormone deficient on formal testing respond well to treatment with intramuscular injections of human growth hormone 5 iu three times a week. Treatment should be continued throughout puberty.

Steroid therapy suppresses growth and many children on long-term steroids are short. This effect may be due to a combination of steroid effect plus the underlying chronic disease, but when steroid therapy is discontinued these patients show catch up growth.

Psychosocial deprivation can present as short stature. Investigation will show normal thyroid function but growth hormone levels may be low. When placed in a favourable environment the child will gain weight and show catch up linear growth. Growth hormone levels return to normal in the right environment.

During adolescence growth hormone and androgens act synergistically to produce the pubertal growth spurt. Delay in onset of puberty may cause much anxiety due to the relative short stature, but this delay is usually constitutional and ultimately a normal adult height is attained.

Tall stature

Tall stature is a relatively uncommon problem. Tall parents have tall children but parental concern may arise if one child, usually a daughter, appears to be growing excessively tall. Height prediction will often indicate an ultimate height equal to that of the mother and, if this is acceptable no intervention is necessary. The treatment available is to induce an early puberty with oestrogens, but this is not to be undertaken lightly. Most girls present after the onset of puberty and once menses are established growth is almost complete.

Marfan's and Klinefelter's syndromes may present as tall stature. Excess growth hormone production is rare and is usually due to an eosinophilic granuloma of the pituitary.

Obesity

Simple obesity is associated with tall stature, the height often being at or above the 97th centile. In a child presenting with obesity and short stature an endocrine cause is more likely. There is rarely an endocrine cause underlying simple obesity but these individuals seem to have lower calorie requirements, are less active and expend less energy than slimmer people. Treatment depends on re-educating the family to eat a well-balanced diet and support the child in reducing caloric intake. At the same time exercise should be encouraged. Unless the child and family are well motivated to adjust their eating pattern, significant weight loss is not easily achieved. The main endocrine causes of obesity are hypothyroidism, steroid therapy and, rarely, Cushing's syndrome. All three conditions are associated with short stature and other physical features to suggest the diagnosis.

THYROID DISORDERS

Congenital hypothyroidism

This condition affects one in every 4000 infants born and many cases are clinically undetectable at birth. For this reason, neonatal thyroid screening programmes are being introduced to detect cases and institute treatment early. Delay in treatment beyond 3 months of age adversely affects prognosis and may cause mental retardation.

The hypothyroid baby is quiet, lethargic and slow with feeds. There may be prolonged jaundice in the neonatal period. Physical examination may reveal poor peripheral circulation with cool extremities, an umbilical hernia, distended abdomen, dry skin, a poorly sustained cry and widely open fontanelles. A goitre may be palpable. The classical appearance of a cretin may not develop until 6–10 weeks of age by which time irreversible brain damage may have occurred.

Table 20.2 shows the causes of congenital hypothyroidism. Screening programme results suggest

Table 20.2 Causes of congenital hypothyroidism

Non-goitrous
athyrosis
lingual or ectopic thyroid
secondary hypothyroidism
Goitrous
enzyme defect
iodide induced
drug induced

that only one-third of cases are athyrotic, the remainder having lingual thyroids or an enzyme defect. In considering aetiology, details of maternal health and pregnancy are essential, especially family history of thyroid disease or maternal ingestion of antithyroid or iodine-containing drugs. Investigations should include serum T4 and TSH levels and assessment of bone age.

Treatment consists of L-thyroxine 5–7 μg/kg daily (25 μg or 0.025 mg daily in newborns), and increased according to clinical status and weight gain. Close monitoring of clinical state and T4 levels is necessary during the first year of life to avoid excess thyroxine dosage. Treatment is life-long, but whether brain damage sustained in utero can be reversed by early thyroxine therapy remains unknown.

Juvenile or acquired hypothyroidism

Juvenile hypothyroidism may present at any age and is associated with chronic lymphocytic thyroiditis or a lingual thyroid. The onset is gradual and growth retardation the commonest presenting symptom. Other features such as weight gain, constipation and mental slowing may only be elicited while taking the history. On examination these children are short for their age, and body proportions remain infantile with short legs and a long trunk. Pallor and anaemia are often present plus mild obesity and a dry skin. A low T4 level and elevated TSH confirm the diagnosis of primary hypothyroidism. Dental age is often delayed as is the radiological bone age and X-rays may also show epiphyseal dysgenesis. Measurement of antithyroid antibodies and a thyroid scan may help in diagnosing thyroiditis.

Replacement thyroxine is commenced in a dose

of 3–5 μg/kg daily, as older children have lower thyroxine requirements than the rapidly growing infant. Parents should be warned that their child may become naughty and perform less well at school as treatment commences. but will subsequently improve. Efficacy of treatment is assessed by growth response and serum thyroxine levels.

Hyperthyroidism

Hyperthyroidism in childhood is usually due to Graves' disease, there is often a positive family history and the same female predominance as in adults. Initial symptoms are of hyperactivity, emotional lability and tiredness, with weight loss and exophthalmos developing later. On examination there is evidence of a hyperdynamic circulation with tachycardia, raised pulse pressure and warm extremities. The child is restless and fidgety. A goitre is usually present, the thyroid being smooth, soft and diffusely enlarged: a bruit may be audible over the gland. The serum T4 is elevated and T3 resin uptake is low. A serum T3 level should also be checked as this is elevated in T3 toxicosis.

Treatment is medical using either carbimazole 30–40 mg, or propylthiouracil 100 mg three times a day as a starting dose to induce remission. When remission is achieved the dosage is reduced to a maintenance dose and continued for 2 years. Propranalol 10 mg three times a day may relieve severe symptoms until a euthyroid state is reached. Rest is important to minimise symptoms but school attendance should be continued if possible. Where medical treatment fails to control the hyperthyroidism or if relapse occurs then partial thyroidectomy is indicated. Most centres avoid the use of radio-active iodine therapy in children because of potential carcinogenic effects, but this treatment has been used in post-pubertal patients when other methods have failed.

Neonatal hyperthyroidism

This is a self-limiting condition affecting infants born to mothers with active or previous thyrotoxicosis. It is caused by the placental transmission of LATS or other thyroid-stimulating hormone which produces overactivity of the fetal thyroid. After delivery the stimulus is removed but the hyperthyroid state may persist for up to 3 months. The infant is hyperactive, restless and shows poor weight gain despite a voracious appetite. There may be persistent tachycardia at rest and exophthalmos. Severe hyperthyroidism may lead to heart failure and marked weight loss. Treatment with potassium iodide or propranolol will control the condition until it has resolved, but in severe cases carbimazole and digitalisation may be necessary.

Simple goitre

This occurs secondary to excess or inadequate iodine intake and is common in endemic areas, or following drug ingestion. A transient goitre often occurs in adolescent girls but it is essential to confirm that thyroid function is normal.

PUBERTY

There is a wide variation in the time of onset of puberty, and the trigger factor which initiates physical and sexual maturation remains unknown. Pubertal changes occur under hypothalamic control following secretion of LHRH (luteinising hormone releasing hormone), which stimulates increased secretion of the pituitary gonadotrophins, FSH (follicle stimulating hormone) and LH (luteinising hormone). FSH and LH stimulate the gonads to produce testosterone and oestrogen.

Normal puberty

In girls the first signs of puberty are the oestrogenic changes of breast development and change in the vaginal epithelium from red to pink. Adrenal androgens produce growth of pubic and axillary hair, apocrine sweat activity and facial acne. Androgens are also responsible for the pubertal growth spurt which occurs early in girls and is almost complete by the time menstruation commences (Fig 20.1). Irregular menses are common in the first year following menarche and require no treatment.

The earliest sign of puberty in boys is testicular enlargement above the prepubertal size of 2 ml

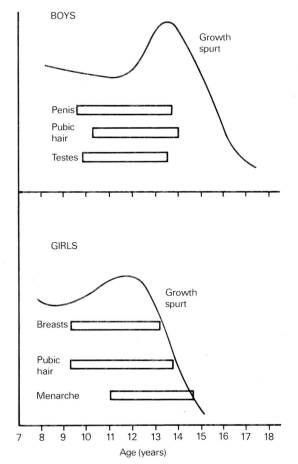

Fig. 20.1 Variation in time of onset of pubertal changes and timing of average growth spurt in boys and girls

volume using the Prader testiculometer. Increased testosterone secretion produces more obvious signs of puberty such as growth of pubic, axillary and facial hair, enlargement of the penis, deepening of the voice and acne. The growth spurt occurs later in boys and is associated with an increase in body size and muscle bulk. Gynaecomastia occurs in 65 per cent of normal boys during puberty and is usually transient. The mechanism is thought to be increased end-organ sensitivity to normal oestrogen concentrations and it is frequently unilateral.

Premature thelarche

Premature thelarche or isolated breast development occurs in young girls under the age of 3 years. Differentiation from precocious puberty depends on the absence of androgenic effects, i.e.

no pubic hair or increased growth and no oestrogenic changes in the vaginal mucosa. The condition is benign and requires no treatment but the patient should be reviewed if other pubertal changes develop.

Premature adrenarche

Premature adrenarche consists of early development of pubic and sometimes axillary hair, without other signs of puberty. It occurs mainly in girls, is due to increased adrenal androgen secretion and may be associated with increased growth. Ultimately, the girl will enter normal puberty and achieve normal adult height. If there is any clitoromegaly or progression in the degree of virilisation then adrenal hyperplasia or other source of excess androgens must be excluded.

Precocious puberty

Pubertal development is regarded as precocious if it occurs before the age of 8 years in girls and 9.5 years in boys, and may be a true or pseudo-precocious puberty. In true precocious puberty there is normal pubertal development with gonadal maturation occurring under hypothalamic control but at an abnormally early age. Pseudo-precocious puberty is the development of secondary sexual characteristics without maturation of the hypothalamic-pituitary-gonadal axis, but as a result of excess oestrogens and androgens produced by a normal or abnormal source. These two forms of early pubertal development may be impossible to distinguish clinically in the female, although the androgenic changes may predominate in pseudo-precocious puberty. In the male testicular enlargement is present in true precocious puberty, but absent in pseudo-precocious puberty suggesting a non-testicular source of androgens.

True precocious puberty is much commoner in girls than boys and in 80 per cent of girls it is idiopathic. Girls with chronic neurological disorders frequently mature early. In boys there is likely to be a serious cause underlying the precocious development such as a cerebral tumour and thorough neurological investigation is essential. Children with precocious puberty have an increased growth rate but become short adults due to early epiphyseal fusion.

Treatment in the idiopathic cases depends on reassurance of the parents and, in young girls, menses can be suppressed with progesterone. The main problems are social and behavioural as the child's mature physical appearance belies their emotional immaturity.

In pseudo-precocious puberty, testosterone or oestrogen levels may be significantly elevated and possible sources are tumours of the ovary, testis or adrenal gland. Rarely, a gonadotrophin-producing tumour may produce signs of early puberty. Specialist investigations are necessary utilising hormonal assays, ultrasound and radiological techniques to localise the tumour.

Delayed puberty

Puberty is delayed if there are no pubertal changes in a girl at 13 years of age and in a boy at 15 years, and such delay causes much anxiety in parents and their children. Chronic disease may delay puberty, e.g. cystic fibrosis or Crohn's disease. In the majority of cases delay is physiological but examination and investigation is justified to exclude hypogonadism. The presence of testicular enlargement in boys is reassuring that a normal puberty and growth spurt will follow. Chromosomal studies will exclude Turner's and Klinefelter's syndromes, both of which are examples of primary gonadal defects with normal hypothalamic pituitary function, i.e. hypergonadotrophic hypogonadism. Those patients with low gonadotrophin levels need detailed investigation of hypothalamic-pituitary function.

Whether the defect is due to primary gonadal failure or secondary to a hypothalamic-pituitary disorder, the patient needs hormonal therapy to produce sexual development. In Turner's syndrome oestrogen therapy should be delayed as long as possible to ensure maximal attainment of height before epiphyseal fusion, provided the patient is not distressed by her lack of development. The oestrogen dosage should be slowly increased to promote gradual maturation as in normal puberty, and the patient advised as to the emotional and physical effects of treatment.

In patients with hypopituitarism, gonadotrophin therapy will stimulate pubertal development, but as this must be given by injection it is not practicable for life-long therapy. Fertility has been achieved in some patients using LHRH or HCG injections. Sensitivity is most important in treating these problems and in providing support for the patients and their families.

ADRENAL PROBLEMS

The adrenal cortex produces cortisol, aldosterone and androgens which are metabolised from cholesterol, and the adrenal medulla produces the catecholamines adrenaline and noradrenaline. Both parts of the gland are under hypothalamic control, the cortex being stimulated by ACTH and the medulla by neural control via the splanchnic nerve.

Congenital adrenal hyperplasia

Congenital adrenal hyperplasia (CAH) is an important and life-threatening condition which may present as a neonatal emergency. These infants are unable to produce cortisol due to an enzyme defect inherited as an autosomal recessive. The commonest enzyme affected is the 21-hydroxylase which is required for the synthesis of both cortisol and aldosterone. Inability to produce cortisol results in ACTH stimulation of the adrenal gland with accumulation of the metabolite 17-hydroxyprogesterone, and excess androgen production via the intact pathway (Fig. 20.2).

Lack of cortisol and aldosterone can lead to a salt-losing crisis and death. The excess androgens cause masculinisation of the developing fetus and, at birth, the male infant may have enlargement of the phallus and increased pigmentation of the nipples and scrotum. The female infant may show marked virilisation of the external genitalia with clitoral enlargement, rugose and partially fused labia but normal female internal genitalia. On initial inspection an infant with this degree of masculinisation may resemble a male child with severe hypospadias. Dehydration and salt loss can occur between one and 4 weeks of age, or only at times of stress if the aldosterone deficiency is partial. The presenting features are unexplained

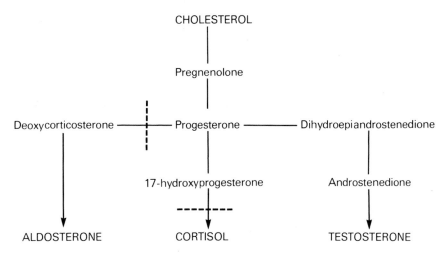

Fig. 20.2 Diagram showing biosynthesis of cortisol, aldosterone and testosterone. The dotted lines indicate the blocks in the pathway occurring in the 21-hydroxylase deficiency

weight loss greater than 10 per cent body weight in the neonatal period, vomiting and diarrhoea, and poor feeding. Severe dehydration and death can follow within 24–48 hours. The diagnosis should be suspected in any infant born with ambiguous genitalia or when there is a history of sudden unexplained neonatal death in a previous sibling.

Essential investigations are chromosome studies and plasma 17-hydroxyprogesterone level, which if elevated confirms the diagnosis. A 24-hour urine collection should be commenced for measurement of 17-ketosteroids and pregnanetriol. During a salt-losing crisis serum electrolytes will show hyponatraemia and hyperkalaemia. Treatment of the acutely dehydrated infant depends on rehydration with 0.9 per cent saline and 5 per cent dextrose in amounts calculated to correct the sodium deficit. Hydrocortisone 1–2 mg/kg body weight must be given intravenously plus the mineralocorticoid, one deoxycortone pivalate (Percosten) 1 mg daily. Once stabilised, maintenance therapy consists of oral hydrocortisone or cortisone acetate 20–25 mg/m² daily and fludrocortisone 0.05 mg-0.2 mg/day. If replacement therapy is adequate added salt should not be necessary. Treatment is monitored by measuring growth velocity, progression of bone age, plasma 17-hydroxyprogesterone and urinary metabolite levels. If growth velocity is accelerated then cortisone dosage is inadequate to suppress ACTH. Cortisone and fludrocortisone

are necessary as life-long therapy and parents must be warned to triple the dosage of cortisone at times of stress, e.g. febrile illnesses or surgery. For the child's safety a Medicalert bracelet should be worn. In the female child clitoroplasty should be performed by the age of 2 years but further surgery deferred until sexual maturity to avoid scarring.

Those patients who produce adequate amounts of aldosterone may not present until adolescence. Girls present with primary amenorrhoea and hirsutism, and the boys with precocious development of external genitalia, tall stature but with small prepubertal testes. Both sexes with untreated or inadequately treated CAH will be short adults as the excess androgens promote early epiphyseal fusion.

Adrenal insufficiency

Adrenal insufficiency is rare in childhood but may result from autoimmune Addison's disease. More commonly, a child with adrenal suppression is precipitated into adrenal crisis by abrupt withdrawal of steroids; gradual reduction in dosage is essential after more than 2 months therapy.

Early signs of cortisol lack are increasing fatigue, lethargy and weight loss. The diagnosis is confirmed by measuring serial cortisol levels during a 24-hour period and cortisol response to synthetic ACTH.

Adrenal tumours

Excess cortisol production is extremely rare in childhood. Steroid therapy for some other condition such as nephrotic syndrome produces the short, obese, cushingoid child.

Adrenal neoplasms may present as postnatal virilisation in girls, and Cushing's syndrome or pseudo-precocious puberty in boys. Investigation is required to identify the tumour and, if malignant, treatment consists of surgical removal and chemotherapy.

THE INFANT OF UNCERTAIN SEX

The problem of ambiguous genitalia at birth is rare but may have profound consequences if unrecognised. In utero, chromosomal sex determines gonadal differentiation; in the presence of a Y chromosome the gonads become testes which secrete Mullerian inhibition factor and testosterone and promote development of male internal and external genitalia. With an XX karyotype the gonads become ovaries which have no endocrine function but allow the fetus to develop as female (Fig. 20.3). Intersex disorders are caused by sex chromosomal anomalies, abnormalities of gonadal differentiation or defective hormonal synthesis due to inherited enzyme defects.

Any infant born with ambiguous genitalia should be investigated immediately. The parents must be told of the uncertainty regarding the baby's sex and to choose a name suitable for either sex. Family history and details of the pregnancy are important, including maternal ingestion of progesterone or other androgens. On physical examination, the external genitalia may show partial labial fusion, clitoromegaly or hypospadias with a small phallus. Inguinal or labial gonads are invariably testes, as ovaries remain in the pelvis.

Chromosomal analysis must be performed to ascertain genetic sex, and indicate whether the child is a virilised female (female pseudohermaphroditism) or an incompletely masculinised male (male pseudohermaphrodite). Very rarely true hermaphroditism occurs where both ovarian and testicular tissue exist in the same individual.

Female pseudohermaphroditism

This condition commonly results from congenital adrenal hyperplasia which must be excluded immediately by appropriate investigations (see adrenal disorders). Progesterone therapy in early pregnancy can also produce virilisation of female external genitalia.

Male pseudohermaphroditism

This is a more complex condition caused either by enzyme defects affecting testosterone biosynthesis e.g. 3β-hydroxylase dehydrogenase deficiency in CAH, or end-organ insensitivity to testosterone

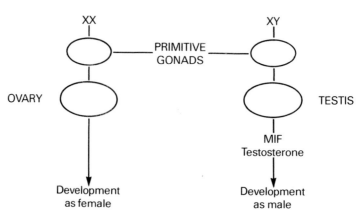

Fig. 20.3 Differentiation of fetal testis and ovary, and control of sexual development *in utero*

which produces incomplete virilisation as in partial or complete testicular feminisation. Investigation includes measurement of testosterone levels and assessment of response to HCG and exogenous testosterone. In both male and female pseudohermaphroditism retrograde urography will define vaginal and urethral openings or a common urogenital sinus.

On completion of investigations the sex of rearing must be decided as soon as possible. Female infants with CAH must be raised as girls. In other cases which are usually infertile the decision is based not on karyotype but on the functional anatomy of the external genitalia, the size of the phallus and the individuals ability to function satisfactorily in a male or female role. The majority are reared as girls, as experience has shown those raised as boys are infertile, require multiple urological operations and later suffer profound psychosexual difficulties. Any decision to change the sex of rearing must be made early, preferably before the age of one year, and is made only after informed discussion between the family doctor, paediatrician and urologist. The parents must be fully involved, and long-term follow up with family support is essential.

DISORDERS OF CALCIUM METABOLISM

Calcium absorption from the gut depends on vitamin D, the pH of the upper intestine, and binding by dietary substances e.g. phytates. In serum, 40 per cent of calcium is bound to serum albumin and the remainder exists in the ionised and metabolically active form. The level of ionised calcium is controlled by vitamin D, parathormone and calcitonin. Calcium is essential for normal muscular activity and hypocalcaemia leads to muscular irritability, tetany and convulsions. Vitamin D or cholecalciferol is found in fish, eggs, butter and margarine, and is also formed in the Malpighian layer of the skin. The most potent metabolite of vitamin D is 1,25-dihydroxycholecalciferol which is generated exclusively in the kidney.

Hypocalcaemia

Hypocalcaemia occurs in the neonatal period in full-term infants fed with cow's milk preparations containing a high phosphate load. These infants are jittery when handled but otherwise behave normally. In preterm infants with perinatal problems a more prolonged form of hypocalcaemia may occur. This is thought to be due to lack of parathormone (PTH) in the neonate following fetal dependence on high maternal PTH levels, and may be associated with hypomagnesaemia. Treatment of both forms consists of oral calcium gluconate but, if hypomagnesaemia is present, the calcium level will not respond until the magnesium deficiency is corrected.

In the older child hypocalcaemia results from deficiency of PTH, either post-thyroidectomy or autoimmune, or from end-organ insensitivity to PTH as in pseudohypoparathyroidism. Deficiency of PTH causes hypocalcaemia, hyperphosphataemia, tetany and generalised convulsions. Examination reveals a positive Trousseau's sign and muscular excitability. The bones remain well mineralised and alkaline phosphatase levels are normal. The autoimmune form of hypoparathyroidism may be associated with diabetes mellitus, alopecia, Addison's disease, hypothyroidism and chronic candidiasis. Treatment consists of control of symptomatic hypocalcaemia using a slow i.v. infusion of 2 per cent calcium gluconate if necessary. Longterm treatment requires vitamin D in doses far in excess of physiological requirements e.g. 50 μg/kg (2000 iu/kg) daily. Response to treatment is evaluated by monitoring plasma calcium and phosphate levels, and avoidance of hypercalcaemia due to excess dosage.

Hypercalcaemia

Hypercalcaemia occurs secondary to excess vitamin D intake or as mild or severe idiopathic hypercalcaemia. The presenting symptoms are vomiting, constipation and failure to thrive. Cardiac anomalies are associated with the severe form. Treatment is based on dietary reduction of calcium and vitamin D plus steroid therapy.

Vitamin D deficiency

Deficiency of vitamin D occurs secondary to poor dietary intake, malabsorption, inadequate skin synthesis and in renal disease. It results in rickets which occurs in infants, toddlers and adolescents. Preterm infants are predisposed to rickets because of rapid growth. Between 6 months and 3 years of age the presenting signs are skull bossing, delay in closure of the anterior fontanelle, swollen wrists and a rickety rosary due to swelling of costochondral junctions and bowing of the legs. The serum calcium is normal or decreased and the alkaline phosphatase elevated. X-rays of wrists and knees show cupping, fuzzing and spreading of the ends of the long bones. In adolescent rickets, limb pain may be the presenting symptom. Treatment requires vitamin D in doses of 75 μg (3000 iu) daily for 6 weeks followed by a maintenance dose of 10 μg (400 iu) daily, or the use of vitamin D analogues or metabolites (alphacalcidiol, calcitriol).

INBORN ERRORS OF METABOLISM

Inborn errors of metabolism are genetically inherited enzyme defects resulting in the accumulation of toxic metabolites which may cause neurological damage and death. Early detection after birth is important both for treatment and future genetic counselling. Phenylketonuria is routinely screened for the UK, and screening for neonatal hypothyroidism is now nationwide (Only 25 per cent of cases of neonatal hypothyroidism are due to an inherited enzyme defect; absence or maldevelopment of the thyroid gland account for the remainder.)

Antenatal diagnosis has been successfully carried out in disorders of lipid metabolism e.g. Tay-Sachs disease, the mucopolysaccharidoses, urea cycle defects and glycogen storage disease. For successful prenatal diagnosis the specific biochemical defect for which the fetus is at risk must be known and the phenotypic expression of the metabolic abnormality in the particular family. Screening for a number of possible diseases is impracticable unless an index case has been identified or heterozygosity of the parents is known.

The possibility of a metabolic disturbance should be considered in any infant with an unexplained illness or acidosis, especially if there is a family history of fetal or neonatal death. Children presenting with delayed development or neurological abnormality should be screened for possible metabolic abnormality.

Treatment of these conditions is based on dietary restriction eliminating the offending aminoacid or sugar, e.g. phenylalanine in phenylketonuria, and galactose in galactosaemia. Of the more common inborn errors of metabolism few are known to benefit from dietary control and these are listed in Table 20.3. In phenylketonuria the diet must contain all aminoacids essential to

Table 20.3 Common inborn errors of metabolism which benefit from diet

Disorder	Frequency	Toxic agent/process	Dietary treatment	Hazards of diet
Phenylketonuria	1 in 10000	Phenylalanine and metabolites	Diet low in phenylalanine with supplements of all other essential aminoacids	Phenylalanine deficiency causes growth failure
Galactosaemia	1 in 50000	Galactose	Rigid exclusion of galactose or lactose in early life	
Maple syrup urine disease	1 in 250000	Leucine, isoleucine, valine	Diet low in branch-chain aminoacids valine, leucine and isoleucine with supplements of all other essential aminoacids	Very restricted diet causes growth failure and aminoacid imbalance
Urea cycle defects		Ammonia	Diet low in protein with supplements of aminoacids when necessary	Growth failure and aminoacid imbalance
Glycogen storage disease		Hypoglycaemia	Frequent high calorie feeds/glucose drinks throughout 24-hour period	–

growth including small amounts of phenylalanine. Girls of child-bearing age need strict dietary control throughout pregnancy as retarded growth, microcephaly and cardiac anomalies have been reported in association with high maternal phenylalanine levels. If low levels are maintained the infant should be normal.

General management of inborn errors of metabolism includes close monitoring of blood metabolite levels and early treatment of infections to minimise catabolism and acidosis. Patients with these disorders benefit greatly from the team approach available in specialist centres with appropriate laboratory facilities and physicians, nurses and dieticians familiar with the individual problems. This is a rapidly changing field with new diseases being discovered and much of the treatment is experimental.

FURTHER READING

Baum J D, Smith M A 1976 The diabetic child. Hospital Update 2: 4, 159–167

Forfar J O, Arneil G C 1978 Textbook of paediatrics. Churchill Livingstone, Edinburgh

Glasgow F T, Campbell S L 1976 Hospital Update 2: 1, 9–17

Lissauer T 1980 Paediatric emergencies — diabetic ketoacidosis and hypoglycaemia. Hospital Update 6: 10, 943–961

21

Oncology

EPIDEMIOLOGY AND AETIOLOGY

Malignant diseases are rare in childhood. They occur in one in 10 000 children per year; from birth to 15 years a child has a one in 600 chance of developing a malignancy, compared with a one in 5 chance in adult life. The types of malignant disease in childhood are very different from those in adults. Embryonic tumours of mesenchymal origin, central nervous system tumours and reticuloendothelial malignancy predominate in childhood in contrast to the carcinomas of adult life. The incidence of the different types of childhood cancers seen in the UK is shown in Table 21.1.

There are significant differences in the tumours seen in Africa and the Far East. Some of these differences are probably. environmental while others are more likely to be of genetic or racial origin. There are, for example, very few cases of Ewing's tumour in African children or in American blacks, but the high incidence of Burkitt's lymphoma in certain areas of Africa is not seen in the American black population. Despite these differences the majority of childhood tumours remain sporadic in origin.

There are, however, certain factors which carry an increased risk of malignancy in childhood, hemihypertrophy carries an increased risk of Wilms' tumour, adrenocortical carcinoma and liver tumours. The actual risk factor is unknown as the true incidence of hemihypertrophy is difficult to ascertain. Congenital aniridia usually occurs as an autosomal dominant trait but, when it occurs sporadically, the risk of Wilms' tumour in the child is increased to 1000 times above normal. Chromosomal banding techniques have shown that these children, who are usually mentally retarded, have a small deletion of chromosome 11. Certain constitutional chromosome disorders carry a known excess risk of cancer and these are shown in Table 21.2. The banding techniques have also shown acquired chromosome

Table 21.1 Average annual incidence of different types of malignancy in childhood (per million children) (Manchester children's tumour registry)

Acute lymphoblastic leukaemia	25.6
Acute non-lymphoblastic leukaemia	5.1
Other leukaemias	1.8
Non-Hodgkin's lymphoma	4.3
Hodgkin's disease	3.6
Astrocytoma (all grades)	9.3
Medulloblastoma	4.6
Ependymoma	2.8
Other CNS tumours	6.0
Rhabdomyosarcomas	4.1
Other soft tissue sarcomas	2.1
Osteosarcoma	2.5
Ewing's tumour	2.0
Wilms' tumour	5.0
Neuroblastoma	6.6
Retinoblastoma	3.2
Hepatoblastoma	0.5
Gonadal and other germ cell tumours	1.9
Other tumours	8.9

Table 21.2 Constitutional chromosomal abnormalities associated with increased tumour susceptibility

Chromosomal anomaly	Cancer type
Trisomy 21 (Down's syndrome)	Acute lymphoblastic leukaemia
Trisomy 18	Wilms' tumour
Turner's syndrome	Neurogenic tumours
XY gonadal dysgenesis	Gonadoblastoma
Klinefelter's syndrome (XXY)	Acute leukaemia, teratoma, breast carcinoma
D deletion (13q -)	Retinoblastoma

changes in malignant cells; these include the Philadelphia chromosome in chronic myeloid leukaemia, trisomy 8 in acute myelogenous leukaemia and translocations of chromosomes 8, 11 and 14 in lymphomas. Approximately 10 per cent of known single gene traits have malignancy as a complication. The better known of these include familial polyposis of the colon, von Recklinhausen's syndrome, tuberous sclerosis and several of the immunodeficiency syndromes.

The only malignant disease which is certainly inherited is retinoblastoma. This tumour occurs in two forms: unilateral when it is rarely inherited, and bilateral when it is inherited as an autosomal dominant trait, in these cases, the tumour is frequently multifocal in origin. Bilateral and multifocal forms of Wilms' tumour and neuroblastoma may also be inherited.

Very few environmental factors have been identified as a cause of childhood cancer. Prenatal exposure to diagnostic radiation does increase the risk but this is really only important when exposure is in the first trimester. Stillboestrol given during pregnancy has been shown to increase vaginal and cervical adenocarcinoma in the daughters and hypotrophic testes and low sperm counts in the sons. Other possible transplacental carcinogens include diphenylhydantoin and barbiturates.

ACUTE LEUKAEMIAS

Diagnosis

Approximately 85 per cent of all children who develop leukaemia have the acute lymphoblastic type; the majority of the remainder have acute myeloid, myelomonocytic or monocytic disease. The peak incidence of acute lymphoblastic leukaemia (ALL) in childhood is between 2 and 6 years, but it can occur at birth and is seen throughout childhood. The non-lymphoid leukaemias show no peak. Children with Down's syndrome (trisomy 21) have a 15 times greater risk of developing leukaemia and develop the disease at an earlier age.

Most children with leukaemia present with vague non-specific symptoms; pallor, lassitude, irritability and bone pain are common. Lymphadenopathy, hepatosplenomegaly and a petechial rash are frequently found on examination. Hypertrophy of the gums is common in acute myelomonocytic and monocytic leukaemias. The association of these findings with anaemia, thrombocytopenia and circulating blast cells usually makes the diagnosis simple. Some children with leukaemia do not have organomegaly or abnormal cells in the peripheral blood and a bone marrow examination is necessary to differentiate the disease from aplastic anaemia. Infectious mononucleosis has many features commonly seen in leukaemia, but the atypical lymphocytes characteristic of the disease are heterogeneous in appearance, and significant anaemia or thrombocytopenia are rare. Idiopathic thrombocytopenic purpura is usually seen following a viral infection in an otherwise healthy child and a low platelet count is the only abnormality of the peripheral blood.

Once the diagnosis of leukaemia is made, the child should be referred to a major paediatric oncology unit. This is to allow optimum therapy by using a more detailed and complex classification of the disease; the majority of children with acute lymphoblastic leukaemia have small cells known as L_1. In the L_2 sub-group the blast cells are large, they account for about 10 per cent of childhood cases. The L_3 group have very primitive cells which carry surface markers characteristic of B-lymphocytes and account for about 1–2 per cent of childhood cases. T-cell surface markers can be demonstrated in about 10–15 per cent of children with lymphoblastic leukaemia. Most of these children are boys and in older age groups; they have high white cell counts and anterior mediastinal masses. The majority of cases of childhood leukaemia (70 per cent) have receptors for a specific ALL antigen and are classified as having common ALL; they usually have L_1 cells and the best prognosis. Another group without cell markers (null cells) have an intermediate outlook. In all there are six sub-groups of acute non-lymphocytic leukaemia.

Treatment of acute lymphoblastic leukaemia

Treatment can be divided into three phases:

1. Induction of remission. This is usually achieved by use of steroids, in conjunction with vincristine sulphate and asparaginase or an anthracycline such as doxorubicin (Adriamycin). The term remission means that the child's symptoms and clinical signs have regressed and that the bone morrow contains less than 5 per cent of blast cells and other normal marrow elements are present in normal proportions. This phase is usually complete by the end of 4 weeks of treatment.

2. Consolidation and central nervous system prophylaxis. This involves further cytoreduction and may use other drugs or further courses of those used in the induction phase. Treatment of the central nervous system is essential to prevent the later overt development of leukaemic disease there. Some authorities advocate the use of intrathecal drugs alone, usually methotrexate, but more frequently it is combined with cranial irradiation.

3. Maintenance. This consists of repeated cycles of treatment using several drugs. The mainstays are 6-mercaptopurine and methotrexate often combined with pulses of cytosine arabinoside, vincristine and steroids. Treatment with these drugs is usually continued for 2–3 years; the optimum length of maintenance therapy has not yet been established.

Many protocols have been devised which have been shown to be very successful in the management of ALL and 5 year disease-free survival rates in excess of 50 per cent are common. A proportion of children relapse while still on therapy; the majority of these will respond to further therapy but usually relapse again and median survival time after relapse is approximately 9 months. Of the remainder who come off therapy, about 10 per cent will relapse in the first year and decreasing numbers relapse in the next few years. Few relapses have been described after 4 years off therapy. With more detailed sub-classification, it has been possible to delineate prognostic factors; the majority of failures occur in children:

1. Under the age of 2 and over the age of 10 years
2. Presenting with high white cell counts at diagnosis
3. With anterior mediastinal masses — who usually also have T-cell markers
4. With CNS disease at diagnosis
5. Who are black
6. Who are boys and develop isolated testicular disease.

Patients falling into the first three of these categories will probably benefit from the use of treatment programmes involving even more intensive therapy and the use of more drugs. Whether or not it is possible to eradicate central nervous system leukaemia without inflicting late damage on the central nervous system is not yet known, certainly the repeated use of intrathecal drugs and irradiation produce a deterioration in mental function.

The treatment of acute non-lymphocytic leukaemias (ANLL)

The general principles of management are similar to those of ALL. The most widely used and useful drugs are, the anthracyclines (daunorubicin and doxorubicin, cytosine arabinoside and thioguanine). Remission induction can be obtained in about 70 per cent of patients. Consolidation is given with the same agents, including central nervous system prophylaxis. Remission is not achieved without a period of severe hypoplasia and these children need special supportive care if they are not to succumb to uncontrolled bleeding, coagulation problems and severe infections. They should not be treated outside special units.

Whether or not maintenance therapy has any part to play is patients with ANLL is questionable and, indeed, in patients with a suitable donor that bone marrow transplant is the treatment of choice once remission is obtained.

DIAGNOSIS AND TREATMENT OF THE CHRONIC LEUKAEMIAS

Adult-type chronic granulocytic leukaemia

This type of leukaemia shows the Philadelphia (Ph[1]) chromosome; it accounts for approximately 1.5 per cent of childhood leukaemias. The clinical presentation in childhood is varied; signs and symptoms may be insidious in onset. The symptoms are related to anaemia, marrow hyperplasia and splenomegaly and give rise to malaise, pallor, bone pain and a feeling of upper abdominal fullness. There is usually a mild anaemia, an associated marked leucocytosis usually greater than 100

$\times 10^9/l$ and a normal platelet count. The majority are mature cells.

There is a group of children with Ph_1 chromosome leukaemia who present as acute lymphoblastic leukaemia and, if cytogenetic studies are not available, may be suspected on the basis of failure to respond to usual therapy. Another group may present in blast cell crisis with morphology suggestive of acute myeloid leukaemia.

The most appropriate method of treatment depends on the findings at presentation. Busulphan is the drug of choice in the chronic phase, while the other forms show better response to similar therapy for acute disease. None of these patients have a good long-term prognosis.

Juvenile chronic myeloid leukaemia

There is a skin rash, hepatosplenomegaly, lymphadenopathy, thrombocytopenia and a significantly raised fetal haemoglobin. The disease runs an acute course and is unresponsive to chemotherapy.

TUMOURS OF THE CENTRAL NERVOUS SYSTEM

These tumours make up the largest group of solid tumours in childhood, approximately 20 per cent. They differ from those of adult life in that 70 per cent of them occur in structures below the tentorium. The histological subtypes also differ; almost half the malignant tumours in adults are glioblastomas while they only account for about 10 per cent of childhood tumours; high grade astrocytomas considered by many to be a variant of glioblastomas account for another 5 per cent. There is also a group of astrocytic tumours arising in the brain stem in which, because of the site, histological verification is difficult; most of these are probably malignant and they account for 10 per cent of the total. Medulloblastomas are a common group in childhood, about 20 per cent of the total, while they are very rare in adult life. Ependymomas, most of which occur infratentorially, are also more common in children than adults. Teratomas, pineal tumours, craniopharyngiomas and pituitary tumours are rare but, nevertheless, important diagnostically as they may present initially with precocious puberty, diabetes insipidus, growth failure or the diencephalic syndrome.

Diagnosis and Treatment

Most children with brain tumours present with symptoms and signs directly related to raised intracranial pressure and to the focal effects of the mass. The rise in intracranial pressure is usually due to cerebral oedema or to a block in the cerebrospinal fluid pathways and only rarely to the volume of the lesion itself. Symptoms include headache, vomiting and impaired vision.

A common false localising sign is a sixth nerve palsy. Enlargement of the cranium may occur in young children, but convulsions are rare. As so many childhood brain tumours arise in the cerebellum and brain stem, a disturbance of gait and balance is common. Children may be noticed to become clumsy, to walk into furniture or to have deteriorating handwriting. Many of these tumours are benign astrocytomas amenable to surgical removal but delay in diagnosis may lead to permanent impairment of vision from raised intracranial pressure. Pontine tumours produce similar symptoms and, in addition, defects in the lower cranial nerves with palatal weakness and swallowing difficulties. Spinal tumours, if intramedullary, produduce symmetrical weakness and wasting, while extramedullary tumours produce nerve root effects.

Computerised axial tomography has made the diagnosis of brain tumours much simpler as it has removed the need for invasive techniques and, in those children with suggestive symptoms and signs, this investigative procedure should be carried out.

At the present time surgery is the treatment of choice for all central nervous system tumours. Total removal is rarely possible except in the case of cerebellar astrocytomas and the occasional supratentorial low-grade glioma. With improved surgical techniques, the use of the dissecting microscope and better supportive care, the surgery is improving and more aggressive surgery holds out the best chance of cure.

Radiation therapy is effective is dealing with small residual portions of the more benign gliomas, but there is no significant evidence of its effect in malignant gliomas. It plays a very important role in the management of medulloblastomas in which whole central nervous system irradiation is essential to obtain a cure as the tumour tends to seed the meninges. The dose is critical and unfortunately the level of radiation necessary is associated with subsequent growth hormone deficiency and learning problems. X-ray therapy is also essential for the treatment of ependymomas which, because of their site, can rarely be removed surgically. The brain-stem tumours diagnosed only radiologically show an approximate 25 per cent long-term response to radiation.

Chemotherapy has, as yet, not been fully evaluated in the treatment of brain tumours. There is no doubt that the majority of the tumours do show a response; this has been demonstrated most frequently in recurrent disease. Some patients have had long-term second remissions with clinical and radiological evidence of regression of disease.

There are problems inherent in the use of chemotherapy but the often quoted one of the need for the drug to cross the blood-brain barrier is probably not significant with brain tumours, as the barrier is usually non-functional. It is hoped that with a more optimistic approach by neurosurgeons that adjuvant chemotherapy will be used more frequently.

THE LYMPHOMAS

Hodgkin's disease

Most children with this disease present with painless enlargement of one or more lymph node groups, with giant binucleate cells, known as Reed-Sternberg cells, and distorted lymphoid architecture. There are four histological subtypes:

1. Lymphocyte predominance
2. Nodular sclerosis
3. Mixed cellularity
4. Lymphocyte depletion

The degree of malignancy increases from type 1–4 and there is a decreasingly good prognosis. It is essential, once the diagnosis has been made, to establish the histological subtype and the extent of disease, as these determine appropriate treatment. Four stages (I–IV of disease have been delineated and subdivided into A and B dependent

on the absence or presence of constitutional disturbance, 10 per cent weight loss in 6 weeks, fever, or night sweats.

Stage I disease is limited to one lymphatic region or extranodal site other than liver, bone marrow, skin or lungs. Stage II is involvement of two or more lymph node regions on the same side of the diaphragm. Stage III disease includes involvement of nodes or extranodal sites on both sides of the diaphragm, and Stage IV disease means diffuse involvement of liver, spleen, lungs, skin, bone marrow or central nervous system with or without nodal involvement.

Investigations used to establish the stage of disease include lymphangiography, staging laparotomy and splenectomy. Lymphangiography may be technically very difficult in young children and is not without complications. Staging laparotomy and splenectomy also have serious implications and there is a high rate of infectious complications. Computerised tomography scans do not provide very accurate indication of splenic disease; in view of these problems it is considered justifiable to defer or omit splenectomy in young children.

Chemotherapy is probably the preferable treatment in children under the age of 8 years irrespective of stage, as there is less interference with growth of bone and soft tissue. The commonly used combinations of drugs do, however, have the disadvantage of possibly inducing sterility. In older children with unequivocal stage I disease the treatment of choice at present is involved field radiation. Radiation and chemotherapy or chemotherapy alone are best in stages II and III and chemotherapy with consideration of radiation to areas of bulky disease for stage IV. Various combinations of drugs have been shown to be effective, the majority include nitrogen mustard, procarbazine and a vinca alkaloid; other drugs which have been used are adriamycin, cyclophosphamide and bleomycin.

Five-year survival rates of more than 90 per cent have been achieved for stage I disease, 70–90 per cent survival rates are possible for stages II, III and IV.

Non-Hodgkin's lymphomas

This term includes all the malignant solid tumours

of the lymphoid system other than Hodgkin's disease. They are a difficult group of disorders to categorise satisfactorily; there are nodular and diffuse forms. The diffuse form is the commoner non-Hodgkin's lymphoma in childhood and also has the worse prognosis.

Children with these tumours present in a wide variety of ways. Cervical lymph node enlargement is common but is rarely the only site of disease. Mediastinal involvement is often seen, the child presenting with cough, superior vena caval syndrome or airways obstruction; tumours arising in this site usually carry T-cell markers and tend to progress to marrow involvement at an early stage. Primary gastrointestinal disease accounts for about 30 per cent of patients, the tumour is usually in the ileum, caecum or ascending colon and the child frequently presents with intussusception. Other sites include retroperitoneal and mesenteric nodes, tonsil, adenoid, bone and gonad.

Burkitt's lymphoma is characterised by a particular histological picture and, when it occurs in Africa, presents with clinical symptoms of primary jaw lesions, abdominal disease or a paraspinal mass causing paraplegia. The same histological picture is found in non-African children but is not associated with jaw lesions, an abdominal tumour is then the commonest.

No truly effective staging system has been evolved for non-Hodgkin's lymphoma in childhood as the different histological types have different patterns of spread. There is some doubt as to whether stage I disease ever really occurs and, for this reason systemic chemotherapy is the primary form of therapy and radiation is used for treatment of bulk disease. Spread to the central nervous system is so frequent that prophylactic therapy is probably indicated in all cases except localised abdominal disease. The most effective chemotherapy programmes are now achieving 2 year disease-free rates of 50–70 per cent. They involve intensive cyclical treatment with several drugs to minimise the development of resistance.

HISTIOCYTOSIS

Controversy continues about the exact aetiology of this group of disorders. They show infiltration of normal tissues by histiocytes and include: histiocytic medullary reticulosis; familial haemophagocytic reticulosis; and the spectrum of histiocytosis X which includes Latterer-Siwe disease, Hand-Schüller-Christian disease and unifocal eosinophilic granuloma. Most of these disorders carry a very poor prognosis and it is only the localised disease without evidence of organ disfunction occuring in the older child in which the outlook is good. Various treatment regimens have been tried; children with Letterer-Siwe disease may respond to combinations of vincristine, steroids and alkylating agents, but the disease often recurs. Single eosinophilic granulomas may regress spontaneously or respond to currettage or low-dose irradiation. Chemotherapy is the treatment of choice for multiple lesions and careful evaluation of pituitary function is necessary as these patients often have growth hormone failure and diabetes insipidus from involvement of the pituitary.

NEPHROBLASTOMA

Nephroblastoma accounts for around 4 per cent of childhood malignancy; the tumours are bilateral in about 10 per cent of cases. The peak incidence is between the ages of 2 and 6 years. Most children present with an increase in abdominal size, but haematuria is also common and children with this complaint who do not have a urinary tract infection should always be further investigated. Once the diagnosis is suspected the treatment of choice is surgery and there are very few children in whom total nephrectomy with removal of tumour is not possible. The histology of the tumour should be carefully assessed as it is now established that there are some pathological types of tumour which carry a bad prognosis. It is also important to stage the extent of spread of the tumour. Without this knowledge it is not possible to continue with optimum therapy. Tumours of good histology which are confined to the kidney do not require radiation therapy and probably need only short courses of chemotherapy, while those with rupture of the capsule, regional node involvement or poor histology need radiation therapy and at least two-drug chemotherapy. With these methods of treatment between 85 and 90 per cent of these children should survive.

Patients with metastatic disease to lungs are still curable and, using three or four drugs, usually vincristine, actinomycin and Adriamycin, and radiotherapy, about 50 per cent can be expected to survive. Liver metastases have a less favourable outcome. Bilateral tumours are often very responsive to chemotherapy and surgery is either used primarily to remove the worst affected kidney or after drug treatment to resect residual disease.

NEUROBLASTOMA

These tumours of the sympathetic nervous system have so far defied response to the advances in treatment seen in other childhood tumours. They are primarily tumours of young children and arise most often in the adrenal gland, mediastinum or coeliac axis, with smaller numbers in the cervical ganglia or the pelvis. A high proportion present with evidence of widespread metastases to bone; there may be periorbital haemorrhage making non-accidental injury one of the differential diagnoses. There is a group (stage IVS) which presents at birth or in the first few months of life with a small primary tumour, and spreads to liver, bone marrow or skin, but there are no frank bone lesions. These babies usually have spontaneous regression of their disease and require no treatment.

Patients who present with localised disease have best chance of cure if their tumour can be completely excised. Localised residual disease often responds to X-ray therapy. Chemotherapy will achieve considerable regression of tumour but there is little evidence of its long-term effect. New methods of therapy using drugs to achieve regression, removal of bone marrow prior to further intensive therapy and replacement of marrow after treatment, are now being investigated. The results are encouraging but as yet no long-term cures have been achieved.

Soft tissue sarcomas

Soft tissue sarcomas originate in embryonic mesenchymal tissue and arise in many different sites. The commonest type in childhood are the rhabdomyosarcomas which arise in muscle and although not all tumours exhibit rhabdomyoblasts they tend to behave in the same clinical way. Treatment of this group of tumours is one of the success stories of paediatric oncology. They have a tendency to metastasise early and to spread locally by infiltration so, at diagnosis, they are rarely confined to the tissue or organ of origin. Metastases are present at diagnosis in about 25 per cent of patients and bone marrow involvement is found in about 20 per cent. Four pathological sub-groups are recognised: embryonal; pleomorphic; alveolar; and mixed. The alveolar histology is primarily seen in extremity lesions and carries a particularly bad prognosis. The wide variety of sites of origin of rhabdomyosarcomas makes it difficult to generalise about therapy; 30 per cent arise in the head and neck and many of these are in structures adjacent to the meninges where there is a tendency to spread to the central nervous system. Other common sites are the orbit (15 per cent), genito-urinary system (30 per cent), and the extremities and trunk (15 per cent). Initial investigations should include a very thorough search for both local spread and metastatic disease. Computerised axial and body tomographic scans are very helpful.

The major advance in therapy has occurred since adjuvant chemotherapy has been introduced. It has been particularly effective in the pre-surgical reduction of tumour mass, and has enabled surgeons to carry out conservative resections with retention of normal function, as opposed to massive mutilative surgery. This makes it particularly important that children with these tumours should be referred to specialist centres for full evaluation before treatment rather than after surgery. Radiation therapy has an important role, particularly in the treatment of residual disease after chemotherapy in sites not amenable to surgery. The combination of vincristine, actinimycin D and cyclophosphamide has been shown to be the most effective. Adriamycin also has an effect in these tumours but is probably not essential to the optimum management of stage I and II casses.

Other soft tissue sarcomas in childhood, such as fibrosarcomas, liposarcomas, leiomyosarcomas, synovial sarcomas and haemangiopericytomas are very rare and no standardised treatment programmes have been evolved. They should undoubtedly be referred to specialised centres and therapy similar to that for rhabdomyosarcomas is probably the best.

BONE TUMOURS

Osteogenic sarcomas and Ewing's tumours account for about 5 per cent of childhood malignancy. The former is a tumour of bone-forming mesenchymal cells while the latter is a non-osseous small cell sarcoma. Both tumours have a maximum incidence in the second decade but while 70 per cent of all Ewing's tumours are seen before the age of 20 years, 50 per cent of osteogenic sarcomas occur in adults. Both tumours are commoner in males. The commonest site for both is in the long bones, but osteogenic sarcomas tend to occur in the metaphyseal region, while Ewing's tumour is more often found in the shaft and is also relatively more common in the pelvic bones. The two tumours present with pain and swelling, pain usually preceding other symptoms and signs by several weeks. The radiological appearances of osteogenic sarcoma include loss of normal trabecular pattern, lytic lesions and new bone formation, and soft tissue extensions often show calcification. Ewing's tumours produce localised rarefaction and periosteal reaction resembling onion skin layers from layers of new bone formation. Both tumours require biopsy to confirm the diagnosis.

The treatment of osteogenic sarcoma has undergone several changes in the last 10 years. There are increasing data indicating that several cytotoxic agents are effective in preventing or diminishing the number and frequency of metastases. Very high dose methotrexate, adriamycin, cisplatinum and bleomycin have all been shown to cause regression of lung metastases and are now used in addition to amputation. A small number of orthopaedic units are now undertaking wide excision of the tumour and prosthetic replacement of the involved bone. The early functional results are very encouraging and do not seem in any way to undermine cure, providing full chemotherapy is also given. Single centre studies have produced 40 to 70 per cent 5-year survival rates.

The most effective treatment of Ewing's tumour involves radiation therapy to the primary site and then adjuvant chemotherapy with vincristine, cyclophosphamide, actinomycin D and adriamycin. The tumour is radiosensitive providing sufficient dose can be delivered, but Ewing's tumour, like osteogenic sarcoma, has a great tendency to develop metastases. In about 20 per cent of cases metastases are present ot diagnosis and many others become overt within a year but some can be delayed for periods of up to 10 years.

GERM CELL TUMOURS AND MALIGNANT TERATOMAS

Germ cell tumours originate in those cells which eventually differentiate into the ovum and sperm. Tumours of these cells can therefore arise within the gonads or anywhere along the migration path during fetal life. The histology of the tumour depends on the point in maturation at which the abnormal growth occurs, pure yolk sac tumours (endodermal sinus tumours) can occur both in the gonads and in extragonadal sites. These tumours are always associated with an elevation of α-feto protein concentrations; the measurement of this marker is an excellent guide to the complete removal of the tumour and to the development of metastases. When the germ cells have already differentiated and matured along somatic pathways then the resulting tumour is a teratoma; the tumour comprises a variety of different tissues foreign to the part and may be benign or malignant. All these tumours are best treated by surgery when complete removal is possible and then by chemotherapy. The vinca alkaloids, cyclophosphamide, actinomycin D, bleomycin and cisplatinum have all been shown to be effective in various combinations.

Non-germ cell gonadal tumours of childhood include dysgerminomas, seminomas, Leydig and Sertoli cell tumours, granulosa cell and theca cell tumours and adenocarcinomas.

RETINOBLASTOMA

Retinoblastoma is the commonest ocular malignancy of childhood. Significant cure rates for this tumour have been possible since the beginning of the century. Bilateral cases have the inherited autosomal dominant form of the disease and their offspring have a 50 per cent chance of developing retinoblastomas. The majority of children present in the first 2 years of life. The abnormal white pupil so often described as the common presentation is really an indication of a large tumour unless it arises in the macula. A squint is often present at an early stage. Treatment varies according to the extent of disease; enucleation is usually the treatment of choice in unilateral cases unless the disease is diagnosed at an early stage when radiotherapy may be curative without loss of vision. In bilateral disease, careful evaluation of each eye is necessary and the therapeutic decision is based on the size and location of the tumours.

One should note the chance of second malignancies in these children; there is a well-documented association between retinoblastoma and osteogenic sarcoma. This second tumour may arise in the site of previous irradiation or in bone remote from the orbit.

TOXICITY OF THERAPY

Immediate effects

There are many immediate complications of the modern treatment of childhood malignancy. Severe and rapidly spreading infections are a major problem, so unexplained fever in these patients requires immediate investigation and treatment with intravenous broad spectrum antibiotics. Viral infections such as measles, chicken pox and herpes simplex can be fatal; fungal infections and *Pneumocystis carinii* are also quite common.

The children run a considerable risk of nutritional deficiency which may be due to: anorexia associated with the disease or the drugs; vomiting again due to disease or therapy; or malabsorption. Every effort should be made to induce the patients to take normal foods by mouth but it may be necessary to supplement with high-calorie liquid foods and total parenteral nutrition may sometimes be required.

Long-term effects

As more children have survived childhood malig-

nancy, it is clear that a considerable price has to be paid. In order to achieve a cure, certain side effects are inevitable, most of these are due to interference with normal growth by surgery and radiation, endocrine deficiencies produced by radiation and chemotherapeutic effects on the gonads, pituitary, and thyroid glands, and developmental and learning problems produced by cranial irradiation. Many of these problems can be minimised or treated by appropriate replacement therapy, but vigilance is necessary in detecting further problems generated by the newer aggressive treatment programmes. Primary neoplasms have been shown to occur with 10 per cent greater frequency in patients cured of one malignancy in childhood. These have been reported within a few months of the first to as long as 30 years later. Approximately 50 per cent of the reported cases have arisen in sites of previous irradiation, 30 per cent in patients with known tendencies such as retinoblastoma and basal cell carcinoma syndrome, and the remainder where no single underlying cause can be determined.

Psychosocial problems

A family with a child with cancer is under great stress, the chronic nature of the diseases, the disruptive pattern of prolonged chemotherapy and the long-term insecurity associated with the uncertain future take a very significant toll. Those families in which psychosocial problems pre-exist are particularly vulnerable and require constant support. Community services are not geared to provide this and new methods of help need exploration. Considerable progress has been made in the eradication of cancer in childhood and at the present rate of cure, one in 1000 20-year-olds will soon be survivors of childhood cancer. If they are to be considered truly cured, all services concerned with their care must be aware of their needs. At the moment their general care lags behind the advances in cure. Too many survivors of malignancy are sentenced to be classified as handicapped, because the community will not accept them as normal adults.

FURTHER READING

Altman A J & Schwartz A D 1978 Malignant diseases of infancy, childhood and adolescence. Vol. XVIII Major problems in clinical paediatrics. W B Saunders Company, Philadelphia

Fraumeni J F (ed) 1975 Persons at high risk of cancer: an approach to cancer aetiology and control. Academic Press, New York

Marsden H B & Steward J K (eds) 1976 Recent results in cancer research : tumours in children, 2nd edn. Springer Verlag, Berlin

Morris Jones P H (ed) 1979 Topics in paediatrics I, haematology and oncology. Pitman Medical, Tunbridge Wells

Mulvihill J J, Miller R W & Fraumeni J F (eds) 1977 Genetics of human cancer Vol III. Raven Press, New York

Sutow W W, Vietti T J & Fernback D J (eds) 1977 Clinical paediatric oncology, 2nd edn. C.V. Mosby, Saint Louis

Waterhouse J, Muir C, Correa P & Powell J (eds) 1976 Cancer incidence in five continents, Vol III. IARC scientific publication No. 15, Lyon: International Agency for Research on Cancer

22

Neurology

Common neurological disorders causing referral to paediatricians and neurologists include central nervous system infections, epilepsy, headaches, blackouts, developmental delay, neurological handicap and learning problems; disorders such as myasthenia gravis and degenerative disease are rare. It is important for the general practitioner to recognise deviations from normal rather than know neurological diseases in detail.

CENTRAL NERVOUS SYSTEM INFECTIONS

Infections of the central nervous system include meningitis, encephalitis, myelitis (spinal cord), or rarely, brain abscess; the clinical and pathological features depend on extent of involvement and type and virulence of the infecting organism.

Meningitis

Meningitis is inflammation of the meninges; it may be due to infection, leukaemia (leukaemic meningitis), tumour (carcinomatous meningitis) or penetrating injuries of the skull (traumatic meningitis). Infectious meningitis may be due to bacteria, viruses, mycoplasma, tuberculosis, fungi, spirochaetes, leptospira or protozoal organisms. Spread to the meninges is either haematogenous through the choroid plexus, or from localised infection, such as otitis media or sinusitis.

Recurrent bacterial meningitis is often due to anatomical continuity between the meninges and the external environment; congenital defects such as midline (cerebral or spinal) dermal sinuses.

Rarely, recurrent meningitis is due to an immunodeficiency disorder.

Bacterial meningitis (purulent meningitis, septic meningitis)

The predominant infecting organisms causing meningitis vary with age in childhood (Table. 22.1). Bacterial invasion causes inflammation and

Table 22.1 Bacterial meningitis at different ages

Under 28 days (neonate)
Group B streptococcus
Escherichia coli (K strains)
Listeria monocytogenes
Pseudomonas aeruginosa

1 Month–2 Years
Haemophilus influenzae
Neisseria meningitidis (meningococcus)

2 Years–5 Years
Neisseria meningitidis
Haemophilus influenzae

Over 5 Years
Streptococcus pneumoniae
Neisseria meningitidis

hyperaemia of the meninges, followed by neutrophil migration into the subarachnoid space and pus formation. The pus may block the outflow of CSF causing hydrocephalus.

Clinically, there is sudden onset of fever, headache, photophobia, nausea and vomiting, and nuchal or spinal rigidity. Infants usually are irritable with a high pitched cry and have a bulging fontanelle. Convulsions and coma are bad prognostic signs. On examination the child is irritable, drowsy, and has neck stiffness (inability to passively dorsiflex the neck, to touch the chest with the chin on dorsiflexion or the knee on body flexion), a positive Kernig's sign, Brudzinski's sign and tripod sign (when asked to sit up the child may adopt a tripod position with both hands stretched aside and head in extension to avoid a leptomeningeal traction). Some of these signs may be present with causes of meningism such as subarachnoid haemorrhage or painful cervical adenitis. Sixth, third and fourth cranial nerve palsies may also be present. Papilloedema is rare.

The diagnosis is confirmed by laboratory examination of the cerebrospinal fluid (CSF); raised intracranial pressure should be excluded before lumbar puncture. The CSF findings in several infective conditions are shown in Table 22.2. In bacterial infection, neutrophils and organisms may be identified on microscopic examination of the CSF, CSF protein is raised and the sugar is low. Thirty per cent of children with meningitis have positive blood cultures; culture of lumbar fluid confirms the infection and determines antibiotic therapy. The white to red cell ratio allowed in CSF is 1 : 500; peripheral counts and blood sugar should be determined at the time of lumbar puncture.

Countercurrent immunoelectrophoresis (CIE) is a new method which demonstrates the presence of bacterial antigen using specific antibody; pneumococcus, meningococcus ABC, haemophilus and group B streptococcus can be identified. The test is useful if bacterial cultures are negative (example with pre-treatment) or as rapid diagnosis. Urine should also be screened as this may be source of infection.

Antibacterial chemotherapy should be given as soon as the diagnosis is confirmed. The drugs chosen depend on the likely organisms or on proven culture and sensitivity. The current drugs of choice are benzylpenicillin (300 mg/kg daily in 4–6 divided doses, ampicillin (100 mg/kg daily in 4 doses) and chloramphenicol (100 mg/kg daily in 4 divided doses) intravenously. Treatment is given for 10–14 days; the need for repeat lumbar puncture is open to debate. In the newborn period the place of chloramphenicol (25 mg/kg daily) is controversial; a penicillin and aminoglycosede, or cephalosporin are often used.

Meningitis is contagious and it is important to provide antibiotic prophylaxis to close contacts especially with *Haemophilus influenzae*, type B, or meningococcal meningitis. Pre-school, nursery children, household contacts and medical staff should be considered for chemoprophylaxis. The drug given is usually rifampicin; this approach has been shown to prevent secondary cases and spread

Table 22.2 CSF findings in infective conditions

Diagnosis	Cell type/ml	Protein (g/l)	Glucose (mmol/l)	Smear	Comments
Normal	0–5 (lymphocytes)	0.1–0.45	2.8–4.8	Negative	–
Bacterial	200–2000 (mostly polymorphs)	Increased	V. low	Positive	CIE (countercurrent immunoelectrophoresis)
Viral	100–1000 or more (mostly lymphocytes)	Normal or slightly raised 0.45–0.85	Normal (low in mumps)	Negative	Viral isolation Paired sera for antibodies
Tuberculosis	100–1000 or more (mostly lymphocytes)	Increased 0.6–5	Low 0.5–2	Prolonged examination	Ziehl-Neelsen and immunofluorescence
Lesions outside subarachnoid space	Often increased 50–1000 (both lymphocytes and polymorphs)	Normal or increased	Normal	Negative	Cultures usually negative

in a susceptible community. Vaccination against some strains of meningococcus (A and C only) is possible; this is done in the USA where these serotypes predominate; in the UK most infections are due to serotype B. There is currently no satisfactory vaccine against *Haemophilus influenzae*.

Complications of bacterial meningitis

These include ventriculitis. This is the commonest problem encountered in young infants especially in neonates, and is difficult to treat. Ventriculitis should be suspected in any young child who responds poorly to therapy and in whom CSF pleocytosis persists despite therapy. The mortality is high and, if untreated, severe mental and physical handicap is inevitable. Diagnosis is often established by an enhanced CT scan which demonstrates dilated ventricles together with marked periventricular enhancement. Dilatation of the ventricles may also be demonstrated by ultrasound.

Intraventricular antibiotics and surgical drainage are required; this is achieved by the insertion of a Rickham reservoir through which CSF may be obtained and antibiotics instilled. Intrathecal antibiotic therapy is not adequate.

Subdural effusion is not uncommon in young children with meningitis due to *Haemophilus influenzae* and pneumococcus but is less common with meningococcus. The diagnosis should be suspected if the temperature persists, if CSF cultures continue to be positive despite adequate therapy, or if there is a focal or persistent convulsion with positive neurological signs. Diagnosis is now established by CT scan. Surgical drainage is required.

Electrolyte disturbances are common complications of meningitis. They are often only transient and may be due to vomiting alone or development of inappropriate antidiuretic hormone secretion.

Meningococcal meningitis

This is a serious disease which affects any age but preschool children are most susceptible. If the organism which resides in the upper respiratory tract invades causing a septicaemia the child characteristically develops a purpuric or petechial rash together with signs of meningitis. Meningo-coccaemia without meningitis has a worse prognosis than meningococcaemia with meningitis. Why this should be is not clear. Haemorrhage into the adrenal glands or Waterhouse-Friderichsen syndrome is a well-known complication with a high mortality despite the use of steroids. The syndrome is due to disseminated intravascular coagulation. There may also be embolization and fibrin thrombi to the lungs (causing pulmonary odemea) and kidney, or septicaemic shock due to bacterial endotoxin.

The organism can be isolated on lumbar puncture, blood culture or from the purpuric rash. The rash is punctured with a sterile needle and a smear is Gram-stained; intracellular Gram-negative diplococci is often seen. Treatment in meningococcal disease is 10–14 days intravenous benzylpenicillin (penicillin G). Children who are allergic to penicillin may be treated with chloramphenicol. Both drugs may be used in combination. Exchange transfusion and infusion of fresh frozen plasma may be needed while steroids are used if Waterhouse-Friderichsen syndrome is suspected. Meningogococcal disease is a medical emergency. In general practice, if the disease is suspected, i.m. or i.v. penicillin should be given early and often prior to transfer to hospital.

Chronic meningococcaemia without meningitis is a different disease process; this is an autoimmune complex disorder in which there is an intermittent fever an purpuric rash, chronic arthritis, and pneumonitis, with or without serous effusion. Penicillin is still the treatment of choice.

Pneumococcal meningitis

Pneumococcal meningitis is not uncommon in children especially if there is sickle cell disease. The organism enters the meninges by direct spread from the upper respiratory tract (otitis media, mastoiditis, sinusitis) or by haematogenous spread from primary pneumococcal pneumonia. The organism is readily identifiable in the CSF; penicillin is the drug of choice. The disorder has a high relapse and complication rate, subdural effusion and hearing loss are often seen.

Pneumococcal polysaccharide vaccines against B and C serogroups are available and at risk children (sickle cell disease, splenoctomy) can be immunised. Recurrent meningitis should alert the doctor to the possibility of an abnormal connection between the upper airway or ear and the meninges or an immune deficiency.

Haemophilus meningitis

This is the common form of meningitis in children between the age of 6 months and 5 years with a peak age incidence of 1–2 years. There is generally a preceding upper respiratory tract infection. Chloramphenicol and high dose ampicillin are used in treatment; ampicillin resistance is becoming a serious problem. Subdural effusion is a common complication; persistence of fever, irritability, vomiting or a bulging fontanelle should alert the doctor to this possibility and neurosurgical referral should be considered. This form of meningitis has a 5 per cent mortality and variable long-term morbidity.

Neonatal meningitis

The signs and symptoms of meningitis in neonates and young infants are not always clear-cut; they may be vague (e.g. unstable temperature, hypotonia, apnoea) and the diagnosis should be considered in any baby with suspected or proven septicaemia or urinary tract infection. The infants at risk are those born preterm or small-for-dates, babies of diabetic mothers and those born after a complicated delivery, prolonged rupture of membranes or maternal infection; long lines for intravenous feeding, umbilical catheters and endotracheal tubes also increase the risk. A possible cause of meningitis is spina bifida (Fig. 22.1). Diagnosis of meningitis is by lumbar puncture. The newborn with meningitis is at particular risk of disseminated intravascular coagulation (DIC) and septicaemic shock.

Treatment is with antibiotics, often given empirically at first, and then changed depending on results of culture; fresh frozen plasma and exchange transfusion may have to be considered. Any electrolyte disturbance or hyporglycaemia should be corrected and convulsions treated with anticonvulsant drugs. Ventriculitis or subdural effusion should be suspected if there is no response to standard treatment.

The mortality with newborn meningitis is high; long-term morbidity is also high with hydrocephalus, mental retardation and spasticity often encountered.

Cerebral Abscess

An abscess in the brain may occur as a complication of bacterial meningitis, especially following a septic focus such as otitis media, sinusitis with osteomyelitis of the skull, face lesion, or a skull fracture through the sinus or mastoid, it may also occur as a complication of cyanotic congenital heart disease. Clinical features and signs are variable depending on the size and site of the abscess; there

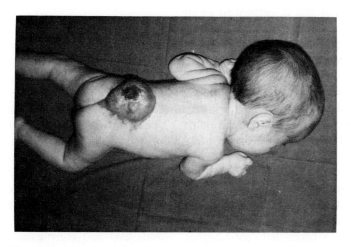

Fig. 22.1 Newborn baby with spina bifida and hydrocephalus

may be fever, malaise, headache, vomiting and focal fits. Localising signs such as hemiplegia, visual defects or evidence of raised intracranial pressure may be present. A high index of suspicion is required to make the diagnosis, confirmation is by CT scan. An EEG may locate an abscess by showing slow wave activity. Lumbar puncture is dangerous if there is raised intracranial pressure.

Management is supportive (treat convulsions), with antibiotics and surgical drainage. Prognosis is variable and depends on delay in diagnosis, the size of the abscess and response to therapy.

Tuberculous meningitis

Children are at risk of developing TB meningitis from contact with open tuberculosis (usually from a relative). The onset is usually gradual, a primary tuberculous complex may not be suspected; miliary TB develops with generalised clinical features and eventual meningitis. The child may initially have personality change, irritability and headache; vomiting, marked constipation and prolonged anorexia then develop followed over a week or so by increasing drowsiness, photophobia and worsening headache. There may be neck stiffness, opisthotonus, sixth nerve palsy, squint, papilloedema, choroidal tubercles or nystagmus. If the diagnosis is missed the child goes on to coma and convulsions with decerebrate rigidity, markedly raised intracranial pressure and often death.

A high index of suspicion is required to make a diagnosis. A tuberculin test is performed in all children in whom the disease is suspected although it is important to remember that in 25 per cent of established cases there is anergy and a negative test. Examination of the CSF confirms the diagnosis; if this is allowed to stand it forms a web which contains tubercle bacilli. The CSF pressure is often raised, there is a lymphocytosis with increased protein and decreased sugar. Acid-fast bacilli may be seen on Ziehl-Neelsen training. If spinal tuberculosis is suspected, an X-ray of the spine with tomography and a bone scan should be sought. A chest X-ray may show miliary tuberculosis.

Antituberculous treatment should be started as soon as the diagnosis is confirmed (see Chapter 17). Cerebral oedema may also need to be treated.

The infection is mainly basal; communicating hydrocephalus and raised intracranial pressure are recognised complications. If the child develops intermittent coma or drowsiness a CT scan should be is advisable. A Rickham reservoir may need to be inserted so that CSF may be removed to reduce pressure, or streptomycin may be instilled into the lateral ventricles. The prognosis has improved with medical and neurosurgical management; long-term morbidity is considerable with visual and hearing deficits, hydrocephalus, mental retardation, spasticity and post-meningitic epilepsy occurring.

Partially-treated meningitis

During the early stages of bacterial meningitis, symptoms and signs may not be obvious and oral antibiotics may have to be prescribed for suspected otitis media, tonsillitis, pneumonia. There may be some suppression of the central infection but only incomplete treatment; lumbar puncture may suggest meningitis (but often there is a lymphocytosis rather than an increase in neutrophils). A child who has had antibiotics and presents with borderline CSF findings should be treated as for bacterial meningitis until it is proved otherwise. Countercurrent immunoelectrophoresis of CSF, blood and urine may be helpful in the situation.

Aseptic (viral, lymphocytic) meningitis

The virus enters the meninges directly or retrograde via peripheral nerves as in poliomyelitis and herpes simplex, or by haematogenous spread as in mumps and varicella. The epidemiology of viral illness in the child's school and community should be noted; the viruses which often cause meningitis include mumps, measles, enteroviruses, herpes simplex, varicella and Epstein-Barr virus.

Clinical onset is often gradual with fever, headache, vomiting, anorexia and neuralgia leading to meningitic features; around 10 per cent of children have associated features of encephalitis (marked drowsiness and convulsions). The clinical examination is as for bacterial meningitis; there may be parotid swelling in mumps meningitis, or diarrhoea and rash in enteroviral meningitis.

The diagnosis depends on CSF findings; CSF may be clear, the pressure is normal, protein is only mildly elevated, the sugar is normal, except in mumps meningitis where it is low, lymphocytes predominate and no organisms are seen on staining. Electron microscopy of a spun CSF specimen may show viral particles; diagnosis is often only established later with culture or in retrospect by serology.

No specific treatment is usually required; there is often confusion between viral meningitis and partially-treated bacterial meningitis and, if in doubt, assume bacterial meningitis and treat appropriately. Initial diagnostic lumbar puncture often serves as a therapeutic measure and the child improves. The mechanism for this is not fully understood but may be related to CSF dynamics. Antiviral therapy should be considered in severe cases, particularly if signs of focal encephalitis supervene. Headache may require medication; often paracetamol is adequate.

Recent evidence suggests a significant number of children have some residual handicap following viral meningitis. This is in the form of easy tiredness, behaviour changes, headache and permanent marked weakness.

Encephalitis

Encephalitis is an infection of the brain substance, encephalopathy refers to inflammation of the brain due to non-infective causes (metabolic or toxic). In encephalitis, there may be direct invasion by the virus or an immunological perivascular response. Acute encephalitis is usually due to a virus and is more serious than viral meningitis as it often results in permanent brain damage. The viruses which cause meningitis can also cause encephalitis. The herpesvirus group is an important cause in children. Clinically there is altered consciousness, disorientation, confusion, convulsions, coma, delirium, headache and vomiting. In herpes encephalitis the intial symptomatology may be non-specific and includes fever, vomiting, a refusal to feed, mild coryza, lethargy and behaviour disturbance. Skin lesions or cold sores may be present 3–6 weeks prior to the onset of symptoms or at the same time. Focal convulsions occur between the second and fourth day of the illness, together with focal neurological signs such as flaccid or spastic hemiplegia, unilateral cranial nerve involvement and unilateral choreiform or dystonic movements. There is a typical EEG in herpes encephalitis which aids the diagnosis. Management includes treatment of cerebral oedema and anti-viral drugs (adenine arabinoside or acyclovir). The prognosis is poor with late treatment, many children die or are left with permanent handicap; early treatment with antiviral drugs may improve the prognosis.

HEADACHE

Headache is a common symptom in children; in infants it may manifest as irritability and screaming; an older child can describe the pain. The pain is due to irritation, pressure or traction on pain sensitive structures in the head or neck. The brain itself is relatively insensitive to pain. The main causes of headache are shown in Table 22.3.

Acute headache

Acute headache may be severe. In many cases, the child has a fever with a virus infection, but a neurological cause needs to be considered especially if there is associated vomiting or alteration in consciousness. Meningitis, encephalitis, acute hydrocephalus, subarachnoid, intracranial or acute subdural haemorrhage need to be considered in the differential diagnosis. If there is a suggestion of meningitis (see p. 244) hospitalisation and a lumbar puncture are necessary to exclude it.

Children with concussion following head injury may also have severe headaches. Analgesics may be given but sedation should be avoided. If there is progressive deterioration in the conscious level then immediate neurosurgical referral is indicated. Dexamethazone should be avoided until an intracranial bleed is excluded by a CT scan.

Table 22.3 Causes of headaches

Acute		Chronic			
With vomiting	*Without vomiting*	*Progressive with vomiting and fits*	*Without vomiting (no fits)*	*Persistent with vomiting*	*Without vomiting*
Simple febrile illness	Simple febrile illness	Raised intracranial pressure	Trigeminal neuralgia	Migraine	Tension headache
Meningitis	Poisoning and intoxication e.g. glue sniffing	Space occupying lesions, tumour abscess, cyst, chronic subdural haemorrhage	Glosso pharyngeal neuralgia		Malocclusion Poor head or neck posture
Encephalitis	Hypoglycaemia		vasculitis		Referred pain Sinusitis
Subarachnoid, intracranial or acute subdural haemorrhage		Pseudotumour cerebri (benign intracranial hypertension)			Rhinitis
Concussion of the brain		Hypertensive encephalopathy Lead poisoning			Toothache
					Cervical spondylosis

Acute headache without vomiting is rare and may be due to drug intoxication (e.g. glue sniffing), or to unrecognised recurrent hypoglycaemia.

Chronic headache

Chronic headaches are distressing to both child and parents and are a common cause for missing school. Doctors are often unable to give a clear-cut explanation. The headaches may be progressive, gradually increase in frequency and duration, or persistent, remaining unchanged in frequency and duration over a period of time.

Progressive headache

Increased intracranial pressure may present as progressive headache with vomiting; there may be focal neurological signs or papilloedema and a space-occupying lesion such as tumour or abscess should be suspected. Early morning headaches or those which wake the child are usually serious, however, migraine can also cause this form of headache. A skull X-ray may show suture separation or calcification while a CT scan may show the lesion. Hypertension, chronic disease and lead poisoning must also be excluded. Progressive headache without vomiting is generally due to local irritation or pressure; trigeminal or glossopharyn-geal neuralgia are good examples. The problem should be recognised as the pain may respond to analgesic agents or to carbamazepine.

Persistent headache

Headaches which are recurrent are unlikely to be due to raised intracranial pressure; migraine and its variants are relatively common. The incidence of migraine is 50 per 1000 which is eight times more frequent than epilepsy. There is often a positive family history (in 80 per cent). Migra-inous attacks are rare under the age of 2 years but do occur in early childhood; they are more common in the pre-pubertal period and boys are affected twice as often as girls. In adolescents and adults migraine is commoner in females. Where there is a strong family history, attacks may begin early in life. Infants may present with crying and vomiting and they are often labelled as windy or colicky babies. The vomiting and abdominal pain persist in childhood and become more pronounced; the child is often then diagnosed as periodic syndrome. Migraine is only diagnosed when the headache becomes the main feature. Young infants are not able to complain of headache but are usually irritable or pale during an attack. Older children often have a history of travel sickness or sleep disturbance and nightmares.

Various factors may act as a trigger; food (milk and milk products, egg, chocolate, tea, coffee, nuts), food colouring (tartrazine) and additives. Emotional upset, tension, psychosocial deprivation, learning problems, intercurrent mild illness, severe exercise, mild head injury, exercise and bright sunshine are also known to precipitate an attack in a susceptible individual.

There are four types of migraine: classical migraine and common migraine, which have a preceding aura, and cluster headache and complicated migraine which may not. The type of aura depends on which arteries are involved and on the degree of vasoconstriction. The commonest is a visual hallucination due to ophthalmic artery involvement, these include flashing lights, field defects (blind spot), microscopia (objects looking smaller than they are), and scotomata. Mesenteric artery constriction causes gastrointestinal aura (nausea, vomiting, sensation of fullness), while hemianaesthesia and aphasia occur if the cranial arteries are involved.

Classical migraine

The headache in classical migraine is unilateral (hemicrania), often frontal or temporal but bifrontal or occipital headache may also occur. It is described as throbbing and severe. Photophobia or vertigo may be present; the child tends to lie down in a dark room and go to sleep. The duration of the attack is variable; most children improve after sleep but some attacks may last for as long as 2–3 days.

Common migraine

Here the aura is less well-defined than in classical migraine; the headaches are diffuse and the child often has nausea or vomiting. He looks ill and is pale. Vasodilatation of the extra-cerebral vessels causes oedema of the scalp and venous pulsation can be felt over the temple. Headache intensity may be decreased by pressure over the vessels.

Cluster headache

Here the headache may recur daily for several days at a time with prolonged trouble-free periods between attacks. There is no aura nor photophobia. The pain is severe and throbbing but often of short duration (30–90 minutes) and usually occurs in the orbital or temporal regions. Conjunctival redness, oedema, lacrimation, pulsation of the eye, and urinary frequency may be present. Cluster headaches are commoner in males. The headache usually responds to simple analgesics and the child does not seem to prefer a dark room.

Complicated migraine

This form has a varied presentation which may include periodic syndrome, abdominal migraine or rare forms such as ophthalmoplegic, hemiplegic, alternating hemiplegic, basilar artery, convulsive or psychomotor migraine. Complicated migraine may lead to mental retardation especially if it is the alternating hemiplegic type. There is presumably neuronal death secondary to prolonged and frequent arterial vasoconstriction. There may be brain infarction resulting in permanent visual defects, ophthalmoplegia, aphasia or hemiplegia.

Treatment of migraine, especially in classical form is difficult. If there is clear evidence of food intolerance then the offending substance should be avoided; remember that many food products may contain the substance and advice from a dietician may be helpful. In classical migraine the child should lie down in a quiet dark room, analgesia may help but there is no evidence that an ergotamine preparation is useful. Ergotamine is only helpful in common migraine where vasodilatation is the main feature; in children with the complicated form it is contra-indicated as it may increase symptoms due to excessive vasoconstriction. Anti-emetic and anti-vertigo agents are useful as symptomatic adjuncts. Frequent (more than two attacks a month) or severe attacks may respond to continuous migraine prophylaxis; pizotifen may be helpful. Parents and children should be warned that it may take 3–4 weeks before any benefit is seen and the importance of routine therapy should be emphasized. Beta-blockers (such as propranolol) help only in acute attacks but not in prophylaxis. Assurance should be given that migraine tends to improve with age (but may recur in adolescence), that there is no serious disease present and the child should be regarded as normal and otherwise healthy.

Functional or tension headache

Functional or tension headache is usually vague but persistent, non-throbbing and may be diffuse or occur bilaterally into the vertex or occiput. Inquiries should be made about family or school stress, insomnia or depression. Drug medication is not usually of help and often advice from a child guidance clinic or psychiatrist may be indicated.

Referred headache

These are due to excessive muscle contraction as occurs in poor head or neck posture, or dental malocclusion. Non-paralytic squint, myopia and astigmatism are not causes of headaches in children, unlike adults, but may interfere with vision and therefore should be corrected. Detailed examination of the sinuses, eyes, teeth and cervical region may suggest the site of origin. Management involves analgesia and treatment of the cause.

Headaches, regardless of cause, are a significant symptom to the child and a sympathetic approach is required from the physician, family and school for satisfactory management.

SEIZURES

Terminology can be confusing. The terms convulsion, fits and epilepsy are by no means synonymous in the lay mind. It is important to clarify what has been observed by the parent, what preceded it and what the child's condition was like following the episode; their use of the word fit may refer to a genuine seizure or to a temper tantrum, night terror or rigor.

A seizure is characterised by alteration in motor, sensory or autonomic function, with or without loss of consciousness and associated with abnormal neuronal electrical discharges. A convulsion is a symptom of an underlying disorder and is not in itself a diagnosis.

Most individuals can be induced into having a seizure depending on the stimulus and their 'seizure threshold'; the threshold is not measurable but is thought to be reduced in young individuals and by: (1) structural abnormalities of the brain such as hydrocephalus, cysts, tumour or abscess; (2) chemical abnormalities, including hypoglycaemia and hypocalcaemia; (3) stimuli such as fever, causing febrile convulsions, flashing lights, causing photogenic/television seizures and psychogenic factors such as stress. A suitable history, or direct observation, is required to diagnose the presence of convulsions and an electroencephalogram (EEG) may be helpful in characterising the seizure. Telemetric and 24-hour recordings which allow normal activity may be useful.

There are four components to a seizure: (1) prodrome, this may last a few hours or even days. There may be a change in behaviour, mood, appetite or sleep pattern which may be recognisable by parents or the child himself; (2) aura, 50 per cent of children give a history of an aura or warning which may be visual, auditory or olfactory; (3) convulsion (see Table 22.4), the pattern depends on the site of the abnormal electrical discharges, and (4) post-ictal; the child may be confused, drowsy or have automatisms.

Epilepsy

Epilepsy is a condition in which there is a tendency to recurrent seizures. The incidence is roughly 5–7 per 1000. A single convulsion for which there is a correctable cause such as hypoglycaemia is not strictly epilepsy. In 80 per cent of childhood epilepsy no cause is apparent (idiopathic epilepsy); secondary causes include central nervous system malformations or infections, metabolic abnormalities (e.g. phenylketonuria), trauma, cerebrovascular disease, tumours, drugs and drug withdrawals, degenerative disease and the neurocutaneous syndromes (e.g. tuberous sclerosis). Idiopathic epilepsy is frequently familial but with no specific inheritance pattern; several secondary epilepsies are inherited such as those associated with tuberous sclerosis.

Table 22.4 International classification of seizures

Type	Clinical feature	Origin of focus	EEG	Aetiology	Most effective anticonvulsant
1. Partial seizures (those beginning focally)					
a. Partial seizures with elementary (motor or sensory) symptoms	No loss of consciousness	Cortical, single focus	Focal	Focal anatomical lesion — tumour, cyst, abscess, scar (head injury), A–V malformation	Carbamazepine Phenytoin (Phenobarbitone)
b. Partial seizures with complex symptoms (temporal lobe epilepsy)	Loss of consciousness	Cortical temporal lobe focus	Temporal lobe spikes	Temporal lobe sclerosis (Ammon's horn sclerosis) cyst, tumour	Carbamazepine Phenytoin (Phenobarbitone)
c. Partial seizures with secondary generalisation	Initial focal then GM (grand mal), GM with aura	Cortical focus with spread to other cortical parts	Asymmetrical		Valproate Phenytoin Carbamazepine Combination Carbamazepine + Valproate Phenobarbitone
2. Generalised seizures (those without focal onset)					
a. Petit mal	Absences	Cortical	Bilateral, symmetrical 3 c/s spike and wave	Idiopathic (genetic)	Valproate Ethosuximide
b. Grand mal	Tonic-clonic	Cortical, central	Bilateral symmetrical discharges	Idiopathic (Genetic)	Valproate Phenobarbitone Phenytoin Carbamazepine
c. Myoclonic	Often on wakening or drifting to sleep Could be very frequent	Cortical, central	Typical 2 or c/s spike and wave; polyspike complexes	Idiopathic, Degenerative disorders A few may be benign (benign myoclonic epilepsy)	Valproate, Clonazepam Carbamazepine Steroid, ACTH Ketogenic diet
d. Infantile spasms	Salaam fits Lightening spasms	Cortical, multifocal	High voltage disorganized — hypsarrhythmia	Idiopathic or symptomatic (tuberous sclerosis. triple immunisation, birth asphyxia)	ACTH, Nitrazepam Valproate
e. Akinetic	Drop attack	Cortical, multifocal	Atypical spike and wave complexes mixed often polyspikes		Valproate Nitrazepam
3. Unilateral seizures	Unilateral, grand mal	Cortical, unilateral	Unilateral discharges	Focal anatomical lesion — tumour, A–V malformation, cyst	Carbamazepine, Phenytoin
4. Unclassified seizures					

Classification

Epilepsy is classified into:

1. Generalised
2. Partial or focal epilepsy.

In generalised epilepsy the seizures are generalised from onset and originate from both hemispheres, whereas in focal epilepsy there is a single focus within the brain. Generalised epilepsy is further sub-divided into primary and secondary depending on whether the seizures originate from normal cortex (primary) or from cortex which is damaged (secondary). Primary generalised epilepsy is often familial and there is normal intelligence and neurological examination. Children with the secondary form are often mentally retarded and invariably have some neurological abnormality such as spastic quadriplegia, optic atrophy, microcephaly or ataxia. With focal epilepsy intelligence is usually normal and there may be a focal neurological abnormality. The seizure type should be included in describing the type of epilepsy. The international classification is shown in Table 22.4. If there are several seizure patterns then the patient should be classified by the predominant type.

Partial seizures

These originate from a single focus within the brain and may be elementary (focal) or complex (e.g. temporal lobe epilepsy). Focal convulsions may be motor or sensory depending on which part of the cortex is involved; motor and sensory components may, however, coexist. Typically, there is no loss of consciousness although if the electrical discharge spreads to involve other areas of the brain then the seizure may become generalised (partial seizures with secondary generalisation).

Partial seizure with elementary motor symptoms (partial motor seizure)

The motor symptoms depend on which part of the motor cortex is involved and are evident in the contralateral limb or body. The thumb is most often affected; in Jacksonian seizures jerking usually starts in the thumb and spreads to the fingers, then to the hand and eventually involves one-half of the body.

Partial seizure with elementary sensory symptoms (partial sensory seizure)

The focus occurs in the sensory cortex and, depending on the area, results in either a somatic or special sensory seizure. The somatic form presents with tingling, numbness or warmth of a part of the body and, because of the proximity with motor cortex, a degree of motor involvement in the form of short tonic spasms or posturing. Special sensory seizures originate in the occipital or temporal lobe and involve the auditory, visual, olfactory or taste area; there may be vertigo, flashing of lights or hallucination of smell, sound (hearing voices, noise, music) or vision (objects looking larger than normal).

Partial seizures with complex symtpoms (complex partial seizures)

These were previously known as temporal lobe epilepsy or psychomotor epilepsy and form about one-quarter of all, and 50 per cent of focal seizures. The convulsion starts in the temporal lobe but can spread to involve other parts of the cortex. Temporal lobe damage may be due to: (1) chronic neurological disease or an illness damaging the brain (e.g. birth asphyxia, meningitis, tuberous sclerosis, head injury); (2) prolonged seizures, including febrile convulsions, lasting more than 30 minutes in young children may cause neuronal damage of the hypocampal areas of the temporal lobe; and (3) space occupying lesions in the temporal lobe (e.g. cysts, tumours, or tuberous sclerosis). These convulsions present in various ways: (a) with an aura which may include visceral or special sense experiences such as nausea, vertigo, olfactory (unpleasant smell) or auditory (hearing voices, music) hallucinations, or the well-known déjà vu (a sense of familiarity in an unfamiliar setting) or jamais vu (a sense of unfamiliarity in a familiar setting) phenomena. Mood upsets in the form of fear or anxiety are common. If the dominant hemisphere is involved then speech may be affected (dysphasia or aphasia); (b) staring attacks which may resemble petit mal epilepsies where the child stops what he is doing; there may be impairment of consciousness, the attack usually lasts 2–5 minutes and the child often experiences post-ictal confusion; (c) automatisms which may be simple or complex and may last a few minutes or hours. Simple automatisms include grimacing, lip smacking, chewing, sucking, picking at clothes, toys or hair. Complex automatisms include violent running, undressing, walking about aimlessly, screaming and scratching.

The diagnosis may be difficult if only an aura in the form of sensory phenomenon or automatisms occur; usually there is a combination. These seizures are of short duration and begin and end abruptly. An EEG may be helpful in confirming the diagnosis. Children who do not respond readily to anticonvulsant therapy should be further investigated with a CT scan to exclude a space-occupying lesion or scar.

Partial seizures with secondary generalisation

These are focal seizures which become generalised, and the child loses consciousness. The EEG often shows an asymmetrical discharge involving one hemisphere more than the other, the hemisphere with the initial focus shows more spikes.

Therapy of partial seizures

Both elementary and complex forms often respond well to carbamazepine or phenytoin. Intractable temporal lobe epilepsy may require surgical removal of the temporal lobe. Partial seizures with a secondary generalisation respond well to sodium valproate alone, or in combination with carbamazepine.

Children with partial complex seizures may have psychological disturbances, personality disorders, memory loss and reduced learning ability; parents and schools should be appropriately counselled and in severe cases psychiatric or child guidance clinics involved.

Generalised seizures

Epileptic discharges originate in both hemispheres or a deep-seated focus and results in a generalised convulsion (see Table 22.4).

Petit mal or absence attacks

These are frequent, abrupt in onset and brief (5–20 s) episodes of unconsciousness associated with cessation of activity and are more common in girls aged 5–12 years. During the attack the child may show motor or aural automatisms such as staring, blinking, chewing or lip smacking. There is no post-ictal phase and the child is usually unaware of the seizure but may be embarrassed by an associated incontinence. Petit mal status is uncommon. The seizures are associated with EEG bilateral symmetrical spike and wave complexes occurring at a rate of 3 per second and which can be provoked by hyperventilation. The prognosis of petit mal is unfavourable if it develops before 5 years or after 12 years of age, or if there is a pre-existing neurological abnormality or mental retardation; these children later develop other seizures such as grand mal.

Drugs of choice is petit mal are sodium valproate or ethosuximide. Sodium valproate is given orally at 20–30 mg/kg daily in divided doses; some children may require up to 50–60 mg/kg daily. Treatment should be continued for two symptom-free years; withdrawal after prolonged therapy should be slow (3–4 months).

Grand mal (generalised motor tonic-clonic seizures)

Approximately 80 per cent of children with epilepsy have grand mal seizures. The seizure begins abruptly and usually without warning; there is a loss of consciousness and the child falls to the ground; a generalised tonic (rigid) phase then occurs, during which time there is apnoea, cyanosis and deviation of the eyes, followed by a clonic phase. There is rapid generalised jerking movements of all four limbs, the child may bite his tongue, respirations are irregular and pharyngeal secretions are increased with frothing of saliva. Urinary and faecal incontinence and a short period of tachycardia and hyperventilation may occur. A phase of relaxation occurs; the child is limp, respirations and heart rate become normal and then post-ictal sleep of variable duration follows. After this the child may be irritable, confused, may complain of headache or tiredness and there may be paralysis, ataxia and slow speech. There may be only a tonic or clonic phase.

The pharamacological management of grand mal involves anticonvulsant drugs (sodium valproate is the drug of choice; phenobarbitone, carbamazepine and phenytoin are also used). The side effects of sodium valproate include transient hair loss, obesity, enuresis, thrombocytopenia and, rarely, disturbance of liver metabolism with raised blood ammonia concentration and encephalopathy. Side effects with phenytoin are common and include ataxia, nystagmus, gum hypertrophy, hirsutism, and interference with immunological function. Carbamazepine and sodium valproate are a useful combination in difficult cases. Duration of drug therapy is arbitrary; usually a 2-year seizure-free period is felt to be necessary before slowly discontinuing drugs. This should be done one drug at a time and over several months. The EEG does not provide an adequate guide to discontinuation.

Myoclonic epilepsy

This is a brief. involuntary, single or multiple jerk of an extremity. Sleep myoclonus is a normal phenomenon and occurs when drifting to sleep or when awakening. Myoclonic epilepsy may be idiopathic (primary) or more complex (secondary); secondary causes include metabolic abnormalities (e.g. uraemia). neuroallergic reactions (such as post-encephalopathy or immunisation) and hypoxic brain damage. Infantile spasms, benign myoclonus of early infancy, myoclonus of early infancy, myoclonic astatic epilepsy or Lennox-Gastaut syndrome, progressive myoclonic epilepsy of childhood, myoclonic epilepsy of adolescence and eyelid myoclonia with absences are sometimes lumped into this group; the international classification of seizures puts infantile spasms and akinetic attacks under a separate heading.

1. Lennox-Gastaut syndrome: a form of infantile spasms which occurs in older children. There may be associated grand mal and petit mal seizures. The EEG shows a slow spike and wave discharge. This is one of the most severe forms of epilepsy and the attacks are often intractable to conventional therapy; sodium valproate alone or in combination with carbamazepine, nitrazepam or acetazolamide may be helpful. If the attacks are resistant then a ketogenic diet or steroids should be tried. The prognosis is poor and good control is achieved in only 20 per cent; the remainder become progressively mentally retarded.

2. Benign myoclonic epilepsy of childhood: children between 3 and 8 years are usually affected; myoclonus occurs in the upper limb and there are frequently violent falls. The EEG in this condition shows 3 per second spike and wave, or polyspike wave complexes. This form of epilepsy responds well to sodium valproate with a good prognosis. Therapy should be continued until adult life.

3. Myoclonic epilepsy of adolescence: this is similar to the benign myoclonic form in childhood but appears in puberty and is more common in females particularly at period times. There may be sleep myoclonus and frequently grand mal seizures. The prognosis is good. Sodium valproate is the drug of choice.

4. Myoclonic absences: these are rare and consist of a brief interruption of consciousness as in petit mal absences together with myoclonus and automatisms. A combination of sodium valproate and ethosuximide is used.

5. Eyelid myoclonia with absences: this is a rare form of myoclonic epilepsy with typical absences, jerking of the eyelids and upward deviation of the eyes. The attacks are photosensitive and are induced by bright light or repetitive blinking. They can be confirmed by EEG and respond to a combination of sodium valproate and ethosuximide.

Minor status epilepticus

This is considered by some authorities to be a variant of myoclonic epilepsy. It may be suspected in children with predominantly grand mal epilepsy who despite adequate control continue to show a fluctuating deterioration in intellectual or motor function. There is often head nodding, eye flickering, dribbling, slurred speech and confusion. A pseudodementia or pseudoataxia may be present and disappear when the attacks are relieved. The EEG shows a marked abnormality with prolonged electrical storms of 1.5–4 cycles per second and waves, mixed sharp elements or spikes, together with ill-defined complexes. Treatment is difficult; steroids and ketogenic diets have been used. Intravenous chlormethiazole or continuous clonazepam may need to be tried in resistant cases.

Akinetic epilepsy

In this form of epilepsy the child has sudden loss of muscle tone and falls but recovers quickly. These attacks are socially embarrassing and may cause physical trauma, bruises and haematomas. Loss of consciousness is absent or minimal and there is no post-ictal phase. The attacks occur alone or in combination with other forms of seizure. Treatment is difficult; clonazepam, sodium valproate, ketogenic diet and steroids can be tried alone or in various combinations.

Infantile spasms (salaam attacks or West's syndrome)

This affects young children, aged 3 months to 1 year. The parents first notice brief, but frequent, flexor spasms. The child gives a short cry, shoots out his arms and flexes his body and legs giving a salaam or greeting posture. The attacks last a few seconds but recur in succession with about 15–30 attacks a minute. The parents often describe the episodes as colic. There may be fit-free periods of several minutes or hours. The child shows failure in developmental progression and even regression. Infantile spasms may be secondary to a pre-existing neurological abnormality such as severe birth asphyxia, metabolic disease, infection or tuberous sclerosis. In the majority, however, no pre-existing neurological abnormality is obvious. The EEG shows a typical chaotic pattern with a total disorganisation of cortical activity which is termed hypsarhythmia (hyps means mountain-like).

Treatment should be started at diagnosis; untreated attacks may burn out leaving the child severely retarded and with other types of seizures. The treatment of hypsarrhythmia is i.m. ACTH with or without nitrazepam in combination. The prognosis is variable.

Epilepsia partialis continua This is a rare type of epilepsy in which the discharges originate in an isolated area of the motor cortex so that prolonged focal epilepsy without loss of consciousness occurs.

The attacks may be prolonged and difficult to treat; ACTH or steroids, or lobectomy may have to be considered.

Unclassified seizures

Reflex epilepsy

Attacks begin in childhood or early puberty (age 6–15 years) and are more common in females. Grand mal or petit mal seizures are precipitated by certain sensory stimuli (especially visual or auditory); an example is television or photosensitive epilepsy which is induced by flickering light. The attacks are induced by sitting close to a poorly adjusted television set, or by lights in discothèques. The EEG with photic stimulation may induce attacks; spike discharges may be seen. The photosensitive child should be advised to watch television from a distance of at least 3 m and the room should not be darkened. They should be advised to cover one eye when approaching the television set to adjust the channel, when suddenly facing a bright light or entering a discothèque. Tinted sunglasses may be helpful in bright sunlight. If drug treatment is required sodium valproate is used.

Benign focal epilepsy of childhood (benign Rolandic epilepsy)

This form of partial epilepsy starts at 7–10 years of age, disappears by 15 years and is commoner in males. A family history is present in 15 per cent of cases. Attacks occur during sleep or often on awakening; during the attacks the child wakes up, salivates and may have mild jerks of limbs, lips or tongue. He may be unable to speak but is conscious. Some children have tonic-clonic seizures. The EEG is characteristic with unilateral or, rarely, bilateral spikes over the Rolandic or Sylvian region. The attacks may respond to carbamazepine.

Status epilepticus

A series of seizures without recovery of consciousness between attacks, or any seizure lasting more than 30 minutes should be considered as status epilepticus. This is a medical emergency as continuous seizures cause brain hypoxia, cerebral oedema, hyperpyrexia and dehydration; the cause (e.g. encephalitis) needs to be determined.

Status epilepticus is also seen if there is a sudden withdrawal of anticonvulsants in children who have had long treatment with these drugs; the drugs should be recommenced.

The present treatment of choice for status epilepticus is a diazepam preparation given intravenously or by the rectal route. Drug absorption from the rectum is good and control of convulsions is achieved quickly. Each dose is 0.5 mg/kg up to 10 mg maximum or 1 mg per year of age plus 1 mg. Continuous diazepam and a dose of 0.5 mg/kg h^{-1} may be given as continuous rectal or continuous intravenous infusion. There is no place for intramuscular diazepam as it is slowly absorbed.

Other drugs which may be helpful include phenobarbitone and rectal or intramuscular paraldehyde. Rectal paraldehyde is given preferably mixed with equal volumes of an oil (e.g. arachis oil). The modern plastic syringes are resistent to paraldehyde but, to be safe, the drug should be administered soon after drawing it up.

If the convulsion lasts more than 6–8 hours the child should be treated for cerebral oedema with intravenous mannitol, phenobarbitone and dexamethazone. Intravenous chlormethiazole may be effective in resistant cases. Supportive care includes an adequate calorie and fluid intake by the nasogastric or intravenous route, control of body temperature, and chest physiotherapy if prolonged sedation is required. Resistant cases becomes comatose due to brain cell death or coning.

General management of epilepsy

The parents should be taught principles of maintaining the airway and appropriate posture to prevent aspiration of vomit. During ambulance transfer oxygen therapy should be given.

At home the parents can be taught to administer rectal diazepam in selected cases. Medical advice should be sought with any prolonged convulsions. For drug treatment by the doctor see status epilepticus.

Long-term anticonvulsant medication depends on the seizure type rather than the epilepsy classification (see previous sections). The aim is to use a single drug, but occasionally combinations are necessary. Compliance should be monitored by occasional blood or salivary levels, especially if a child on anticonvulsants is admitted to hospital with seizures, or to check for toxicity (e.g. phenytoin or phenobarbitone excess may precipitate seizures). Parents should be advised of known drug side effects.

Clinical (school) medical officers and teachers should be kept informed about progress and drug therapy. Both drug treatment and the disorder may affect school performance. A child on anticonvulsants can be encouraged to participate in all school activities, including sports; swimming is allowed if epilepsy control and supervision on site are adequate.

Parents should be counselled and reassured that most epileptics are able to lead normal lives. Overprotection should be discouraged. Convulsions are common in mentally retarded children and in those with behaviour problems (which comes first?). Advice from a child psychiatrist and child guidance clinic may be helpful, particularly with temporal lobe epilepsy. Maladjusted children can induce seizures; some children may improve with operant-conditioning techniques such as denial or reward, or with hypnosis.

Febrile convulsions

A febrile convulsion is a seizure occurring in a child between 6 months and 6 years in association with fever and in the absence of intracranial infection, without previous evidence of cerebral pathology or history of convulsion in the absence of fever. The incidence is 3–5 per cent. The typical febrile convulsion is a brief, single and generalised grand mal seizure. In some children the convulsion may be prolonged (more than 30 minutes) and present as status epilepticus. Post-ictal sleep is common.

Any infection may provoke a febrile convulsion; viral upper respiratory tract and urinary tract infections are the most common. In the young child (under 18 months) many authorities advocate routine lumbar puncture as it is difficult to exclude meningitis.

Febrile convulsions are thought to occur because of a genetically (autosomal dominant) determined low seizure threshold; if either parent or a sibling has had febrile convulsions the risk is 50 per cent. In monozygotic twins the concordance of febrile convulsions is 80 per cent. Males are affected twice as frequently as females. The trigger in the susceptible child is the rate of rise and height of fever; a child with a low threshold may convulse with a minimal rise in temperature whereas those with a higher threshold may only have seizures after a marked rise. Children with a history of cerebral problems at birth have low seizure thresholds and the incidence of convulsions associated with temperature in these children is 20 per cent.

Febrile convulsions are often recurrent and 50 per cent of affected children may have more than one, while approximately 20 per cent may have as many as four; recurrence is more common in girls. The recurrence risk is as high as 50 per cent if the first fit occurred under 18 months of age, while it is only 10 per cent if the first occurred after 3 years. Five to 10 per cent of children with febrile convulsions develop later recurrent unprovoked convulsions or epilepsy.

The aim of management is to stop the acute convulsion and prevent recurrence. Temperature control is important; this may be achieved by antipyretic drugs and simple measures such as undressing the child and tepid sponging. The parents should be instructed about first aid, temperature control and possibly the use of rectal diazepam. Parents should contact their doctor after every convulsion; hospitalisation may be indicated. The long-term management is still controversial. The following plan is reasonable: (1) A child whose first fit is short and uncomplicated, and for whom there is a family history requires no investigations or prophylaxis; (2) (30 minutes or more) or in whom there is an association with a Todd's paralysis should be investigated and prophylactic anticonvulsants considered. For a child who has had his first febrile convulsion which is prolonged; (3) the child who has had many febrile convulsions with, or without, a family history should also be considered for investigations and prophylaxis.

Preliminary investigations include search for an infection site, metabolic screen, skull X-ray for evidence of calcification or raised intracranial pressure, and an EEG. The EEG should be performed 2 or 3 weeks following the seizure in order to obtain a baseline; this may be normal but mild abnormalities may be seen. EEG abnormalities suggest a poor prognosis and the need for careful follow-up. The anticonvulsant chosen for prophylaxis may vary; oral phenobarbitone (5 mg/g daily) is effective and cheap, but may cause severe and unacceptable hyperactivity, sodium valproate has been shown to reduce recurrent convulsions, but is not suitable because it may occasionally cause fatal liver failure. The duration of prophylactic therapy is also controversial; it should probably be given until the child has had at least one seizure-free year. Compliance is important; if a dose is omitted for a day or two, a double dose can be given and then regular prophylaxis continued. Drugs should be discontinued slowly. The prognosis for febrile convulsions is good and most children grow out of the problem.

Neonatal convulsions

Convulsions in the newborn period occur in 1 per cent of all live births. In the majority, the cause is perinatal hypoxia or birth trauma as these cause brain ischaemia, cerebral oedema and haemorrhage. Other causes include metabolic conditions (hypoglycaemia, hypocalcaemia, inborn error of metabolism) and infection (meningitis, septacaemia). The convulsion may present as generalised or focal tonic-clonic seizures or apnoea and cyanosis. Management is symptomatic with anticonvulsant drugs and specific drugs depending on the cause. Prognosis both short and long-term depend on the cause.

Benign familial neonatal convulsions or 5-day fits

This is a rare autosomal dominant form of convulsions. They usually begin in the first week and require anticonvulsant drugs. The prognosis is good.

MIMICS OF EPILEPSY

Several conditions may be misdiagnosed as epilepsy. These include breath-holding attacks, forms of migraine, vertigo and syncope.

Syncope

A prolonged syncopal attack may rarely be followed by a convulsion. Syncope is more common in adolescent girls and should be distinguished from vertigo. Prolonged standing, fasting, emotional upset, the prospect of an unfavourable procedure (e.g. dentistry) or viewing a distressing spectacle (e.g. blood in life or on the screen) can induce syncope.

Observations of pallor, sweating and a slow pulse reinforce the diagnosis. Such children should receive dental treatment in a supine position and can be taught to move their leg muscles if they feel such an attack coming on (feeling faint, distortion of sound or vision). The attack of unconsciousness can be precipitated by hyperventilation when distressed or excited. There may also be awareness of a distorted sound or vision and the child may experience tingling of the extremities and around the mouth. In the infant or toddler, regurgitation or vomiting of food, an unexpected noise or bump, or a painful state, can precipitate a syncopal episode, often with eye rolling and stiffening but little twitching. This has a reflex cardiovascular cause, is benign, self-limiting and of no serious significance. Anticonvulsants are unnecessary, ineffective and potentially harmful.

Types of syncope include

1. *Vasomotor:* a sudden generalised peripheral vasodilation in muscles with peripheral vasoconstriction in skin. The blood pressure falls precipitating a faint.

2. *Carotid sinus syncope:* sudden vagal stimulation causing bradycardia and a faint

3. *Postural hypotension:* rare in children. The child should avoid sudden changes in posture

4. *Hypoglycaemia:* not to be forgotten as a cause and it may follow prolonged fasting

5. *Cardiac:* uncommon in chiloren, examples include a prolonged QT syndrome, hypoxic episodes in children with Fallot's tetraology

6. *Cough syncope:* increased intrathoracic pressure which reduces venous return. This is seen in children with whooping cough and cystic fibrosis

7. *Hyperventilation.*

INVOLUNTARY MOVEMENTS

Tics are the commonest involuntary movements in childhood, although they are not common in the pre-school years. They are habit spasms which are brief, repetitive, involuntary and involve movements of the eyes, face and limbs such as repetitive blinking or shaking of the head. They tend to be stereotyped, increased by anxiety and often have a genetic basis. They are best ignored as far as possible, although some parents find this difficult, especially if there are other tensions in the household or the child has other problems (e.g. with learning). Psychological techniques such as relaxation exercises, mass practice or operant conditioning have been used with varying degrees of success but they are at least harmless. Drug treatment is often unsatisfactory but moderate doses of diazepam, haloperidol with benzhexol to prevent dystonic reactions, or tetrabenazine can be used. Placebo treatment is worth considering.

A severe form is Gilles de la Tourette's syndrome where the tics are uncontrollable and multifocal. During these tics the child makes a grunting, coughing or barking noise. Self-mutilation and aggressive behaviour may be troublesome. The syndrome is most commonly seen in boys aged 5–10 years. No cause for the disorder has been identified. Haloperidol can be tried.
of metabolism. Haloperidol can be tried.

Pathological chorea is most commonly seen in patients with cerebral palsy. Sydenham's chorea is now rare but does occur. The associated hypotonia is usually marked. Serial samples of handwriting will show deterioration and the child may show emotional lability. When Huntingdon's chorea presents in childhood (which is unusual) there may be no choreiform movements, instead a progressive dystonic disorder may occur. Slight choreiform movement (chorea minima) is commonly seen in otherwise normal primary school children. Drug treatment of chorea is usually unnecessary. Tetrabenazine is the most effective agent but can cause depression or Parkinsonian features.

Central tremor is a fine oscillating movement of the hands present throughout the full range of movement. A slight tremor may be seen in children when anxious or fatigued; some, however, show a marked exaggeration of this to an extent which may impair manipulative activities and handwriting. The condition may be familial. Treatment is often unnecessary but primidone or propranolol are the most effective drugs. Weighted bracelets can also be helpful.

MOTOR DISORDERS

The normal variation in motor development can be misleading; many preterm babies show an extended posture in early infancy but few have serious motor disorders later; 7 per cent of normal children do not crawl, but move about by rolling, creeping or bottom shuffling and tend to be more hypotonic than children who crawl, however, they generally walk normally 4–5 months later. There are pathological causes of hypotonia and delayed walking and these include forms of mental handicap, hypotonic cerebral palsy, the hypotonic phase of ataxical choreoathetoid cerebral palsy, or disorders such as muscular dystrophy. At least one-quarter of boys with Duchenne dystrophy are late to walk (after 18 months). The importance of genetic counselling for affected families is clear.

There are a large number of rare neuromuscular disorders and their precise diagnosis requires a specialist opinion; usually serum creatinine kinase, electromyelography, nerve conduction studies and biopsy of muscle (sometimes also sural nerve) may be necessary to allow a diagnosis and permit genetic counselling (dystrophy, spinal muscular atrophy. congenital neuropathy or myopathy). Occasionally, a treatable condition may be found (polymyositis, carnitine deficiency, organic aciduria) by such investigation. Children affected by neuromuscular diseases are weak, hypotonic and hyporeflexic. In Duchenne dystrophy the mean IQ is 85 and affected boys may present with delayed language development.

The commonest motor disorders in childhood are the perceptual motor, balancing, agnosic and apraxic disorders of so-called clumsy children. These are children whose motor abilities lag behind their general abilities by 2 years or more. Their problems and the cause of their dysfunction are heterogenous. Only a minority have had perinatal problems or a genetic predisposition. The subject has not received as serious discussion as have impairment of language, vision or hearing, yet motor skill is important for children in everyday activities, play and writing.

The interested clinician will observe impaired motor performance amongst many children with speech or learning difficulties, behavioural problems or functional symptoms as well as more specific diagnosis such as epilepsy and hydrocephalus. The subject is controversial and approaches to such children are diverse (minimal brain damage, minimal cerebral dysfunction, hyperactive, maladjusted, dyslexic).

It is true that there is no clear cut-off point between normal and clumsy children. Different children, families and teachers react differently to similar degrees of motor incompetence. It is also true that the prognosis is good for most young, clumsy children who have merely a maturational lag. Even they are better managed if their movement difficulties are appreciated. The outcome, however, for more severely clumsy children especially older ones is less clear. Some retain the difficulties in adult life and some run into significant conduct disorders or other psychiatric illness. There can be misperception of some clumsy children if motor competence is not considered; they can become difficult, frustrated or depressed. Parents or teachers may be wrongly blamed. Remedial techniques require further evaluation and will never be sufficiently available to meet the needs of all such children. Widely discrepant abilities present great problems to class teachers and parents. Hospital services neither could nor should, provide the solution apart from expectional cases. Acceptance of each child's strengths and weaknesses is important for the child, who should be encouraged to find activities (e.g. swimming, chess) which may be enjoyable, successful and relaxing. Children with greatest difficulties on testing may need a specialist opinion to exclude specific neurological disorders. Thereafter, a plan of management using existing resources has to be worked out between the school or family doctor, the teacher, the educational psychologist, the parents and the child. There are no medical solutions.

HEAD INJURIES

Head trauma is a common cause of death in childhood, while the sequelae of head injuries such as post-traumatic epilepsy, abnormal behaviour or impairment of intellectual performance may be permanent. Injuries occur at home, in the playground, as a result of traffic accidents or may be non-accidental. The majority are due to falls from a height (trees, windows). or against an object. The skull in infants is relatively thin and elastic and thereby protects the brain and reduces the concussive effects of trauma; over 5 years of age the effects are similar to those of adults as the skull is now a rigid structure with little capacity to expand if there is haemorrhage or oedema. Contrecoup injury is common in children. This is when an injury, usually a blow or blunt injury on one side of the head, causes the brain to hit against the opposite skull vault.

Several types of head injury exist:

1. Contusion, where there is only a bruise on the head with the brain unaffected. There is no loss of consciousness, the child may have dizziness, nausea or vomiting. Skull X-rays are not necessary. The parents however should be given a head injury observation chart.

2. Concussion, here there is loss of consciousness, often brief, but may be prolonged for hours or days. Irritability, dizziness, nausea and vomiting are associated. Headaches may be severe and persist for several days or even weeks. Retrograde and post-traumatic amnesia are often present; prolonged retrograde amnesia may suggest a poor prognosis. A child with concussion should have a skull X-ray and requires admission to hospital for observation. If there is progressive deterioration, particularly in consciousness, severe concussion with brain oedema or intracranial haemorrhage should be suspected. Progressive bradycardia with increasing hypertension suggests raised intracranial pressure whereas a falling blood pressure or unequal pupils may indicate bleeding. Urgent neurosurgical referral is required. Every patient with deterioration should be assumed to have bleeding until proven otherwise (by CT scan) as it is not possible to separate the two clinically. Medical therapy for oedema is theoretically contraindicated with bleeding, although in practice dexamethazone is often used.

3. Brain contusion, bruising of the brain is often a result of contre-coup or coup injury. Microscopic haemorrhages are seen in the brain substance; with severe contusion marked damage occurs. Contusion of the brain is difficult to diagnose clinically; in contre-coup injuries the signs and symptoms are on the opposite side of the head to that which was injured. There may be a hemiplegia or convulsion.

4. Cephalhaematomas and laceration of the scalp, are common and clinically visible. Profuse bleeding from small lacerations is often frightening to the parents and to the child; simple cleaning and suturing is required. In infants, large haematomas, or cephalohaematomas of birth, may be associated with depressed skull fractures.

Skull fractures

These may be simple and linear, depressed or compound. Simple fracture is common and usually of no major clinical significance, although skull X-ray is indicated to confirm the fracture and admission to hospital for observation is advisable. The haematoma subsides spontaneously; routine antibiotic cover is not necessary. Depressed fractures need surgical correction; the cause is often a blow or fall on a sharp object. The depression may be clinically apparent but is confirmed on X-ray. Compound fractures are serious; they may be open or closed (occult). A compound basal skull fracture is accompanied by cerebrospinal fluid leak through the nose or ears which can be confirmed by finding glucose in secretions (by Clinistix), and by evidence of haemorrhage around the eyes. There is a risk of central nervous system infection.

Penetrating head injuries and open head injuries are easy to diagnose, the point of penetration may be obvious and the brain may occasionally be exposed through the wound. There is a risk of infection and damage to the brain substance; the prognosis in most cases is surprisingly good. Neurosurgical referral is important.

Indications for skull X-ray in children include head trauma with unconsciousness, penetrating injury, less than one year of age, cephalohaematoma, depression palpable in the scalp, visible brain, injury with haemorrhage around the eyes, CSF otorrhoea or rhinorrhoea, blood in the middle ear, focal neurological signs and fits, coma or marked lethargy.

Subdural collection

This may occur as a result of trauma or as an effusion associated with meningitis. The child may present with focal convulsions, raised intracranial pressure, or in infants with enlarging head circumference. The history gives a clue. Diagnosis is confirmed by skull X-ray, CT scan (not reliable), angiography, or subdural taps. Management is symptomatic, but surgical drainage may be necessary; if there is raised intracranial pressure. Prognosis is variable and depends on the cause and the result of the pressure effects of the subdural collection.

PROGRESSIVE DEMENTIA IN INFANCY AND CHILDHOOD

Here there is a progressive deterioration in either mental or physical function, or both, as a result of progressive central nervous system pathology. The cause may be an inborn error of metabolism. neurodegenerative disease, persistent encephalities, infiltrative tumour, or chronic drug intoxication (e.g. toluene or lead poisoning); minor motor status, hypothyroidism. and low pressure hydrocephalus may present as pseudodementia which disappears with therapy.

Most children with this group of disorders are normal at birth; a history of arrest or regression of development and loss of skills or progressive dementia is present. It is important to establish the diagnosis so that appropriate genetic counselling can be given. Therapy may be available such as a diet for phenylketonuria; new treatments such as bone marrow transplantation are being developed.

INBORN ERRORS OF METABOLISM
(see chapter 20)

These are recessive inherited disorders where enzyme deficiencies cause either the deficiency of an essential metaboloite or the accumulation of a toxic one. Eight major subgroups exist: disorders of amino acid metabolism (phenylketonuria, homocystinuria, hiştidenaemia, alicaptonuria); disorders of carbohydrate metabolism (galactosaemia, glycogen storage disease); mucopolysaccharidosis, colipidosis and disorders of glycoprotein metabolism (fucosidosis, mannosidosis); organic acidurias (proprionic acidaemia, methylmalonic acidaemia, lactic acidaemia); disorders of lipid metabolism (gangliosidosis); disorders of metal metabolism (Wilson's disease); and disorders of purine metabolism (Lesch-Nyhan syndrome, porphyrias).

THE HEREDODEGENERATIVE BRAIN DISEASES

These are genetically determined; the pathological process is biochemical but, in many, the precise biochemical abnormality is not fully understood. Classification of these disorders is based upon the region of the brain preferentially affected. These are:
1. The basal ganglia (e.g. Huntingdon's chorea, dystonia musculorum deformans (torsion dystonia), Hallervorden-Spatz disease)
2. Cerebellum, brainstem and spinal cord (e.g. Friedreich's ataxia (spino-cerebellar degeneration). ataxia-telangiectasia (Louis-Bar syndrome), olivo-ponto-cerebellar atrophy, hereditary cerebellar ataxia, familial spastic paraplegia (progressive), Ramsay-Hunt's syndrome (dentatorubral atrophy), Charcot-Marie-Tooth disease (peroneal muscular atrophy), familial amyotrophic lateral sclerosis)
3. Peripheral and cranial nerves (e.g. hypertrophic interstitial neuritis, giant axonal neuropathy, hereditary optic atrophy (Leber's optic atrophy), hereditary sensory neuropathy, familial dysautonomia (Riley-Day syndrome)
4. Cerebral degenerative diseases; a. white matter degeneration (leucodystrophies) (e.g. metachromatic leucodystrophy, Krabbe's leucodystrophy, Alexander's leucodystrophy, spongy degeneration of white matter (Canavan's disease), Pelizaeus-Merzbacher disease, sudanohilic cerebral sclerosis; b. grey matter disease or Alper's disease.

23

Surgical disorders

THE NEWBORN

Congenital abnormalities of all systems are the major cause of surgical problems in the newborn period.

The gastrointestinal tract

Oesophageal atresia

Oesophageal atresia has an incidence of one in 3000 to 5000 live births. In the commonest form (85 per cent) the upper oesophagus ends blindly in the upper mediastinum while the lower oesophagus arises by a fistula from the trachea. Atresia without fistula accounts for a further 8 per cent and fistula without atresia 5 per cent. Of these babies, 50 per cent will also have anomalies in other systems and most are of low birth-weight; these two features adversely affect management and survival.

Diagnosis. Polyhydramnios is present in one-quarter to one-third of mothers with babies with oesophageal atresia. After birth, the baby is unable to swallow saliva, drools from the mouth and may choke on a feed. Spill-over of saliva into the trachea may cause choking and cyanosis. Air forced into the distal oesophagus through the fistula produces abdominal distension and may lead to acid reflux into the trachea. The diagnosis is confirmed by an inability to pass a 10–12 gauge catheter into the stomach; if the tube is held up at 10–12 cm the diagnosis is established. Plain X-rays show the site of arrest of the tube while the presence of gas in the abdomen suggests a fistula.

Treatment. In the majority of situations primary surgical correction is possible. For those babies unsuitable for primary repair, the alternative management includes delayed primary anastomosis at 2–3 months, or oesophageal replacement with colon or a tube formed from the stomach, performed at around one year of age. The majority (75–80 per cent) of babies with oesophageal atresia now survive.

Intestinal obstruction

The signs and symptoms in the newborn are: bile-stained or persistent vomiting; abdominal distension; or delayed passage of meconium.

Green vomit in the newborn must be assumed to be secondary to intestinal obstruction until proved otherwise. The level of the obstruction may be indicated by the degree and type of abdominal distension; in high small-bowel obstruction it is upper abdominal, in low small-bowel obstruction it is central, and in large-bowel obstruction in the flanks and across the epigastrium. Over 90 per cent of term babies pass meconium within 24 hours of birth. Delay is associated with prematurity and birth asphyxia but if longer than 48 hours an obstruction should be suspected. In proximal obstructions the distribution of the gas in the gut on plain abdominal X-rays is usually diagnostic.

Duodenal obstruction

Duodenal obstruction, which is seen in one in 5000–6000 live births, may be due to atresia, stenosis, diaphragm or associated with an annular pancreas. The obstruction is commonest in the second part of the duodenum distal to the ampulla of Vater. Other congenital abnormalities are common and 30 per cent have Down syndrome.

Diagnosis. Maternal polyhydramnios is present in about 30 per cent; an ultrasound examination of the mother can identify the dilated fetal stomach and duodenum. After birth vomiting, usually but not always bile-stained, frequently precedes feeding. All feeds are vomited. Abdominal distension varies with the fullness of the stomach. The passage of meconium is delayed. Plain abdominal X-rays show the classical double bubble sign of gas in the stomach and the dilated proximal duodenum.

Treatment. If the diagnosis is delayed, loss of acid gastric contents leads to a metabolic alkalosis which will require correction. The dilated duodenum is then anastomosed, either to the duodenum immediately distal to the obstruction, or to the first loop of jejunum. Delayed transit across the anastomosis is common, but may be overcome by passing a trans-anastomotic tube at the time of the anastomosis. The survival rates in intrinsic duodenal obstruction should be around 70–75 per cent.

Jejunal, ileal and colonic atresias

These are probably due to some intrauterine accident occuring in previously normal bowel. All the signs of obstruction are present. The incidence is about one per 6000 live births with colonic atresias accounting for 10 per cent. Plain X-rays show multiple fluid levels in increasingly distended gut ending in one very large loop.

Treatment. The operation should include resection of the most dilated loop and an end-to-oblique anastomosis. Usually bowel function returns rapidly and survival rates are around 80 per cent. Cystic fibrosis should be excluded by a sweat test in all babies with small bowel atresia or evidence of meconium peritonitis as these may be secondary to meconium ileus.

Meconium ileus

Meconium ileus is the earliest and the most acute intestinal complication of cystic fibrosis. The obstruction, seen in 15 per cent of such babies, is due to impaction of a bolus of abnormally viscid meconium in the distal small bowel. Volvulus, meconium peritonitis or a small bowel atresia may complicate the disorder.

Diagnosis. The uncomplicated case often often has marked abdominal distension present at birth; bile-stained vomiting occurs early and no meconium is passed. Plain abdominal X-rays show evidence of obstruction with stippling in the right iliac fossa or dilated loops with relative absence of fluid levels. A gastrografin enema will outline a tiny colon containing small plugs of mucus, a narrow terminal ileum and a proximal dilated segment. The obstruction is relieved by the enema in about one-half of the uncomplicated cases; complicated cases and those not relieved by the enema, require surgery, in which the most dilated meconium-containing gut resected. The anastomosis should allow the gut to deflate and the colon to return to normal. Full treatment for cystic fibrosis should be started at once and the diagnosis confirmed by a sweat test. Early surgical survival rates of 80 per cent are now possible.

Malrotation and volvulus neonatorum

The essential features of malrotation of the gut are failure of rotation of the duodenum with the duodeno-jejunal junction lying to the right of the midline, and non-rotation of the colon with the caecum lying in the epigastrium. A narrow unstable mesenteric isthmus with a pedicle, around which the bowel can twist, is left causing an obstruction in the second part of the duodenum and may be rapidly followed by strangulation of the mid-gut loop.

Diagnosis. Volvulus should be suspected in those babies who, after initial normal progress, suddenly develop a duodenal obstruction. In doubtful cases, a barium meal will show the level of the obstruction or the abnormal position of the duodenum.

Treatment. Urgent surgical untwisting of the volvulus is required, followed by a derotation of the gut and widening of the mesenteric root. Serious postoperative problems should only be seen when resection for infarction is required.

Hirschsprung's disease (congenital intestinal aganglionosis)

This can present at any stage in childhood. The incidence is one in 5000–6000 live births.

In over 90 per cent, symptoms start in the first week of life. The underlying abnormality is the absence of parasympathetic ganglion cells from the wall of the gut; this is probably due to a failure of migration of ganglion cells which explains the constant involvement of the terminal rectum, the variable proximal extent, and the absence of skip lesions. The condition is conventionally divided into short-segment disease, where the aganglionosis does not extend proximal to the junction of sigmoid and descending colon (65–75 per cent of all cases), and long-segment disease where more proximal colon is affected. The picture may be complicated at any stage by necrotising enterocolitis.

Diagnosis. The commonest early symptom is delayed passage of meconium which occurs in 90 per cent of cases. Abdominal distension follows and there is a reluctance to feed and reflex vomiting. Bilious vomiting usually occurs later. Rectal examination may lead to an explosive decompression or merely disclose an empty distal rectum. The differential diagnosis includes functional obstruction, seen in prematurity or after a traumatic labour and asphyxia, the meconium plug syndrome or the hypoplastic left colon syndrome. Where there is total colonic aganglionosis it must be distinguished from other small bowel obstructions.

Plain abdominal X-rays and a barium enema will confirm the diagnosis in 80 per cent of cases but must be followed by a rectal biopsy. It is essential that at least 12 hours should elapse between a rectal washout or rectal examination and the barium studies. The barium enema will show essentially normal distal bowel (the narrow segment) expanding rapidly at the point of transition (the cone) into the dilated proximal ganglionic gut. This gives both the diagnosis and length of the aganglionic segment.

Treatment. The initial treatment is a colostomy in an area of ganglionic gut. At the age of 6 months to one year a pull-through operation is performed, resecting the aganglionic segment and bringing ganglionic bowel down to the anal canal by one of the techniques described by Swenson, Duhamel or Soave. Biopsy control is necessary at each stage to confirm the diagnosis, confirm that the colostomy is ganglionic, and to confirm the accuracy of the final operation. Following surgery most children will gain adequate bowel control but at a later date than their peers. A few have problems with failure of relaxation of the internal sphincter and require later dilatation or sphincterotomy. Final survival rates should exceed 80 per cent; most deaths are related to an enterocolitis.

The meconium plug syndrome

A few neonates have an apparent obstruction which is relieved by a contrast or saline enema. It is important to exclude Hirschsprung's disease by biopsy and cystic fibrosis by a sweat test.

Ano-rectal anomalies

Ano-rectal anomalies are generally obvious at the initial newborn examinations. Lesions can be divided into low or high, depending on the level at which the rectum ends; if the rectum ends above the pelvic floor the lesion is supralevator or high, if below it is translevator or low. In most of these babies the rectum ends as a fistula joining the posterior urethra (high lesions) or the perineal skin (low lesions) in the male and the upper vagina (high lesions) or the vaginal introitus or perineal skin (low lesions) in the female. Two further variants occur in the female. In the most severe form, the persistent cloaca, the urethra, vagina and rectum all reach the perineum through a common channel. Intermediate lesions also occur. Associated anomalies, particularly oesophageal and duodenal atresia, are common and abnormalities of the renal tract are seen in 40 per cent.

Diagnosis. The initial assessment should be made by examination of the perineum and gentle probing for the fistula. Plain abdominal X-rays are essential to exclude other gut anomalies and obstructions and a lateral view of the sacrum gives some indication of the state of the pelvic floor and innervation of the rectum. In high, and most intermediate lesions, a preliminary colostomy relieves the obstruction and allows time for full investigation. The distal gut is outlined with a water-soluble contrast introduced through the colostomy, and an intravenous pyelogram and micturating cystourethrogram outline the renal tract. Low anomalies can be corrected by an immediate perineal operation. High anomalies are repaired by a pull-through operation when the baby is around 6–9 months of age.

Necrotising enterocolitis

Necrotising enterocolitis is seen in pre-term babies, after birth asphyxia or shock, in cyanotic heart disease, particularly after surgery, after umbilical vein catheterisation and exchange transfusion, in Hirschsprung's disease, and sometimes for no obvious reason. The underlying pathology is an area of necrosis of the gut wall which varies in its extent in length and depth of the wall. Multiple separate lesions occur. The aetiology, apart from general agreement that ischaemia and secondary bacterial infection are involved, is obscure. The organisms associated with mini-epidemics include *Escherichia coli*, Salmonella, Klebsiella, pseudomonads, Bacteroides and clostridial species.

Diagnosis. The condition should be suspected in any at-risk neonate who becomes less active, has temperature instability, gastric retention or abdominal distension. Blood in the stools increases the probability and plain abdominal X-rays are usually diagnostic. The early X-ray signs are those of bowel-wall oedema and increased fluid between dilated loops. Intramural gas (pneumatosis intestinalis), which may progress to free gas or gas in the portal veins in the liver, confirms the diagnosis.

Treatment. The treatment is initially medical and includes: stop oral intake and start nasogastric suction; intravenous fluids and i.v. feeding; i.v. antibiotics such as gentamicin, penicillin and metronidazole; close monitoring of vital signs, haemoglobin, platelets, because of the risk of disseminated intravascular coagulation, acid-base balance, and daily abdominal X-rays.

Surgery is reserved for patients who fail to respond or develop a perforation or obstruction.

On recovery, late stricture formation is seen in at least 20 per cent of cases.

Exomphalos

Exomphalos is a useful term to cover all congenital abnormalities with herniation of gut at the umbilicus. These should be subdivided into:

1. Hernia into the cord: here there is only a small defect at the base of the umbilical cord. The amount of herniated gut varies from a single loop or adherent Meckel's diverticulum to most of the small bowel. Reduction of the hernia and surgical repair usually present no problem.

2. Omphalocele: this is a defect of the muscle of the abdominal wall where the sac has a wide base and frequently contains liver. Associated anomalies such as cardiac defects or extroversion of the bladder are common. Minor defects can be repaired but large defects present a major surgical problem. Cover by mobilised skin flaps or simple conservative management by painting with antibacterial agents are often effective. After healing, a late ventral hernia repair is required.

3. Gastroschisis: here there is a short transverse defect alongside the umbilicus through which the gut prolapses. The cause is probably an early antenatal rupture of hernia into the cord. Treatment is complicated by the difficulty of returning the bowel to the contracted abdomen and delay in return of function of the gut.

Diaphragmatic hernia

Congenital diaphragmatic hernias occur at three sites, oesophageal hiatus, which is discussed under gastro-oesophageal reflux, posterolateral or Bochdalek's hernia, and retrosternal or Morgagni's hernia.

The posterolateral hernia, most frequently (80 per cent) on the left side, allows gut into the chest during intrauterine development. The lung on the affected side fails to develop and, in the most severe forms, displacement of the mediastinum causes underdevelopment of the opposite lung. This is the most urgent of neonatal emergencies. As air is swallowed the gut in the chest expands and progressively compresses the lungs. The diagnosis should be suspected in any newborn with respiratory distress, cyanosis and apparent dextrocardia, particularly if the abdomen is scaphoid.

A plain chest X-ray will usually give the diagnosis. Bowel loops are seen on the affected side, the mediastinum is displaced, the opposite lung collapsed and the abdomen is empty.

Treatment. Emergency treatment is directed at deflating the gut with a nasogastric tube and positive pressure ventilation through an endotracheal tube. Ventilation through a face mask will only force more air into the gut and increase the pressure on the lungs. Early surgery is mandatory. At laparotomy the gut is withdrawn from the chest and the diaphragm repaired. Survival depends on the amount of lung present and complications such as persistent fetal circulatory pattern; around 60 per cent of babies survive. Long-term lung function in survivors is usually normal.

Neural tube defects

These comprise spina bifida, anenecephaly, encephalocele and hydrocephalus and have an incidence of between 5 and 6 per 1000 live births. The term spina bifida covers all defects of the vertebral neural arch.

Spina bifida occulta, where the defect is a split in the bony arch without meningeal or skin protrusion, is most often discovered as an incidental finding during X-ray examination of the lumbosacral spine. The presence of a hairy patch, capillary haemangioma, or dermal sinus may point to the underlying defect which is then not strictly occult, and may rarely be associated with spinal cord involvement, a tethered filum terminale or diastematomyelia — splitting of the cord. A true dermal sinus must be distinguished from the common post-anal dimple or pit which is skin-lined, lies over the tip of the coccyx, and apart from the uncommon complication of local sepsis from retained stool, is of no significance. A dermal sinus is situated more cranially in the midline and has a lining of modified pink skin which leads down to or into the spinal theca; this always requires full investigation and excision.

A meningocele, the least common form of spina bifida, is a skin-covered lesion with cystic protrusion of the meninges, but without underlying neurological involvement. With lipoma of the cauda equina, a similar bulge over the spine occurs and is filled with fatty tissue intimately involved with the cord, nerve roots and often meningeal distension. There is often both a primary neurological defect and a risk of deterioration secondary to differential growth of the spine stretching a fixed cord.

In meningomyelocele, an abnormal cord is adherent to the surface of the sac often at a raw plaque; in the most severe form myeloschisis or rachischisis, the whole cord lies open on the surface for several segments. The neurological deficit varies with the level and nature of the lesion from pure sacral lesions with only bladder and anal involvement to total paralysis caudal to the defect. Mixed upper and lower motor neurone lesions are common. Most (70–80 per cent) of the severe defects develop progressive hydrocephalus secondary to an associated Arnold-Chiari malformation, where there is displacement of the hind brain and fourth ventricle through the foramen magnum into the vertebral canal and prolapse of the cerebellar tonsils. Defects in the midline of the skull (cranium bifidum), most commonly frontal or occipital, may similarly be meningoceles without underlying brain damage or contain abnormal brain tissue and are then known as encephaloceles. These lesions are also often associated with hydrocephalus.

Hydrocephalus is also caused by other blockages of the cerebrospinal fluid pathway; in the cerebral aqueduct, at the exit foraminae of the fourth ventricle, or secondary to intracranial bleeding or meningitis with blockage of the basal cysterns, and most rarely by posterior fossa tumours.

Management

There is now general agreement that the treatment should be planned in the light of the probable immediate and late outcome. In spina bifida there is a policy of selection of those children most likely to benefit from immediate surgery, i.e. within 24 hours of birth. Adverse factors against surgery include: severe paralysis of the lower limbs, total paraplegia or hip flexors only acting; severe hydrocephalus, a head circumference 2 cm above the 90th centile corrected for weight and gestational age; gross kyphosis; or other associated major abnormalities of severe cerebral birth trauma.

These criteria will exclude about 60 per cent cases from early surgery. After early closure, even of the less severe defects, 70 per cent develop hydrocephalus requiring control by one of the valve systems (Holter, Pudenz, Hakim) with ventriculoatrial or ventriculoperitoneal shunting.

The management of severely affected babies without operation is more controversial. If fed normally, but given no other treatment apart from dressing of the back, 20–30 per cent survive. The spinal lesion epithelialises in one to 3 months but most develop hydrocephalus. These survivors can be later transferred to the full treatment regimen without disadvantage.

The immediate orthopaedic assessment is confined to determining the degree of fixed deformity and the extent of voluntary and reflex muscle activity. Passive manipulation of fixed deformities, e.g. talipes, should start at once. Splints must be used with care to avoid damage to anaesthetic skin.

Early urological investigation, similarly, is limited to assessing bladder function from the pattern of micturition and the extent of bladder filling. Outflow obstruction is recognised by a persistently full bladder and constant dribbling. Total bladder and bladder neck paralysis, in which the bladder is either easily expressible or never full, is the safer lesion. Regular expression is only of value for babies with flaccid bladders without outflow obstruction.

Long-term management

Even the less severely affected children, who now form most of the survivors, have life-long medical problems.

Valve complications. (i) *Blockage*: All valves block eventually. Some children will no longer be valve dependent when this happens, but many of these lead a precarious existence with permanently increased intracranial pressure and are liable to acute problems following minor head injuries or intercurrent infection. The blockage is equally common at upper and lower ends; in the ventricle, choroid plexus or brain may plug the catheter while at the lower end, as growth proceeds, the

catheter becomes too short and is pulled out of the atrium with blockage in the venous system. In the peritoneum the catheter may simply retract from the cavity or a CSF pocket may become walled-off from the general peritoneal cavity. The signs and symptoms of blockage are headache, altered state of consciousness, convulsions, vomiting, squint and down-turning of the eyes, increased tension in the anterior fontanelle and over the spinal defect, dilated scalp veins and papilloedema. Acute blockage must be treated urgently by the appropriate operative revision.

(ii) *Valve colonisation*: Up to one in three valves become colonised by organisms of low pathogenicity, most frequently *Staphylococcus epidermidis*. The signs of this are a general malaise, low-grade pyrexia, anaemia and, when a vascular shunt has been used, splenomegaly, proteinuria and haematuria. Colonisation may cause blockage of the shunt system especially in the peritoneum. Treatment involves control of systemic infection by appropriate antibacterial agents and replacement of the infected valve by a new clean system.

Urological management. The renal tract is at risk from disordered bladder and sphincter contraction, which lead to incomplete bladder emptying with infected residual urine, ureteric reflux and back pressure on the kidneys. Regular urine culture is essential, and intravenous pylograms or isotope renograms should be repeated every 2–3 years or more frequently if there are problems. Micturition cystourethrography is useful to demonstrate reflux and bladder-outflow obstruction. Around 30 per cent of these children can achieve acceptable levels of urinary continence. Cystomanometry is probably the most valuable means of assessing the prospects and deciding the methods of treatment. Overactive detrusor contractions can be damped by imipramine, and sphincter obstruction may respond to phenoxybenzamine. Bladder expression by an adult, or for older children by themselves, with or without drugs, helps to get complete emptying.

Sphincter obstruction not responding to drugs should be relieved by external sphincterotomy. Contrary to expectations, by permitting complete emptying of the bladder, this may improve continence. For the remainder, diversion by conduits of ileum or colon to the anterior abdominal wall is much less favoured than in the past. Alternatives include penile applicances for males, and intermittent non-sterile self catheterisation for both sexes and indwelling catheters for girls.

INGUINO-SCROTAL PROBLEMS

Hernia and Hydrocele

Inguinal hernias in childhood are almost always of the indirect type and due to the persistence of the processus vaginalis. Direct hernias are rare, but may be seen in association with lower abdomen muscular deficiencies. Femoral hernias are rarer still. Indirect hernias occur in 1–2 per cent of boys and in about one in 500 girls; approximately 60 per cent are right-sided, 25 per cent left-sided and 15 per cent bilateral.

Primary hydroceles similarly are often secondary to patency of the processus vaginalis. In some cases, this is obvious as the hydrocele is reducible, that is a communicating hydrocele or fluid hernia while, in others it is valvular and although there are fluctuations in size during the day, fluid cannot be returned to the abdomen. Hydroceles of the spermatic cord are also collections of fluid in persistent loculi of the processus and communicate with the peritoneal cavity.

Diagnosis

The commonest presenting symptom is a swelling which may be confined to the inguinal region or extend down the spermatic cord into the scrotum. In the first year of life the swelling usually appears after a bout of crying or coughing and may become irreducible, even at first presention; irreducibility or strangulation becomes less common as the child gets older. If the swelling is present at the time of examination and reduces, the diagnosis is easy; if the swelling is irreducible the differential diagnosis is between an obstructed hernia, a hydrocele, an incompletely descended testis, and inguinal adenitis or abscess. An obstructed hernia is tender, may surround the testis, and always extends up to the external inguinal ring. Inguinal lymph nodes lie lateral to the external inguinal ring and are often multiple; there may be an obvious primary septic lesion in the drainage area. A hydrocele of the spermatic cord presents as a swelling in the cord above and separate from the testis. If in doubt, it is usually safest to presume that an irreducible lump is either a strangulated hernia or a torted, undescended testis. When no swelling is present at the time of examination, careful palpation of the cord, rolling it over the pubic bone, will reveal the thickening due to the sac and the walls of the sac slipping on each other may be felt. For an experienced examiner this, together with the history, is adequate for surgical intervention. Children over 4 years are able to cooperate by coughing, lying down and standing up, making the diagnosis easier.

Management

Non-communicating hydroceles are common in the first few months of life. Their fine valvular communications close spontaneously and do not require treatment. Those still present by the first birthday require exploration. Inguinal hernias do not recover spontaneously and, provided an experienced paediatric surgeon and anaesthetist are available, the only reason to delay operation in an otherwise fit baby is extreme prematurity. It is best to wait until a weight of 2500 g is reached before surgery. The operation for inguinal hernias and hydroceles is essentially the same involving simple division of the processus vaginitis at the internal inguinal ring; no repair is required. In the UK, bilateral explorations are usually restricted to children who have definite signs on both sides. The operation on an irreducible hernia in a baby is one of the most difficult in surgery; fortunately full strangulation of the gut with the risk of perforation is rare. The greatest risk is to the blood supply of the testis. It is usually best to sedate the child, nurse him in the head-down position and as soon as he is relaxed, either spontaneous reduction will occur or, gentle to firm pressure will achieve reduction. After a successful reduction, operation should be delayed by 2–3 days to allow the oedema to subside. When reduction fails an urgent operation is required.

Undescended testis

The testis normally descends into the scrotum before the end of the eighth month of pregnancy; incomplete descent is seen at birth in only 2.7 per cent of full-term boys, but in 21 per cent of preterm boys. Most of these testes descend in the course of the subsequent 9 months. Spontaneous descent after the age of one year, when the prevalence of incomplete descent is only 0.5–0.7 per cent, probably occurs only rarely.

The incompletely descended testis must be differentiated from the ectopic, the retractile and the absent testis. The ectopic testis lies in a position outside the normal line of descent, most commonly lateral to the external ring, the inguinal ectopic testis, and only rarely in the femoral, perineal or penile positions. A retractile testis has descended normally, but is pulled out of the scrotum by the action of the cremaster muscle. Testes may be congenitally absent or disappear following torsion.

Diagnosis

The testis is most easily felt in the neonatal period, and most difficult to feel around ages of 3–5 years, with palpation becoming easier again towards puberty as the organ enlarges and the cremaster relaxes. Palpation requires a warm and relaxed patient who is lying down, and a gentle examiner with warm hands. The testis should be milked down towards the scrotum by one hand, stroking along the line of the inguinal canal from the internal to the external ring, where it can be caught by the fingers of the other hand and pulled as far into the scrotum as it will come. If there is any doubt, pulling the thighs into the fully flexed, slightly abducted position, like squatting, will usually make a retractile testis descend into the scrotum.

Indications and timing for operation

Spermatogenesis will not occur normally in a testis left undescended until puberty. Changes in ultrastructure can be recognised after the first birthday, and more obvious changes on light microscopy after the fifth birthday. While early placement of the testis in the scrotum has not been definitely shown to improve fertility, it is the only hope. Most undescended testes are associated with an inguinal hernia, and have an increased risk of undergoing torsion, and a slight, but definitely increased risk of the later development of malig-

nancy. The teasing and emotional problems of having only one testis in the scrotum provide a further powerful reason for consideration of orchidopexy.

The operation should, therefore, be performed certainly before the fifth birthday and where there are skilled paediatric services, probably shortly after the first birthday. At operation, absence will be confirmed, any hernias can be corrected and torsion prevented, but there is probably no long-term effect on the development of malignancy.

Torsion of the testis

Testicular torsion may be major or minor. In torsion major, the whole testis and epididymis twists on the spermatic cord, usually within the tunica vaginalis (intravaginal). This is generally secondary to an abnormal anatomical position of the testis, horizontal clapperbell testis or undescended. The underlying abnormality must be assumed to be bilateral. If a torsion is not corrected within 4 hours, some testicular damage is inevitable and this damage increases with time.

Torsion minor, which is commoner than torsion major, is a torsion of the hydatid of Morgagni, a small embryological remnant on the upper pole of the testis or epididymis.

Torsion is a sudden and painful event. The pain is abdominal as well as local, and in the descended testis the swollen and tender scrotum makes the diagnosis obvious. Epididymitis, except in association with other problems, such as a chronically infected bladder associated with spina bifida, is rare in childhood and should be considered only when torsion has been excluded by operation. In torsion minor, the symptoms are less acute and the tenderness may be clearly localised over a tender dark nodule at the upper pole of the testis. Rarely, an acute hydrocele develops in children with a fine patent processus vaginalis in response to an intercurrent infection and mimics an acute scrotal emergency.

Management

External reduction has been suggested but few surgeons have had real success with this and, besides, early fixation is required. Urgent exploration and reduction of the torsion is therefore recommended. It is seldom correct to excise the testis before puberty, but late atrophy is common. Both the affected and the normal testis should be fixed in the scrotum to prevent recurrence. In torsion minor the hydatid is excised. If the diagnosis has been delayed, it is important to remember that the symptoms will subside in about a week even without treatment.

Idiopathic scrotal oedema

This is an acute swelling of the soft tissues of the scrotum. The area is red and oedematous, the swelling extends up into the groin and may be tender, but a normal cord and non-tender testis can generally be palpated through the swelling. The whole condition usually subsides spontaneously within 2–3 days. The cause is obscure and antibiotics and antihistamines have been used in treatment but it is doubtful whether they make much difference.

Testicular tumours

These are rare. Teratoma, orchioblastoma and rhabdomyosarcoma present as painless, testicular swellings. They may be confused with hydroceles. They should be excised urgently.

Circumcision

Phimosis

The foreskin is normally adherent to the glans penis at birth. Separation occurs over the first years of life and, in the majority, the skin can be pushed back freely by the age of 5 years. Provided there is an adequate external meatus no attempt to retract the foreskin should be made before then. The meatus is best assessed by observing the urinary stream or by pulling the skin forwards away from the pubis. A thin or spraying stream suggests obstruction, ballooning of the prepuce during micturition is usually normal and does not of itself indicate obstruction. Fewer than 5 per cent of normal boys require circumcision for these reasons.

Cicatrical phimosis is seen in older children. The prepuce is obviously scarred, the urinary stream is obviously obstructed and often painful, bleeding is common and ballooning unusual. The condition follows forceful retraction of the skin, severe napkin rashes, infective balanitis, balanitis xerotica obliterans, and after inadequate circumcision.

Posthitis and balanitis

Posthitis (or inflammation of the skin of the prepuce), is part of a nappy rash and is a contraindication to circumcision. Balanitis which is infection under the prepuce, occurs with a widely open prepuce as well as with stenosis and obstructed drainage. Immediate treatment includes warm bathing, local antibiotics and rarely a surgical dorsal slit of the prepuce. Circumcision is indicated after healing.

Smegma collections develop during separation of the prepuce. They appear as white swellings over the glans. Left along they discharge spontaneously. The rare true preputial cysts are treated by circumcision.

Other indications

Circumcision is also demanded for religious, cultural, or simply social reasons. It is impossible to prevent its performance for religious and cultural reasons but it should never be recommended on a purely social basis. It is probably best delayed, if possible, until after the child is out of napkins. It should also be avoided in children with hypospadias until it is clear that the skin will not be required for repair, although a tiny amount of skin needs be removed for a ritual Jewish circumcision.

Complications of circumcision include infection, haemorrhage (haemophilia may present in this way), damage to the penis, meatal ulceration and stenosis, and recurrence. Meatal ulceration is rarely seen in a glans protected by the prepuce but commonly follows circumcision. The symptoms are pain and bleeding on micturition and sometimes even acute retention of urine. The diagnosis is obvious on examination of the penis; retention is usually relieved by sitting the child in a warm bath. The ulceration should be treated by a local ointment such as a topical steroid. If healing is associated with meatal stenosis a formal meatotomy is required.

Hypospadias, epispadias, ectopia vesicae

In hypospadias the external urethral opening is on the ventral surface of the penis. It may be glandular, coronal, penile, peno-scrotal, scrotal, or perineal. In epispadias the urethral opening is on the dorsal surface of the penis. There is again a gradation of severity from splitting of the glans, a long dorsal defect of the penile shaft to total extraversion of the bladder (ectopia vesicae).

The aim of treatment is to produce a straight penis with a normal urinary stream and preferably the urethral opening at the apex of the glans. Hypospadias is the commonest of these anomalies. In the most minor degree, glandular hypospadias, there is only a cleft glans associated with a hooded prepuce not united at the fraenum. Provided the urinary stream is straight no treatment is required. There may be a chordee, or ventral bowing of the penis, which must be corrected. The chordee correction is performed at around 18 months of age and the repair of the hypospadias at around 4–5 years, so that the young boy is micturating normally when he goes to school. In this group there is a slight increase in the incidence of upper urinary tract anomalies, but routine intravenous pyelography is probably only indicated in the more severe forms of hypospadias. In the more severe degrees of hypospadias, particularly if the testes are undescended, it is essential to establish the sex of the infant before starting treatment as errors can be made. Hypospadias should be an absolute contra-indication to circumcision until it is clear that the prepuce tissue will not be required for a later repair. Later the hooded appearance of the prepuce in glandular hypospadias may be a cosmetic indication for circumcision.

Epispadias is a much more complex anomaly, often involving deficiencies in the bladder neck, and can occur in both sexes. Female epispadias can be recognised by the bifid clitoris and widely open urethra; it is a rare cause of urinary incontinence. In the male, the penis is short and there is reverse chordee. It is essential to check on the upper urinary tract and bladder neck by an intravenous pyelogram and voiding cystourethrogram. Repair is best delayed until it is possible to say whether the child is continent which is usually by 4–5 years of age. Penile lengthening may be required before the repair. If the bladder neck is deficient it will also require repair, but this is a less satisfactory procedure and continence is not always achieved.

Extraversion of the bladder (ectopia vesicae) also occurs in both sexes. The bladder is open on the anterior abdominal wall, there is a generalised deficiency of the abdominal wall often with an associated omphalocele, the symphysis pubis is widely separated, the anus is anteriorally placed and, in the male, there is epispadias. The upper urinary tract is usually normal at birth but the ureters may become obstructed as their orifices prolapse through the abdominal wall defect. When the bladder is of reasonable size a repair, at around one year of age or earlier, followed by reimplantation of the ureters, tightening of the bladder neck and repair of the epispadias can be attempted. Results, even in specialised units, are still disappointing. For those children where repair fails and those with bladders too small for the attempt, a urinary diversion with bladder excision is required; currently for children with good bowel control, there is renewed interest in ureterosigmoid anastomosis.

BREAST LESIONS

Breast lesions are seen in childhood and include: neonatal hypertrophy with or without secondary infection, prepubertal mastitis, precocious development, absence of one or both breasts, gynaecomastia in boys, and adolescent hypertrophy.

Breast enlargement with secretion is common in the neonatal period. Left alone most cases resolve within a few weeks. Expression of milk predisposes to abscess formation. Abscesses are nearly always caused by a penicillin-resistant staphylococcus and should be treated by a systemic β-lactamase resistant penicillin such as cloxacillin, and by early incision. Extension of the abscess due to delayed treatment may destroy breast tissue and cause large skin defects.

Pre-pubertal mastitis is seen at around 8–12 years of age in both sexes; one or both breast discs become enlarged and painful, simultaneously or sequentially. The condition is usually self-limiting and the breast returns to its normal prepubertal size within a few weeks. Biopsy should be avoided as it is almost certain to cause permanent damage to the breast.

Precocious breast development under 8 years of age should be investigated to exclude the various causes of precocious puberty.

Male gynaecomastia is seen at puberty. It nearly always regresses spontaneously but embarrassment makes many boys request treatment. Simple bilateral mastectomy is sometimes justified.

Absent breasts require plastic surgery early in puberty as the skin must be stretched to accommodate the prosthesis.

Overgrowth of the female breast at puberty develops usually after 15 years of age but is seen earlier and can be sufficiently severe to require reduction mammoplasty.

Breast tumours are almost unknown before puberty.

DEFECTS AT THE UMBILICUS

The umbilical cord contains the umbilical vein, two umbilical arteries and possibly vestigial remnants of the vitello-intestinal duct and the urachus. A discharge may therefore be due to infection in one of the vessels, particularly after therapeutic cannulation, or less frequently bowel content from the vitello-intestinal duct, or urine from a urachal fistula. A persistent vitello-intestinal duct must be excised at a formal laparotomy to ensure that there is no narrowing in the bowel where the duct attaches to the ileum. With a urachal fistula full studies of the urinary tract, particularly to exclude outflow obstruction, are essential before surgical closure.

An umbilical polyp is most often a pyogenic granuloma; this responds to treatment with silver nitrate, simple ligation, or surgical diathermy. The rarer protrusion of a vitello-intestinal remanant of bowel mucosa (often gastric) can be recognised by its velvety appearance, surrounding excoriation, and failure to respond to simple measures. It should be excised.

Hernias at the umbilicus are very common, especially in children of African ancestry. In the true umbilical hernia there is a circular defect under the cicatrix, which varies from the just palpable to the large defects admitting several fingers. The bulge tends to alarm the child's parents but strangulation of gut is unusual and spontaneous rupture very uncommon. As the natural tendency is for the ring to close spontaneously, considerable patience is advised, even for large defects, as reduction in the size makes the operation easier. Operative repair should not usually be considered before 5 years and only very seldom under 2 years of age. The surgical technique should retain the umbilical cicatrix. A few small defects, particularly in older children, may trap omentum or peritoneal fat and cause intermittent acute central abdominal pain.

A supraumbilical hernia is really a form of epigastric hernia. The defect is immediately above the umbilical scar and is transverse. This and epigastric hernias further up the linea alba, do not have a hernial sac, may be painful from trapping of extra peritoneal fat and do not close spontaneously. Operation is therefore recommended.

THE ABDOMEN

Appendicitis

Appendicitis can occur at all ages, but is uncommon before the second birthday. While the cause remains obscure, it is obstruction of the lumen, for example secondary to a faecolith, lymphoid swelling, or previous scarring, which leads to progressive disease, which can be dangerous because of the risk of perforation and local abscess formation and general peritonitis. In the classical presentation, the diagnosis is easy. Abdominal pain, initially central, moves to the right side of the abdomen, the tongue is coated and the breath fetid, and there is vomiting following the onset of the pain. Pyrexia is usual, but in early cases the temperature does not often exceed 38°C except in young children in whom, early in the disease, it can be much higher. Tenderness and guarding in the right iliac fossa are the essential clinical signs in confirming the diagnosis. In children over the age of 5 years, with pelvic appendicitis without definite abdominal signs, a rectal examination will reveal the anterior tenderness. In those with definite abdominal signs, the rectal examination usually adds little to the diagnosis and, in children under the age of 5 years in whom an abscess is not suspected, often very little information is obtained. In cases of doubt, a polymorphonuclear leucocytosis is helpful confirmation of the presence of acute pyogenic infection. A plain abdominal X-ray may also be helpful in difficult cases, showing the evidence of oedematous bowel in the right iliac fossa, localised fluid levels, or even the presence of a calcified faecolith.

Helpful markers to exclude some of the differential diagnoses include:

1. Simple colic — the pain is central and of short duration and abdominal tenderness and pyrexia are absent

2. Mesenteric adenitis — this is usually associated with an upper respiratory infection or tonsillitis. The temperature is often high and the abdominal tenderness central and diffuse.

3. In viral or bacterial bowel infection there is diarrhoea, and any tenderness is over the whole colon

4. In urinary tract infection the pain is either over the bladder or in the loins, there is dysuria, and pus cells are found in the urine on microscopy

5. In pneumonia, there should be chest signs, but if these are obscured there is still flaring of the alae nasi, often tachypnoea, the pain is usually upper abdominal and guarding is absent

6. The predominant symptom in infectious hepatitis is severe anorexia, which precedes jaundice and pain

7. Intussusception is commoner under the age of 2 years and colic is particularly severe

8. Most children who have been starving for over 12 hours have acetone in their breath. In diabetes mellitus, there should be a longer history and blood and urine sugar levels are raised.

The possibility of appendicitis coinciding with an upper respiratory tract infection or measles must always be remembered.

Management

The treatment of acute uncomplicated appendicitis is appendicectomy. Where the diagnosis is delayed and an abscess has formed, simple drainage or conservative treatment followed by appendicectomy 6–8 weeks later may be preferable.

In generalised peritonitis, rehydration with intravenous fluids and control of infection by antibiotics such as metronidazole and gentamicin, should precede laparotomy and appendicectomy. Complications include local wound sepsis, intraperitoneal abscesses, and late adhesion obstruction.

Meckel's diverticulum

Meckel's diverticulum, which is a persistence of the intestinal end of the vitello-intestinal duct, arises from the anti-mesenteric border of the distal ileum. It is present in 2 per cent of the population and most cause no problems. The complications, in order of frequency, are bleeding secondary to ectopic gastric mucosa, intestinal obstruction from intussusception, volvulus around, or an internal hernia behind, a persisting band, and acute inflammation.

Bleeding from a Meckel's diverticulum usually starts in the first year of life, is painless and can be severe. Confirmation of the diagnosis between episodes is difficult, but a technetium-99 pertechnate scan will often show a hot spot over the ectopic gastric mucosa in the gamma camera image. The treatment includes blood replacement, followed by laparotomy with excision of the diverticulum including its base.

Intussusception

Intussusception is an invagination of one segment of bowel into the adjoining, usually distal, segment. In older children the process is often initiated by abnormalities such as polyps, cysts, or a Meckel's diverticulum. The more common form, which occurs in children between the ages of 3 months and 2 years, often has no obvious cause. The apex in the terminal ileum or at the ileo-caecal valve is carried round the gut by peristalsis; with very delayed diagnosis it may appear at the anus.

Clinically, the children are typically previously fit and have recently had an upper respiratory tract infection. The first symptom is violent crying caused by severe colic. This comes in waves and is followed by vomiting of stomach contents and emptying of normal stool from the bowel. In between the spasms of pain, the infant looks pale and anxious. Many babies go on to pass a stool of mixed blood and mucus, redcurrant jelly, or blood may be seen on the examining finger after rectal examination. This is not essential for the diagnosis. Gentle palpation of the abdomen during a quiet interval will usually reveal the mobile sausage-shaped mass lying in the line of the colon. Failure to feel this may be because of its position, such as under the liver, or muscle guarding as the intussusception is tender, or abdominal distension. Delay in diagnosis leads to rapidly progressive signs of small intestinal obstruction with copious bile-stained or faecal vomiting, and pyrexia and dehydration. Plain abdominal radiographs, supine and erect, are helpful; the caecal gas shadow is absent, there are dilated loops of small bowel with fluid levels, the intussusception itself may be seen, and there is evidence of peritoneal oedema in the right iliac fossa.

An intussusception is an acute surgical emergency and the rare deaths are nearly always due to delays in diagnosis and treatment. Intravenous fluid replacement and the administration of antibiotics are often needed. A barium enema will make or confirm the diagnosis in cases of doubt. Where the child is fit and the history short, generally under 24 hours, the enema can also be used to achieve reduction. Surgical reduction is still frequently required. An irreducible intussusception requires resection and a primary anastomosis. Recurrence is seen in 5 per cent of cases. The typical cry generally means that the diagnosis is made early; some of these reduce spontaneously, the others should be managed as above with possibly a freer use of operation to exclude an anatomical lead point.

Chronic inflammatory bowel disease

Ulcerative colitis and Crohn's disease are rare in children. In the majority of cases the conditions are easily distinguished but in about one-fifth the signs and symptoms overlap. Crohn's disease is being seen with increasing frequency.

Ulcerative colitis

This affects the large bowel. There is mucosal inflammation and ulceration; the muscle layers are only affected when there is toxic megacolon. The disease has a long and intermittent course of remission and relapses; as in adults it is premalignant, but the time before the development of malignant change is longer than the 10 years quoted as critical in adults. The symptoms are chronic diarrhoea with blood and slime in the stools. Anaemia and failure to thrive are usual, anal fissures are common, and systemic complications, such as arthritis, iritis and liver disease are sometimes seen. The diagnosis is made from the history and confirmed by sigmoidoscopy and biopsy. Barium enema and colonoscopy show the severity and extent of the disease and are necessary in the long-term follow up to look for malignant change. The drugs of proved efficacy in treatment are steroids to induce remission and sulphasalazine as maintenance.

The indications for surgery include: toxic megacolon as an emergency; chronic disease leading to growth failure, delayed puberty or loss of schooling; and severe local or systemic complications. The usual operation in children is a total colectomy with a terminal ileostomy and preservation of the rectum. In some cases bowel continuity can be restored later by ileo-rectal anastomosis or a mucosal core-out and endo-rectal pull through.

Crohn's disease

Crohn's disease is a chronic granulomatous disease of the gut of unknown aetiology. It affects the full thickness of the intestinal wall with the ileo-caecal region the commonest site, but any part of the gut can be affected, and multiple lesions are common. Perianal lesions and mouth ulcers are also common; systemic lesions do occur but with less frequency that in ulcerative colitis. Finger clubbing is seen in one-quarter of patients.

The disease runs a long and intermittent course. The initial symptoms are often those of vague ill-health with failure to thrive or grow, anorexia, diarrhoea, and abdominal pain. As a result the diagnosis is usually not made until a year or more after the start of symptoms. Once it has been suspected, the diagnosis can be confirmed by barium studies and sigmoidoscopy or colonoscopy with biopsy of an accessible lesion. The typical string sign of a narrowed segment of terminal ileum can be shown by both barium meal and barium enema examinations. Earlier radiological signs are loss of the mucosal pattern and evidence of fissuring and oedema of the bowel wall. Endoscopically the lesions vary from small aphthous-like ulcers to areas of cobble-stone mucosa fissuring and segments of narrowing. The histological features are those of granuloma formation with giant and epithelioid cells.

Neither surgery nor medical management is satisfactory as the disease recurs in 80 per cent of patients. Drugs of proven effect are steroids and sulphasalazine; azathioprine and metronidazole have also been used. The indications for surgical excision of the effected segment are similar to those for ulcerative colitis, but the lesions are frequently multiple and the tendency to recurrence and faecal fistulae and sinuses is high.

Oesophageal varices

Oesophageal varices are rare in childhood. The obstruction to portal blood flow is most often secondary to portal vein thrombosis in early life, usually following dehydration or septicaemia. Liver disease is a less common cause, but is seen in cystic fibrosis, α-1-anti-trypsin deficiency, after operation for biliary atresia, after hepatic necrosis and in congenital hepatic fibrosis.

Haematemesis, often very severe, is the normal presenting symptom; splenomegaly is usual, the liver is often normal, but is enlarged if diseased. The diagnosis is confirmed on oesophagoscopy or by a barium swallow. The first acute bleeds usually stop spontaneously. Treatment includes passing a nasogastric tube and the use of iced-water stomach wash-outs, oral neomycin and lactulose, blood replacement, pitressin intravenously and if this fails propranolol and balloon compression with a Sengstaken tube. When these measures fail oesophageal transection is usually successful. Control of the varices should probably be attempted by injection sclerotherapy, leaving any shunt as late as possible to allow normal liver growth and avoid porto-systemic encephalopathy.

Chronic abdominal pain

Only around 5 per cent of children with recurrent abdominal pain (Apley's little belly achers) have a detectable organic lesion. Management demands a detailed history and careful clinical examination to exclude organic disease. Parental and general practitioner concern is usually centred around the possibility of appendicitis, which in fact is one of the least likely causes. Over-investigation must be avoided as it is unproductive and promotes anxiety as it proceeds. Reasonable routine screening tests include items such as a full blood count, ESR, routine urine testing with microscopy and culture, and a plain abdominal X-ray. After organic disease has been excluded, the child and his family must be reassured and, where appropriate, acceptable alterations in diet and family organisation advised.

Peptic ulceration

Peptic ulceration, gastric and duodenal, is seen only rarely in childhood. There are usually diagnostic pointers in the history: a positive family history, loss of school time, loss of appetite, epigastric pain, relief of pain with vomiting and alkali, waking at night, and association with school or family stress. A barium swallow and meal is probably still indicated as the first investigation, but the diagnosis must be confirmed by endoscopy.

If an ulcer is found, the treatment is similar to that for adults, including drugs such as cimetidine or ranitidine.

Gastro-intestinal bleeding

Bleeding from the upper gastrointestinal tract can present as the vomiting of fresh or altered blood (coffee grounds). More rarely the blood is only recognised in the stool, usually as melaena, but in babies and younger children it can appear as fresh blood; the type of the bleeding, varying from fresh red to melaena, usually indicates the proximity of the source to the anus, but the speed of intestinal transit may make this misleading. It is frequently impossible to determine the cause of minor bleeding from the anus. Most often rectal bleeding is of minimal significance and the first need is to identify those cases requiring fuller investigation. Severe bleeding, as shown by finding a sizeable quantity of blood or clot in the stool or a fall in the haemoglobin level, recurrent bleeding, and bleeding associated with colic or vomiting should be investigated.

The bleeding and clotting times must, of course, be checked to exclude a haemorrhagic tendency. In the newborn, swallowed maternal blood is a common cause of melaena. Swallowed blood from lesions of the nose or throat should be considered at all ages and the presence of blood in the stool confirmed by routine chemical testing (Table 23.1).

Constipation

In children, constipation is a source of complaint

Table 23.1 Gastrointestinal bleeding

Age	Bleed	Cause	Vomit	Investigation
Haematemesis				
Neonate	Minor	Pyloric stenosis	Coffee grounds	Test feed Barium meal ultrasound
		Reflux oesophagitis		Barium swallow
	Severe	'Stress' peptic ulcer	Fresh blood	Barium meal
Older	Minor	Hiatus hernia with Reflux oesophagitis	Coffee grounds	Barium swallow and endoscopy
	Severe	Acute gastric erosions		Barium meal and endoscopy
		Peptic ulcer		Barium meal and endoscopy
		Mallory-Weiss syndrome*		Endoscopy
		Oesophageal varices		Barium swallow and endoscopy

* The Mallory-Weiss ulcer is a longitudinal split in the oesophageal mucosa caused by severe vomiting

Age	Bleed	General conditions	Cause	Stool	Investigation
Rectal bleeding					
Neonate	Minor	Well	Anal fissure	Blood steaked	Local examination
		Well	Haemorrhagic disease of the newborn	Fresh blood	Prothrombin time
			Mucosal erosions	Blood streaked	None
	Major	Ill	Necrotising enterocolitis	Blood and stool mixed	Plain X-ray
		Ill	Volvulus	Fresh blood	Plain X-ray Barium meal Laparotomy
Toddler	Minor	Well	Fissure in ano	Blood streaked	Local examination
	Mixed	Ill	Intussusception	Fresh blood and mucus	Clinical examination Barium enema
	Major	Usually well	Meckel's diverticulum	Fresh blood or melaena	Technetium scan
Older	Minor	Well	Fissure in ano Polyps Infective diarrhoea	Blood streaked Fresh blood Blood and pus Blood and mucus	Local examination Sigmoidoscopy Stool culture
	Mixed		Ulcerative colitis	Blood and mucus	Barium enema Colonoscopy
			Peptics ulcer	Melaena	Barium meal Endoscopy
	Major		Oesophageal varices	Mixed blood and melaena	Barium meal Oesophagoscopy

for the parents rather than the child. Investigation is required when there is a general upset with loss of appetite, severe straining at stool with bleeding, and faecal soiling. The problem often starting around the time of toilet training is variously described as holding back, idiopathic megarectum, obstipation, and it responds well to encouragement and an adequate aperient regimen. A rectal examination is essential to exclude anal stenosis and other obstructive lesions and to confirm that the anal canal is dilated and loaded down to the anal verge. The anal reflex should also be tested to exclude a neuropathic rectum, although this in isolation from bladder problems is improbable. Wash-outs and enemas should be required only rarely. Those children with a history starting in the neonatal period, who fail to thrive, or do not respond to the aperient regimen require investigation to exclude Hirschsprung's disease and anal achalasia. A barium enema is helpful in short-segment Hirschsprung's disease, but when the aganglionic segment is shorter than about 3–4 cm it is not diagnostic. Suction rectal biopsies taken at 3, 4 and 5 cm from the anal verge will establish or exclude the diagnosis of Hirschsprung's disease.

Ano-rectal manometry is essential for the diagnosis of anal achalasia in which there is a failure of relaxation of the internal sphincter as seen in Hirschsprung's disease, but no histological abnormality. This and many of the other less clearly established abnormalities respond well initially to an anal sphincter stretch under anaesthesia, combined with encouragement and aperients. Relpase is probably best treated by a formal internal sphincterotomy.

Hirschsprung's disease in the older child

While most children with Hirschsprung's disease are diagnosed in the neonatal period, a few with less severe symptoms present later and even in adult life. Constipation starting from birth is very suggestive, but attacks of enterocolitis may cause confusion with intermittent diarrhoea. Failure to thrive is usual but not invariable. With short and long-segment colonic disease the clinical signs are chronic large bowel distension with an empty lower rectum. With very short-segment disease the faecal mass is forced distally into the aganglionic segment

and may reach the anal verge with consequent soiling and present a picture very similar to simple rectal inertia.

A rectal biopsy is required for diagnosis. Where the aganglionic segment is less than 5 cm long, an extended internal sphincterotomy may be adequate. For most a formal pull-through operation is required.

Minor ano-rectal problems

Anal fissure

Anal fissures are a common cause of rectal bleeding and pain on defaecation. The blood streaks the stool and the toilet paper. Pain on defaecation is usual but not always present. In the infant, fissures may be multiple and part of a napkin rash. In the older child, the fissure follows tearing of the anal canal from passage of a hard stool.

The diagnosis is made by examination of the anal canal with gentle eversion of the anal verge. Rectal examination should not be attempted while the pain is acute. Very often there is a skin tag or sental pile, marking the outer end of the fissure. Treatment involves keeping the bowel motions soft by aperients. Local anaesthetic ointments are helpful only for older children who can apply them personally before a bowel action. Those few fissures which do not respond to simple measures will heal after a sphincter stretch under anaesthesia. If this is necessary, it is wise to perform a biopsy to exclude chronic inflammatory bowel disease.

Perianal abscess and fistula-in-ano

Perianal abscesses follow infection of a perianal haematoma or in a anal gland and present as painful fluctuant swellings at the anal verge. The treatment is to incise and lay open the abscess under general anaesthesia. Abscesses arising in anal glands tend to recur as the gland opens into the anal canal and a fistula forms. This will only heal after laying the whole track open.

A chronic fistula must always be biopsied as it also may be secondary to chronic inflammatory bowel disease.

Ischio-rectal abscesses

These arise from infection deep in the space lateral to the rectum but are rare in children. They present with pyrexia and a painful, tender mass lateral to the anus, and require antibiotic treatment and early incision to prevent formation of a high ano-rectal fistula.

Rectal prolapse

Rectal prolapse is common in children. It occurs after straining at stool or with acute or chronic diarrhoea. The causes of chronic diarrhoea, especially cystic fibrosis, must be excluded. Most prolapses are of mucosa only and will recover spontaneously. Prolapse of the full thickness of the rectal wall is rarer but occurs particularly in patients with paralysis of the pelvic floor muscles. Simple management includes a mild aperient to keep the stool soft, abandoning potty training, and strapping the buttocks together. Where this is ineffective a submucous injection of phenol in arachis oil will usually suffice, reserving circumferential perianal suture for those few resistant to all other measures.

THE HEAD AND NECK

Congenital defects arise from failures of fusion, inclusion of dermal elements at fusion lines, and persistence of remnants of structures from embryological development.

Pierre-Robin syndrome

A small lower jaw (micrognathia), often associated with a median cleft palate, allows the tongue to prolapse into the nasopharynx obstructing the airway.

If the child is tube-fed nursed fully prone, an adequate airway can be maintained. The growth of the lower jaw usually compensates and after a few months it is found that the airway can be maintained.

Choanal atresia

Babies are obligate nose breathers and obstruction at the back of the nasal airway causes severe distress. Unilateral obstructions are often discovered accidentally or later, but bilateral obstructions cause severe cyanosis, and respiratory distress relieved on crying. An oropharyngeal airway strapped into position will maintain the airway for the few hours necessary for transfer for surgery. The obstruction is excised and the nasal airway kept open by leaving plastic tubes in situ.

Cleft lip (hare lip)

Cleft lip and palate result from failure of fusion of the embryological facial processes. The incidence is about one per 600 live births. Embryologically and functionally clefts are now divided into defects anterior and posterior to the incisive foramen behind the incisor teeth in the hard palate. Anterior clefts are inherited separately from isolated clefts of the hard and soft palate.

In anterior defects the problem is essentially cosmetic, while in posterior defects failure of closure of the oropharynx from the nasopharynx prevents normal sucking and swallowing, and speech. Babies with combined defects have both problems. The aims of treatment are that the child should look well, feed well, and speak well. All plans for treatment are compromises in an attempt to achieve these.

Appearance

Repair of the lip is usually delayed until around 3 months of age as it is technically easier at this age and size, but it can be done in the neonatal period. Until the lip has been repaired reassurance for the parents (photographs of previous repairs are very helpful here) is important. It is relatively easy to get a good cosmetic repair of a unilateral lip defect but in bilateral clefts secondary operations are often required. Correction of the nose is more difficult and this may also require secondary operation.

Feeding

Feeding should not be a problem with lip and alveolar defects as the gums can achieve seal on the nipple or teat adequate for sucking. With palatal defects sucking is not possible. A few babies will require tube feeding initially, but most can be taught to feed from a spoon tipping the milk well back over the tongue. Various modified teats for bottles and palatal obturators have also been recommended and for those determined to breast feed the milk can be expressed either onto a spoon or directly into the baby's mouth.

Speech

Palatal repair, which is essential for normal speech, is usually undertaken around 12–15 months of age. The earlier the successful repair the sooner feeding and speech problems can be overcome, extensive early dissection increases the risk, however, of intereference with the growth of the maxilla.

Throughout management it is essential to control the upper alveolar (gum) arch by orthodontic appliances to improve its position before, and prevent collapse after operation. Speech is not often a problem after a satisfactory palatal closure and minor defects can be improved by speech therapy, but continued failure of closure of the oropharyngeal isthmus or persistent fistulae in the hard palate require later correction by closure of the fistulae and a pharyngoplasty when growth is nearer completion. Abnormalities at the inner end of the Eustachian tube, often aggravated by surgery, increase the risks of middle ear infection and any subsequent deafness will lead to further speech problems. Careful otological supervision and hearing tests are therefore essential.

Other facial clefts

Midline clefts of the upper lip are rare, technically easy to repair and important chiefly for their association with other midline defects such as single nostril, absence of posterior pituitary gland, absent corpus callosum and cerebral cortical defects. Lateral clefts of the face are also rare.

Inclusion dermoids

Inclusion dermoids are epithelial lined cysts occuring at fusion lines. The commonest, the external angular dermoid, lies deep to the lateral end of the eyebrow and above the outer canthus of the eye. It is oval and set in a depression in the bone and rarely may communicate through a defect in the skull with an intracranial extension. Skin and muscle are freely mobile over the cyst which is also mobile over the bone. Other common sites for inclusion dermoids are given below.

Other inclusion dermoids

Orbit — external and internal angular
Ear —posterior to pinna
Nasal — extends deep into the nasal cavity
Scalp — over anterior and posterior fontanelles.

All should be excised at a convenient time, say between 6 months and a year of age as they may increase in size and become infected.

Pre-auricular sinuses

These are common particularly in African babies. The opening is a small pit on the front of the helix of the ear. The deep part ramifies unpredictably in front of the ear. Uninfected sinuses are of no significance. Infection often presents as an abscess over the parotid and will not heal until the sinus has been excised completely.

Thyroglossal cysts and ectopic thyroid

The thyroid gland develops from a downgrowth arising at the site of the foramen caecum on the tongue. Normally, no remnants are left in the line of descent, but any which do persist may develop into cysts at any point along the track. These cysts are tethered to the hyoid bone and therefore move up on protrusion of the tongue as well as on swallowing. A thyroglossal sinus develops from spontaneous rupture or surgical incision of an infected cyst, or after incomplete surgical removal.

Ectopic thyroid tissue can be seen at the base of the tongue or mimicking a cyst in the neck. This is solid, will take up radio-iodine on isotope scanning, and will usually regress on thyroxine therapy. The mass at the back of the tongue should only be excised if the swelling persists after treatment. Ectopic thyroid in the neck should not be excised as it may be the only thyroid tissue present. Many of these children with only ectopic thyroid tissue are bordering on hypothyroidism.

Branchial fistula and cyst

The site of the second branchial cleft is represented in the tonsillar fossa. This cleft may persist throughout its length leaving a fistula from the lower anterior border of the sternomastoid muscle, passing over the hypoglossal nerve and between the internal and external carotid arteries to the tonsil

These fistulae leak saliva, frequently become infected and should be excised. Partial persistence of the track produces a cyst in the anterior triangle of the neck, which can usually only be distinguished from an enlarged lymph node at operation.

Enlarged cervical lymph nodes

Enlargement of the cervical lymph nodes is seen in acute infection, chronic infection and in the rare conditions of leukaemia and Hodgkin's disease. Transient swelling of the nodes is seen with oropharyngeal infections. Pyogenic infection, most commonly staphylococcal, is very common, particularly in the upper deep cervical group including the tonsillar node. The progression to abscess formation is common and very often no obvious focus is found. The infection presents as a red tender swelling below the angle of the mandible in the upper neck. In the most severe cases, there is general malaise and fever and trismus makes swallowing difficult. An antistaphylococcal antibiotic, such as cloxacillin, is indicated. In less severe situations the value of antibiotic

therapy is doubtful and very often it aborts the infections, only for it to flare up again on stopping treatment. When pus is present, surgical drainage is essential. The differentiation of chronic infection such as mycobacterial or fungal infection from neoplasia is best achieved by biopsy. In general, a lymph node which has been persistently enlarged and is not definitely showing signs of regression over a period of 3 months should be excised for biopsy.

Swellings of the salivary glands

Parotid

The commonest cause of parotid swelling is epidemic parotitis (mumps). This should only cause confusion when the swelling is unilateral. Acute pyogenic parotitis is very rare outside infancy. Recurrent subacute parotitis may be associated with stenosis of the duct orifice or dilatation of the duct radicles (sialectasis). Management is difficult as frequently no pathogenic organism can be cultured from the saliva. Despite this, ampicillin is usually given and most cases repond rapidly. Recurrence is common, but the condition eventually burns itself out over a period of years.

Submandibular glands

These are similarly affected by recurrent infection but stone formation in the duct is also seen. This is most easily diagnosed by palpation along the duct in the floor of the mouth. Stones should be removed. Unlike the parotid, the submandibular gland can easily be excised if recurrent infection and swelling become troublesome.

24

Miscellaneous problems

JOINT DISORDERS

Children who present with joint symptoms can sometimes present a difficult diagnostic problem. A careful history and thorough physical examination are, as usual, the cornerstone of diagnosis. The history should reveal the type and pattern of onset of symptoms and the examination should determine exactly which structures are involved (joints, tendons, bursae, pericardium, blood vessels, heart valves, eyes, skin). The age and sex of the patient and the pattern of joint and extra-articular involvement will help to classify the various juvenile chronic arthritides. Symptoms which must be taken seriously include limp, pain on movement or 'loss of function' of any limb or joint and unilateral symptoms. A joint which is hot, swollen or tender might be infected. It is also important to recognise simple post-viral arthropathy and not to label it as a chronic arthritis.

Laboratory investigations, such as the erythrocyte sedimentation rate, should identify those conditions which are inflammatory and simple

radiology can usually separate those conditions due to abnormalities of articular cartilage or the bony epiphyses.

The commoner causes of arthritis in childhood are listed in Table 24.1.

Growing pains

A common symptom in children is a diffuse, vague, recurrent poorly localised ache in the legs, usually worse at night. There is loss of function and in some instances the symptoms suggest attention-seeking. In children with very mobile joints, strenuous exercise may produce these vague symptoms. There are no abnormal physical signs and laboratory tests are normal. Simple reassurance is all that is required.

Traumatic and orthopaedic conditions

Hip pain due to Perthes disease or slipped epiphysis can be diagnosed radiologically. Inflammation of the tibial tubercle (Osgood-Schlatter's disease) causes local tenderness, sometimes with a knee effusion. Overuse of a joint which has an underlying abnormality (e.g. chondromalacia patellae or osteochondritis dissecans) may provoke pain or effusion which is recurrent or slow to resolve. Laboratory tests to exclude active inflammation are normal.

Septic Arthritis

Infection of the joint tissues may occur from either haematogenous spread or from a direct penetrating wound. The joint is hot, swollen and tender and the child toxic and febrile. A similar picture may

Table 24.1 Causes of arthritis in childhood

Trauma	
Infection	Haemophilus, staphylococcus, tuberculosis, viruses
Post-infective	Rheumatic fever, dysenteric
Allergic	Henoch-Schönlein purpura, food and drug allergy
Connective tissue	Juvenile chronic arthritis (see table 24.2)
Blood disorders	Leukaemia, haemophilia, sickle cell anaemia
Malignancy	Neuroblastoma

occur with osteomyelitis in which a sterile sympathetic effusion into a nearby joint can occur. Maximal clinical tenderness over bone outside the joint margins will differentiate this from a septic arthritis. If bone or joint infection is suspected, aspiration of joint fluid for Gram staining and culture is essential. Blood cultures should also be taken. X-ray changes of bone infection are usually absent in the early stages of the disease; bone scanning is more reliable. Delay in diagnosis of joint or bone infection may lead to irreparable tissue damage.

The usual causal organisms are *Stapylococcus aureus*, *Haemophilus influenzae*, streptococci or Pseudomonas. The possibility of gonococcal arthritis in adolescents and the predilection of salmonella, *Streptococcus pneumoniae* and Haemophilus for the bones and joints of children with sickle cell anaemia should be remembered. Antibiotic therapy should be given intravenously for a minimum of 2 weeks and then continued orally until all evidence of joint infection has disappeared and the ESR is normal. Open drainage or repeated aspiration of pus from the infected joint may be necessary. Splinting of joints in the position of neutral function may make the patient more comfortable.

Viral diseases

Joint symptoms occur late in viral diseases such as mumps, rubella or glandular fever. An appropriate history of contact, characteristic physical signs and a rising antibody titre or positive Monospot test will help make the diagnosis. Arthritis may occur after rubella immunisation. Swollen joints may precede the onset of anorexia, liver tenderness and jaundice in infectious hepatitis. Simple analgesia is all that is required as treatment for these self-limiting arthropathies.

Post infective arthritis

Rheumatic fever (arthritis, carditis, erythema marginatum, chorea and rheumatic nodules) may occur 10–14 days after an infection with a β- haemolytic streptococcus. Joint symptoms which accompany a sore throat are, however, unlikely to be due to rheumatic fever. Enteritis

due to salmonella or shigella may be followed by a reactive arthritis (sterile synovitis) which is self limiting.

Allergic arthritis

The purpuric rash of Henoch-Schönlein purpura with its characteristic extensor distribution is the commonest vasculitis of childhood. The associated migratory arthropathy affecting large joints lasts a few days, although in a few cases may be more prolonged. There is usually associated abdomonal pain with or without blood in the stools, haematuria, and patches of urticaria affecting the hands, feet and forehead. Food or drug allergy or urticaria from any cause may also produce a transient synovitis.

Connective tissue disease

There are several sub-groups of juvenile chronic arthritis, distinguished by age of onset, sex, the pattern of joint involvement and extra-articular manifestations, and certain laboratory tests as shown in Table 24.2.

Management of chronic arthritis

1. Suppression of disease activity by aspirin is the most effective treatment; the dosage is 80–90 mg/kg daily. Ibuprofen or indomethacin may be added or substituted if intolerance to aspirin develops. With severe systemic involvement steroids may be necessary.

2. Physiotherapy aimed at maintenance of joint mobility, strengthening weakened muscles and prevention of contractures is an important part of management. The use of a tricycle encourages exercise and mobility without full weight bearing. Hydrotherapy will ease muscle spasm and make movement of stiff joints easier. Night splinting of joints in the neutral position may help prevent deformity.

3. Slit lamp examination to detect early iridocyclitis is vital, particularly in antinuclear antibody positive patients. This should be done every 6 months. Treatment with local steroid drops is usually adequate, but alternate day systemic ster-

Table 24.2 Juvenile chronic arthritis

	Girls: Boys	Age of onset	Joints affected	Other manifestations	Antinuclear antibodies	Rheumatoid factor	Differential diagnosis	Complications Severe arthritis	Iridocyclitis
Chronic arthritis of childhood									
Systemic onset (Still's disease)	4:5	Any	Any	High remitting fever, pink maculopapular rash, splenomegaly, lymphadenopathy, pericarditis	Negative	Negative	Glandular fever, leukaemia, neuroblastoma, rheumatic fever	25%	None
Polyarticular	8:1	Any	Any	Low grade fever, mild anaemia, growth retardation	25%	Negative	Gut arthropathy psoriasis	15%	Rare
Pauciarticular (Type 1)	4:1	Early childhood	1–4 large (hips & sacroiliacs spared)	Few	50%	Negative	Single joint infection TB synovioma	Rare	50%
Juvenile rheumatoid arthritis (IgM rheumatoid factor positive)	6:1	Late childhood	Any but particularly small joints of hands & feet	Low grade fever, anaemia, subcutaneous nodules, vasculitis, erosions on X-ray	75%	100%	Resembles adult rheumatoid	50%	Scleritis
Juvenile ankylosing spondylitis (Pauciarticular type 2)	1:10	Late childhood	Few large (hips & sacroiliac involvement common)	(HLA B27 positive)	Negative 75%	Negative		Some have ankylosing spondylitis on follow up	5–10%

oids may be required to suppress a more active uveitis.

4. Education of the child can usually continue in his normal school, although in some of the more severe cases a sympathetic flexible attitude is required to make life easier for a child who may not be as mobile as his peers. Education of the family about the nature and prognosis of the disease and proper support in more severe cases is another important part of treatment of the child and his family. With early diagnosis and appropriate treatment approximately 80 per cent of children with chronic arthritis may enter adult life with little or no disability.

ORTHOPAEDICS

Borderline orthopaedic abnormalities

There are several variations of normal lower limb postures which cuase anxiety to parents. These are usually related to the position into which the baby was folded in utero. Treatment for these conditions used to be prescribed before it was recognised that a very high spontaneous rate of resolution towards more normal or acceptable posture took place.

Intoeing

Three common causes of intoeing occur:
1. In the foot itself, metatarsus varus
2. In the lower leg, medial tibial torsion associated with lateral bowing of the tibia
3. In the femur, persistent femoral anteversion.

1. Metatarsus varus

Metatarsus varus is an adduction deformity of the forefoot. The heel is always in the normal neutral position and the forefoot, which is frequently highly mobile, can be passively abducted. No treatment is needed.

This condition is sometimes mistaken for a true club foot or talipes equinovarus. In true talipes the heel is high, the Achilles tendon short and the heel in varus deformity. It is usually difficult or frankly impossible to passively correct the abnormal position of the foot and all cases of obvious or suspected talipes should be referred to an orthopaedic specialist for appropriate treatment.

2. Tibial torsion

The foot is normal but rotated medially in relation to the knee, so that when the patellae are pointing directly forwards, the feet are turned in and when the feet are parallel and pointin forwards the patallae point outwards, like a divergent patellar squint! This condition is commonly associated with lateral bowing of the tibiae and normally corrects by the age of 4 or 5. Forward bowing of the tibia is pathological.

3. Persistent femoral anteversion

In this condition the femoral neck remains markedly anteverted in relation to the shaft, with the result that the range of internal rotation of the hip joint is much greater than the more restricted external rotation. The feet and knees are normally aligned, but the child is most comfortable with the hips internally rotated which makes the patellae converge and the feet take up an intoeing position. This position usually corrects by the age of 8. If a particularly ugly posture is still present as a result of failure of spontaneous correction, then a femoral derotation osteotomy may improve the situation, but in very few cases is this justified.

Out toe gait

This is the opposite of intoeing and is due to persistent femoral retroversion. External rotation at the hip is easy and there is little internal rotation.

Knock knees

Provided they are not associated with any other abnormality they will spontaneously correct.

Flat feet

Most children when they first walk have flat feet, but as the medial arch develops this gradually disappears. Providing the feet are pain free, mobile, and the medial arch can be restored by dorsiflexion of the big toe or standing on tiptoe, the condition is benign.

Painful stiff feet are pathological. They may be due to juvenile rheumatoid arthritis or infection of the subtalar joint. Feet of unequal size may suggest an occult spinal dysraphism.

Hip disorders

Each age group has its own likely hip disorder (Table 24.3).

Table 24.3 Hip disorders of various age groups

Age (years)	Disorder
0–5	Congenital dislocation
5–10	Perthes disease
10–15	Slipped epiphysis

Congenital dislocation of the hip (CDH)

This is due to an abnormal development of the acetabulum, femoral head, capsule or other soft tissue; the head of the femur may become partially or completely dislocated. Failure to diagnose and treat this condition early may lead to permanent abnormalities of the hip joint. Every newborn should be examined carefully for signs of unstable hips which include the limitation of abduction of flexed hip, and the ability to dislocate the femoral head over the posterior rim of the acetabulum by pressing downwards and backwards with the thumb, or relocate the femoral head back into the acetabulum by applying pressure forwards with fingers on the greater trochanter (see Figure 7.1).

Asymmetry of the creases on the thigh or unequal leg lengths may also lead one to suspect the diagnosis. A single examination at birth is not sufficient the hips should be flexed and abducted at screening examinations as limitation of abduction may appear after 4 or 5 months of age.

If a child has one or more of the following features which are known to be associated with an increased incidence of CDH, or if he presents signs or symptoms referable to the hip or leg, he should be carefully examined.
1. Family history of CDH
2. Female sex

3. First born child
4. History of oligohycramnios in pregnancy
5. Breech delivery
6. Presence of talipes.

Hips which are dislocatable clunk rather than click. A hip which is completely stable in a dislocated position may not clunk at all and may only be detected clinically by asymmetry of the legs or a high index of suspicion, thus leading to appropriate radiological investigation. Despite careful screening some children with CDH present late. They may present because they walk late with a limp, or asymmetry of the legs, sometimes the CDH is detected on an X-ray taken for other reasons.

Treatment consists of some form of abduction splintage which will usually stabilise the hip. Persistent instability may need an open reduction and the likelihood of this being necessary increases with delayed diagnosis.

Other hip disorders

As mentioned above, Perthes disease and slipped epiphysis usually occur in late childhood or early adolescence; trauma and infection may occur at any age. These conditions may present with symptoms of synovitis: limp, pain in the hip and pain referred to the knee (see Fig. 24.1).

Constitutional symptoms and signs of infection, together with pain, muscle spasm and swelling of the hip joint require aspiration of the joint for a proper bacteriological diagnosis. This is most important as failure to diagnose an infective arthritis early can lead to irremedial damage.

Perthes disease. Perthes disease is due to aseptic necrosis of the femoral head epiphysis which presents with signs of synovitis. There are three stages of the condition each of which lasts for about 9 months.
1. Aseptic necrosis. Initially there are no radiological changes but after a few weeks the epiphysis becomes more dense
2. Revascularisation. The radiological changes become more mottled
3. Reossification. The femoral head is gradually reformed. Avoidance of weight bearing prevents flattening of the femoral head (like a mushroom). If this flattening is masked the incongruity

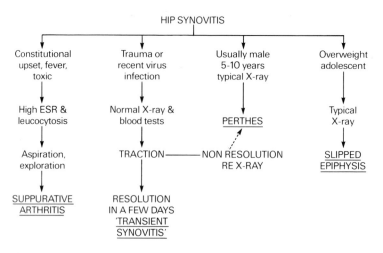

Fig. 24.1 Investigation of a painful hip

between the femoral head and the acetabulum may lead to osteoarthritic changes in the joint in later life.

Slipped epiphysis. This condition affects the adolescent and X-ray appearances of the hip usually show a postero-inferior slip of the femoral epiphysis which is best seen in the lateral projection. Immobilisation may be sufficient to arrest the process, but some form of internal fixation is usually required.

DENTAL EDUCATION AND THE PAEDIATRICIAN

Eruption

The first tooth normally erupts into the mouth at around 6 months of age and the full complement of 20 deciduous teeth is acquired by 5 years. Natal teeth, present at birth, need to be removed if they are loose and in danger of being dislodged and inhaled, if they ulcerate the tongue or if they cause discomfort to the mother during breast feeding.

Teething is the facile excuse given for many symptoms occurring between 6 months and 3 years. Increased salivation and some discomfort in the mouth are understandable; fits, unexplained fever or diarrhoea and vomiting ascribed to teething are not. It is an easy and dangerous excuse for the unwary.

The permanent dentition begins to erupt between 5 and 6 years. The full number of 28 permanent teeth have normally appeared by 13–15 years but the 4 wisdom teeth erupt later, usually by 25 years, making a full total of 32 teeth.

Caries

Dental caries involves the progressive destruction of the calcified dental tissues. Complete destruction of teeth affected by caries can occur if left untreated. By 2 years of age the average child has two carious lesions. In England and Wales, approximately one-third of adults over the age of 16 have no natural teeth at all, largely because of carious destruction. The deposition of salivary polysaccharides matted together with bacteria produces a layer of dental plaque on the teeth. A diet rich in sugary foods and sweets provides the substrate on which the bacteria feed and produce acids in the mouth, which decalcify the enamel and gradually destroy the organic matrix of the tooth.

Prevention

Studies done in the 1940s have shown that if drinking water contains one part per million of fluoride, the prevalence of dental caries is more than halved. This was initially shown by epidemiological surveys in areas with and without natural fluoridation and was confirmed when deficient areas had fluoride added to the water supply. In those ares of the country where the water is not fluoridated, the daily consumption of half a fluoride tablet (each tablet contains 2.2 mg sodium fluoride) between the ages of 6 months and 2 years and one tablet daily until 12 years, will have a significant effect in preventing dental caries. Compliance with this is not usually very good. Fluoridation of the water supply would be preferable; at present, only 10 per cent of the population of the UK drink water containing one part per million of fluoride. Excess fluoride intake can cause mottling of the teeth. The area dental officer will have information about fluoride levels in the local water supply.

Dental care

Fluoride tablets should be allowed to dissolve in the mouth for their topical effect on the teeth. Proper tooth brushing to remove dental plaque should be taught from an early age and a parent should assist in cleaning the teeth until the child is competent to do it by himself. The use of a fluoride contining toothpaste after the age of 4 years is recommended. Children younger than this tend to swallow the toothpaste which contains appreciable amounts of fluoride.

The consumption of highly refined carbohydrate between meals is cariogenic and should be discouraged, but since these snacks are almost part of the daily pattern of eating in children, substitution of low-sucrose foods such as fresh fruit, cheese, nuts or vegetables should be attempted. It is better, if sweets are allowed, to concentrate their consumption to one particular part of the week when the craving can be satisfied ad libitum.

The practice of giving bottles or dummies containing sweetened liquids as a pacifier is to be deplored. This may produce rampant decay of the upper teeth. (The lower ones are usually protected by the tongue).

Regular visits by children to the dentist should be encouraged, if only to watch other members of the family having treatment. The establishment of a good relationship with a sympathetic dentist may be very useful for dental education and save a lot of time and discomfort later in life.

COMMON SKIN PROBLEMS

Napkin rash

This may be caused by:
1. Seborrhoeic dermatitis
2. Chemical irritation (napkin dermatitis)
3. Candidiasis
4. Eczema (atopic dermatitis)
5. Napkin psoriasis
6. Intertrigo

1. Seborrhoeic dermatitis: a transient non-itchy condition seen in babies under 3 months old. It is characterised by greasy scaling affecting the scalp (cradle cap), axillae, flexures, eyebrows, backs of ears, trunk and shoulders as well as the napkin area. It will usually disappear spontaneously, but troublesome cases do respond to 1 per cent hydrocortisone cream or ointment.

2. Napkin dermatitis (ammoniacal dermatitis): this occurs when wet soiled napkins are left unchanged for long periods; it may imply some degree of neglect. Ammonia produced by interaction of stool bacteria and urine irritates the skin. The rash affects only skin in the napkin area; it does not affect the skin flexures such as the groin, and it may lead to severe umbilicate pustules or ulcers. Treatment consists of changing napkins frequently, or if possible not using napkins at all for a day or two and exposing the affected area. Napkins should be rinsed carefully in water containing a small amount of vinegar. Zinc and castor oil cream will usually clear up the dermatitis. If there is associated fungal infection this should also be treated.

3. Candidiasis superimposed on napkin dermatitis is common, particularly if the baby has oral thrush. Initially the perianal skin becomes macerated, then an erythematous sharply defined area involving the genitalia develops. Satellite lesions around the main eruption are typical of candidiasis. Topical application of nystatin, clotrimazole or miconazole, together with oral administration of nystatin suspension to clear up the gastrointestinal candidiasis is usually effective. Proprietary formulations containing nystatin, hydrocortisone and clioquinol are useful when treating infected napkin or seborrhoeic dermatitis.

4. Eczema is uncommon in babies younger than

3 months. It is usually associated with a family history of atopic conditions. The rash is invariably itchy and there are usually widespread lesions involving the face and flexures in the elbows and behind the knees. Topical corticosteroids, anti-histamines for the itching, emulsifying ointment used in the bath instead of soap and avoidance of conditions which will tend to make the child sweat should all be prescribed (See Chapter 13).

5. *Napkin psoriasis* resembles true psoriasis with well defined, slightly raised erythematous scaly plaques in the napkin area, which may spread up the trunk. The flexures are usually involved. The condition usually responds to a weak topical steroid, only some of the affected babies will have psoriasis later in childhood.

6. *Intertrigo* results from constant rubbing together of opposed skin surfaces. This is particularly common in fat babies and easily treated by frequent washing and a sprinkling of dusting powder onto the affected areas to reduce friction. Plastic pants, which encourage sweating, should be avoided.

In all these conditions, if topical steroids are used, 1 per cent hydrocortisone is always sufficient. Fluorinated steroids should *never* be used.

Impetigo

Impetigo is a skin infection caused by a β-haemolytic group A streptococcus or *Staphylococcus aureus*. The portal of entry is usually a crack in the skin and lesions are common around the nostrils and angles of the mouth, or on eczematous skin. Picking and scratching results in further spread of the lesions. The infection starts as small vesicles which rapidly burst, exude and then become covered with characteristic golden 'stuck-on' crusts. Treatment of a small area of localised impetigo can be satisfactorily accomplished with 3 per cent chlortetracycline ointment. The crusts should be removed twice daily by gentle soaking and friction with a mild antiseptic and cotton wool, followed by application of the antibiotic ointment. In more extensive infection local treatment is not usually sufficient and systemic antibiotics are necessary; erythromycin will normally be adequate. If the patient is a nasal staphylococcus carrier, chlorhexidine and neomycin cream

(Naseptin) can be applied nightly. The patient should use his own towel, keep his nails short and refrain from picking or scratching the lesions.

Predisposing factors such as lice and scabies should be sought and treated. Cross infection in schools is particularly common. Nephritis can occasionally occur following impetigo caused by a nephritogenic strain of streptococcus.

Scabies

Scabies is due to infestation with a burrowing mite, *Sarcoptes scabiei*. The female digs into the superficial layers of the skin making a small burrow in which she lays her eggs, one or two per day.

The clinical presentation is with a widespread erythematous papular rash which is intensely itchy, particularly at night when the skin is warm. The diagnostic lesion is the burrow, but these are not always found in the same distribution as the rash. Using an auriscope torch and magnifying lens (but no speculum) burrows can most easily be found in the finger webs and the inner surfaces of the wrists. Fewer burrows will be found in the vest and pants area, the feet and ankles. The face is not normally involved except occasionally in babies. Adult female mites can be lifted from the end of a burrow with a bevelled needle and examined under the microscope.

Treatment is with an emulsion of benzyl benzoate. A single application to all the skin surfaces below the neck will cure 99 per cent of cases. The whole family must be treated simultaneously if reinfestation from an untreated person is to be prevented. Until all the dead mites are shed from the skin, their continued presence may cause itching, but this does not mean that treatment has been unsuccessful.

Fungal infections

Fungal infections account for 3–5 per cent of new referrals to a dermatology clinic. Recognition is important because inappropriate treatment with steroids results in a reduction of the inflammation and irritation, but a more widespread invasion of the skin by the fungus makes proper treatment much more difficult.

The three commonest fungus infections are those due to dermatophytes (ringworm), tinea versicolor and candidiasis.

Dermatophytes

Dermatophytes cause scalp, groin and body ringworm and athlete's foot. Body ringworm is most commonly acquired from animals (cats, dogs, cattle) and is more inflammatory and itchy than the others mentioned. The usual lesion is a ciruclar scaling itchy patch with a raised edge. This is most easily seen on the trunk. Maceration of the skin between the toes with papules and vesicles on the soles of the feet occurs in athlete's foot. In the groin a scaling patch spreading onto the scrotum and inner thigh is seen. In the scalp a typical circular patch occurs in which the hair has broken off close to the scalp. Nail infection causes thickening and separation of the nail from its bed (onycholysis). The nail is discoloured and crumbly.

Diagnosis is confirmed by showing that skin scrapings examined under the microscope contain hyphae. Fluorescence under Wood's light is a useful way of screening large numbers of school children.

Differential diagnosis is from eczema, seborrhoeic dermatitis or psoriasis (which is not usually as itchy as ringworm and does not cause hair loss on the scalp), and compulsive hair pulling (trichotillomania).

Treatment using Whitfield's ointment or specific antifungal agents such as tolnaftate, clotrimazole or miconazole is usually sufficient for localised eruptions provided it is continued for at least 2 weeks. Generalised relapsing or obstinate infections, particularly of the nails and scalp, are best treated with oral griseofulvin.

Tinea versicolor

Tinea versicolor is a mild yeast infection causing a series of hyperpigmented scaling patches usually affecting the trunk, neck and face. There may be more widespread pale fluorescent patches seen under Wood's light. Topical treatment with antifungal agents (clotrimazole) is effective but should continue for several weeks or the condition may relapse.

Warts and verrucae

Warts and verrucae are caused by viruses. Most lesions will disappear if left alone due to the production of immunity in the host. A verruca in a weight-bearing area can be painful and may need to be frozen with liquid nitrogen and curetted by a chiropodist. Providing they are covered with a waterproof plaster, verrucae need not exclude a child from swimming. A number of simple proprietry applications for warts and verrucae are available at the chemist, salicylic acid in collodion or podophyllin paint is as effective as any other method of treating warts.

25

Tropical child health in the non-industrialised world

Three in four children today live in tropical developing countries where malnutrition interacting with infections and parasitic disease contributes to an appalling mortality rate amongst pre-school children, 20–50 times more than in Western Europe. Infants who survive the perils of parturition are likely to die from neonatal tetanus or septicaemia.

MALNUTRITION

Infants and children have greater nutritional requirements than adults because they are growing. Poverty and disasters either natural or man-made, lead to starvation which inevitably affects children most severely. In recent years another factor, the replacement of breast feeding by bottle feeding in developing countries, has led to rampant infantile diarrhoea and malnutrition in the form of marasmus. Malnutrition is responsible for millions of childhood deaths annually, either directly or in combination with infections. These factors are reflected in the causes of death of young children in non-industrialised countries compared with those in the developed world (Table 25.1).

The major forms of malnutrition are marasmus and kwashiorkor with a spectrum of features between the two, in addition to deficiencies of vitamins, iron, folates and trace elements (see Chapter 8).

Marasmus

Marasmus is associated with an absolute deficiency of calories, proteins and other essential nutrients. This stage affects infants and young children who have a marked deficit in both weight and height. Gross wasting of subcutaneous fat and muscles makes these suffering children look wizen but with abdominal distension due to wasting of the abdominal wall through which peristalsis is visible (Fig. 25.1). Marasmic children, in common with others who are malnourished, have impaired immune function of both cellular and humoral systems and succumb to infections. Yet, in spite of these severe changes there is no hepatomegaly, oedema or hair changes, and the child is alert and hungry, (Fig. 25.2). Marasmus is the result of chronic diarrhoea and malabsorption or chronic inadequate food intake.

Kwashiorkor

Kwashiorkor is a syndrome seen in underdevel-

Table 25.1 The main causes of death in children aged 1–4 years in non-industrialised and developed countries (WHO 1976)

Non-industrialised countries	Percentage of deaths	Developed countries	Percentage of deaths
Diarrhoeal diseases	10–40	Accidents	18–37
Respiratory infections	20–30	Congenital defects	8–18
Accidents	1–10	Malignant neoplasms	10–15
Congenital defects	1–5	Respiratory infections	5–12

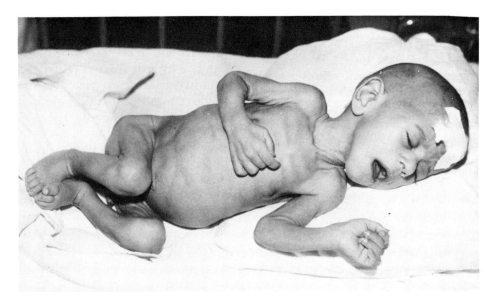

Fig. 25.1 A 3-month Asian infant weighing 3 kg with marasmus after recurrent episodes of diarrhoea. He had been bottle fed since birth

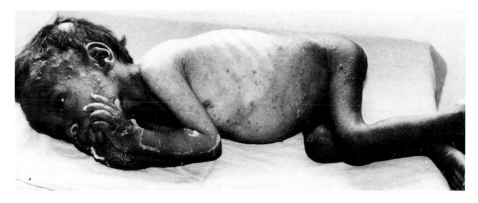

Fig. 25.2 This 2-year-old marasmic child looks alert and hungry, and is suffering from chickenpox

oped tropical countries in children taken off breast milk and given a diet low in protein relative to carbohydrates. Its pathogenesis is incompletely understood, although recent research indicates an association with mycotoxin from contaminated food. Clinical features are related to gross disturbance of protein, water and electrolyte metabolism manifested by oedema associated with hypoalbuminaemia, retarded growth and dermatoses in a miserable apathetic child. Skin changes include hypopigmentation, patches of hyperpigmentation described as 'black paint' that tend to desquamate leaving raw areas similar to second-degree burns, and 'crazy paving' usually on the legs. Hair loses its lustre, falls off easily, becomes sparse and may show the *flag* sign (variation in colour reflecting periods of normal and abnormal nutrition). Visceral organs undergo pathological changes including fatty infiltration of the liver, atrophy of intestinal mucosa and the reticulo-endothelial system, and pancreatic fibrosis.

These severe forms of malnutrition have recently been reported in British children fed on macrobiotic food by their vegetarian parents.

Nutritional anaemias due to iron and folate deficiency, avitaminoses A and rickets are the other manifestations of malnutrition.

Prevention of malnutrition

Children in the underprivileged world are in urgent need of better nutrition, clean water, improved sanitation, and protection against specific infections and parasites to cope with life in a hostile environment, but, the most important health need of children in the tropics is breast feeding. This is the best safeguard against malnutrition and gastrointestinal infection in infants. Unfortunately, breast feeding is being abandoned for artificial feeding and indications are that this trend will continue. Contributory factors to the decline in breast feeding are complex and involve the employment of women outside the home, separation of mothers and babies in hospitals, parental ignorance of infant nutrition, the aggressive sales techniques of milk marketing firms and, changing social values associated with urbanisation. Infant feeding practices in affluent countries also have a significant influence on women in urban areas of the developing world where the trend against breast feeding has been most obvious. It is hoped, therefore, that the present increase in breast feeding being practised in Western Europe and North America, together with the worldwide concern for childhood nutrition will encourage more women in developing countries to breast feed their babies.

Asian rickets

Rickets affects all age groups of Asians from the Indian subcontinent living in the UK. Neonatal rickets occurs in babies born of mothers with osteomalacia, infantile rickets affects toddlers and adolescents have late rickets. Adolescent rickets has been reported in 6 per cent of Asian schoolchildren (5–16 years) in Glasgow. The child complains, of progressively severe pain in the legs, which, if untreated, leads to deformity of the knees (genu valgum) and pelvis. Vitamin D supplements are necessary for Asian children if adolescent rickets is to be prevented (see chapter 8).

DISEASES IMPORTED INTO THE UK

About 4 million passengers arrive from the non-industrialised world each year at London airport and it is estimated that one in 15 persons in the UK is exposed to diseases from the tropics. There are also 1.9 million people from the New commonwealth now living in Britain. Therefore, all doctors in primary health care must be aware of the common childhood diseases which have been imported into this country. These diseases fall broadly into 3 groups: tropical diseases, communicable disease of public health significance and inherited disorders (Table 25.2).

Table 25.2 Childhood diseases imported in the UK

1. *Tropical diseases*
   Malaria — chiefly *P. falciparum* and *P. vivax*
   Intestinal helminths — Ascaris, Tricuris and hookworm
   Nutritional rickets in Asians
   Schistosomiasis
   Leishmaniasis
   Skin infections — fungal and parasitic

2. *Communicable diseases*
   Tuberculosis — pulmonary and disseminated
   Diarrhoeal diseases — Salmonella, Shigella, Giardia and *Entamoeba histolytica*
   Viral hepatitis
   Viral haemorrhagic fevers — Lassa, Ebola and dengue

3. *Inherited disorders*
   Thalassaemias — βthalassaemia and αthalassaemia (haemoglobin H disease)
   Haemoglobinopathaies — sickle cell disease (HbS) and haemoglobin E disease
   Glucose-6-phosphate dehydrogenase (G6PD) deficiency presenting as neonatal jaundice, favism, and drug-induced haemolytic anaemia

Malaria

A worldwide resurgence of malaria occurred during the 1970s, killing a million African children every year. This resurgence was reflected in the UK by the sharp increase of imported malaria from 354 to 1909 cases annually between 1972 and 1978, but the upward trend slackened and declined; 1576 cases were notified in 1981 to the Malaria Reference Laboratory in London. About 220 children in the UK suffered from malaria annually during 1976–78, the majority (75 per cent) being children of immigrants. *Plasmodium vivax* infection contracted in the Indian subcontinent accounted for more than 70 per cent of cases and the remainder were mainly *P. falciparum* malaria from Africa.

Clinical Presentation

Childhood malaria does *not* manifest the periodic fever and rigors so characteristic of malaria in adults. *P.vivax* infection is the usual form of malaria contracted by Asian children born in this country while on holiday in the Indian subcontinent. The incubation period is long, averaging 2 weeks to 9 months because *P. vivax* has an exo-erythrocytic phase in the host's liver from which merozoites can escape, weeks or months after the initial infection to complete the life cycle. Fever (39–40°C) is sometimes accompanied by rigors and vomiting. The child is flushed and hepatosplenomegaly is present. Anaemia is not a feature of vivax malaria. Although distressing, this disease is rarely fatal.

P. falciparum infection, on the other hand, is frequently a fatal disease in young African children living in highly endemic areas. Death usually results from cerebral malaria or acute overwhelming infection. Some children achieve a relative tolerance to the parasite after several attacks of falciparum infection and are asymptomatic in spite of hepatosplenomegaly, parasites in their blood and anaemia. Children suffering an acute attack of falciparum malaria develop a high, continuous fever (38–40°C), anaemia (haemoglobin less than 9 g/dl), an enlarged tender liver and splenomegaly. Febrile convulsions often occur and can be distinguished from cerebral malaria because the loss of consciousness lasts only for a few minutes.

The clinical diagnosis of *P. falciparum* malaria can be difficult to make in white children in this country. Besides the non-specific clinical picture and the low index of suspicion on the part of the doctor, these children have usually taken antimalarial prophylaxis. However, the dosage was either inadequate or the drugs were stopped soon after returning to the UK. These problems are illustrated in the following case.

Case history: A 12-year-old white girl born in Zambia moved to England after her second birthday. Her next visit to the tropics had been a month's holiday in Nairobi and Mombassa. She had taken pyrimethamine 25 mg weekly while abroad but stopped when she arrived home. Two days after the holiday she developed a fever and cough which was diagnosed as pleurisy. She did not improve on penicillin for 10 days after which she attended her doctor presenting with anorexia, vomiting, abdominal pain and fever (38°C). A tentative diagnosis of hepatitis was made and she was nursed at home. Four weeks after her return from Africa she had jaundice (serum bilirubin 90 μmol/l). One week later she was admitted to hospital with drowsiness and vomiting. She was ill with marked pallor and a temperature of 38°C on admission but without jaundice. She had an enlarged spleen 1 cm, a haemic heart murmur, but no abnormal neurological signs and a normal cerebrospinal fluid. Blood investigations showed heavy parasitaemia with *P. falciparum*, and haemolytic anaemia (haemoglobin 3 g/dl), reticulocytes 25 per cent. She was given a transfusion of packed red cells and chloroquine treatment with dramatic improvement; she was discharged from hospital 4 days later.

Malaria can only be diagnosed by blood examination preferably of a thick film stained with Field's stain. This case also emphasises the need for antimalarial prophylaxis to be continued for 6 weeks after leaving a malarious area to ensure the eradication of all forms of *P. falciparum*.

Cerebral malaria is a serious complication of *P. falciparum* infection that can be rapidly fatal and calls for immediate treatment. Capillaries supplying the brain are blocked with parasitised erythrocytes, and produce foci of cerebral necrosis. The child with cerebral malaria presents with fever for a few days followed by repeated convulsions with alteration of the level of consciousness. There are hardly any CNS signs; some children show minimal signs of meningeal irritation, but retinal haemorrhages may be present. The cerebrospinal fluid is usually normal and this distinguishes cerebral malaria from septic meningitis and viral encephalitides. In young children, the mortality rate from cerebral malaria even with the best available treatment is 25 per cent and there is a significant morbidity from neurological sequelae in survivors.

Treatment

The aim of treatment is the eradication of parasites with appropriate drugs. In *acute attacks*, the 4-aminoquinolines, chloroquine and amodiaquine are active agents that will radically cure *P. falciparum*, but will not prevent relapses of *P. vivax* and *P. malariae*. All forms of acute malaria should be treated initially with chloroquine or amodiaquine (Table 25.3). Patients with *P. vivax* and

since this would interfere with development of immunity. Chemoprophylaxis given at the peak of seasonal epidemics will reduce the severity of parasitaemia without interfering with development of immunity, and will assist in promoting normal

Table 25.3 Dosage for oral treatment of acute malaria in non-immune children

Drug	Interval	Age (years)				
		0–1	1–3	4–6	7–11	12–15
		Dosage (mg)				
Chloroquine	*Loading dose* followed	75	150	300	300	450–600
	6 hours later by second dose	75	150	150	150	225–300
	Daily dose for next 2 days	37	75	75	150	150–300
Amodiaquine	*Dose* 1st day	50	100	150	200–300	400–600
	Daily dose next 2–4 days	50	50	100	150–200	250–400

P. malariae infections require the addition of an 8-aminoquinoline to eradicate the exoerythrocytic form of the parasite for a radical cure. Primaquine is of value but has a narrow margin between effective and toxic dosages. Young children are not usually given this drug. Primaquine can be used after a course of chloroquine as follows for a period of 10 days:

Body weight: 10–30 kg — 3.75 mg (base) daily
31–40 kg — 5–7 mg daily
41–40 kg — 11.25–15 mg daily

Non-white children with glucose-6-phosphate dehydrogenase deficiency may develop haemolytic anaemia or methaemoglobinaemia.

In *severe malaria* (coma or persistent vomiting), parenteral therapy with quinine or chloroquine must be given without delay. If the intravenous route is used, the drugs should be infused slowly with a large volume of diluent.

Chemoprophylaxis

Antimalarial drugs should be given to all non-immune people entering an endemic area and to all children in the first 2 years of life when mortality is highest. Older children indigenous to an endemic area do not require continuous therapy

growth. However, continuous chemoprophylaxis is justified in children with sickle cell anaemia in whom severe haemolytic crises are often precipitated by malaria. A simple guide to drug dosages is given in Table 25.4.

Intestinal helminths

The absence of proper sanitation for disposal of excreta and the use of untreated human faeces for manure contribute to the high incidence of ascariasis, trichuris and hookworm in tropical rural communities.

Ascariasis

Ascaris lumbricoides is found in 70 per cent of children, 25 per cent of whom have multiple infestations with other helminths. Adult ascaris worms produce abdominal colic, nausea and vomiting, but heavy infestation may lead to intestinal obstruction, intussusception, peritonitis, cholecystitis, cholangitis and obstructive jaundice. Piperazine citrate in a single dose of 2 g/m^2 body surface area or 3–4 g is effective treatment for ascaris. Multiple doses may cause neurotoxicity with ataxia, hypotonia, incoordination and drowsiness.

Table 25.4 A simple guide to malaria chemoprophylaxis in non-immune children

Drug	Interval	Dosage (mg) Age (years]			
		0–1	1–3	4–7	8–14
Pyrimethamine	Weekly	6.25–12.5	12.5	12.5–25	25
Proguanil	Daily	25	50	75	100
Chloroquine	Weekly	50	100	150	200
Amodiaquine	Weekly	50	100	150	200

In recent years *P. falciparum* parasites have become increasingly resistant to chloroquine in South East Asia, Bangladesh, Eastern India, South America, East Africa and Papua New Guinea. The drugs recommended for the prevention of malaria in these countries are Fansidar (Roche) and Maloprim (Wellcome). One tablet of Fansidar contains 500 mg sulfadoxine and 25 mg pyrimethamine while a tablet of Maloprim contains 100 mg dapsone and 12.5 mg pyrimethamine

Drug	Interval	0–1	1–3	4–7	8–14
Fansidar	Weekly	¼tablet	¼tablet	½tablet	¾tablet
Maloprim	Weekly	Not recommended	¼tablet	½tablet	above 10 years 1 tablet

At least 2 doses should be taken *before* entering an endemic area, and the drug must be continued for 6 weeks after leaving the tropics

Whipworm

Trichuris trichiura (whipworm) infection is common in young children and symptoms are related to the number of worms present in the bowel. Heavy infection presents with abdominal pain, diarrhoea, blood in the stools, tenesmus and rectal prolapse. The worms are attached to the mucosa of the rectum and sigmoid colon and cause bleeding ulcers that lead to iron deficiency anaemia. Complete eradication of trichuris infection is difficult; thiabendazole is fairly effective in a daily dosage of 50 mg/kg for 3 days.

Hookworms

Ancylostoma duodenale and *Necator americanus* exclusively parasitise man. The larvae penetrate the skin of bare-footed children producing a dermatitis *ground itch* at the site of entry and migrate to the lungs where they may cause cough and fever. Adult worms are attached to the jejunal mucosa and live by sucking blood from the host. Iron deficiency anaemia results when the worm load is large. Thiabendazole 50 mg/kg bodyweight up to a maximum of 3 g in a single dose is effective treatment for hookworms and other helminths.

Schistosomiasis

Schistosomiasis is second only to malaria as a major tropical disease affecting 200 million people in the world. The disease is acquired in childhood through exposure to infected streams, rivers and irrigation canals where certain snails, the intermediate host, survive. There are 3 major species of schistosomes (helminthic flukes), *S. haematobium* (in Africa and the Middle East), *S. mansoni* (Africa, Central and South America) and *S. japonicum* (Far East). *S. mansoni* and *S. japonicum* affect the large bowel and liver while *S. haematobium* affects the urinary tract. The development of symptoms depends upon the worm load, the number of ova laid and the immune response of the host. White children are likely to present with anorexia, malaise, prolonged fever, dry irritating cough, urticaria and loss of weight. Investigations show marked eosinophilia and patchy pulmonary infiltration on X-ray in some cases. Children in endemic areas do not present with constitutional symptoms; those infected with *S. mansoni* and *S. japonicum* have diarrhoea with blood and mucus while haematuria and dysuria are symptomatic of *S. haematobium* infection. Chronic infections with

S. haemotobium can cause hydronephrosis which is reversible with early treatment and, later, irreversible fibrosis and calcification of the bladder. Portal hypertension from liver fibrosis is a complication of *S. mansoni* and *S. japonicum* infections. Recurrent salmonella infections are likely to develop in subjects with schistosomiasis, the organisms living in the integument of schistosomes. Niridazole, 25 mg/kg body weight given orally for one week is effective against all three forms of schistosomes.

Leishmaniasis

Leishmaniasis is a parasitic disease due to protozoa spread by sandflies. Two major syndromes are recognised.
1. Visceral leishmaniasis (kala azar) affecting the reticuloendothelial system is a systemic illness
2. Cutaneous leishmaniasis in which skin and sometimes adjacent mucous membranes are attacked.

Endemic areas exist in China, India, the Middle East, Mediterranean countries, Africa and Central and South America. Visceral leishmaniasis attacks children under 8 years, who present with prolonged fever seldom over 39°C, loss of weight, hepatosplenomegaly, and lymphadenopathy. Infants are toxaemic. Anaemia is usually severe (haemoglobin less than 7 g/dl), normochromic, normocytic, associated with leucopenia and thrombocytopenia. Secondary bacterial infection and bleeding are complications. The disease is sometimes mistaken for acute leukaemia when the bone marrow is examined. Visceral leishmaniasis is a diagnosis to be considered in a child with prolonged fever who has been on holiday in the Mediterranean. Pentamidine 4 mg/kg body weight or sodium stibogluconate (Pentostam) 10 mg/kg (maximum 600 mg) given by injection daily for 10 days is the treatment.

Tuberculosis

Tuberculosis is a common and dangerous disease in young children in many developing countries. Haematogenous spread of tubercle bacilli is frequent in poorly nourished children and affects lymph nodes, meninges, peritoneum, bone and joints and rarely, kidneys. In the UK, the estimated annual risk of tuberculosis infection in 1978–79 was 0.07 per cent for children born of British parents, 0.5 per cent for children born in the UK to Asian parents and 1.65 per cent for children born abroad to Asian parents. Tuberculin testing of all immigrant children on arrival is recommended and BCG given to all who have a weak or no reaction. A weak or minimal tuberculin reaction in the presence of active tuberculosis may occur in: very malnourished children; severe disseminated infection; following measles; patients on immunosuppressive drugs; the first weeks of an infection; or faulty technique or inactive tuberculin.

DIARRHOEAL DISEASES

Acute diarrhoea with its serious consequences of dehydration, electrolyte imbalance and nutritional impairment is a major cause of morbidity and mortality in developing countries (Table 25.1). Over 6 million deaths from diarrhoea occur worldwide each year in pre-school children. Viruses, bacteria and parasites have been identified as causal agents of acute diarrhoea in infants and children.

Rotavirus infection is an important cause of acute diarrhoea in some developing countries, e.g. Bangladesh, but its precise role in other countries has still to be established. It is probable that a rotavirus vaccine will be available in the near future and this has raised hopes of effective intervention to control diarrhoeal disease.

Shigellae and salmonellae are the most frequently identified bacterial pathogens. Although enterotoxogenic *Escherichia coli* has been identified in nurseries in industrialised countries and in adults with travellers' diarrhoea, its role in acute infantile diarrhoea awaits clarification. Campylobacter has been cultured from stools of children with acute diarrhoea in tropical Africa. Untreated, the infection tends to persist for 7–14 days with apparent recovery followed by relapse of symptoms mistaken for acute appendicitis.

Giardiasis and amoebiasis are the two major

diarrhoeal diseases caused by parasites. In the highlands of Papua New Guinea, a syndrome of severe abdominal distension, vomiting and diarrhoea in breast-fed infants under 6 months of age has been described in association with heavy infestation of *Strongyloides fuelleborni*. Other features of this infection are ascites and oedema with hypoproteinaemia, and eosinophilia. The disease is rapidly fatal unless treated with mebendazole 25 mg/kg body weight.

Management of diarrhoea in developing countries

In 1978, the World Health Organisation launched a global diarrhoeal diseases control programme with the support of UNICEF. The immediate objective of this programme was to reduce diarrhoea-related mortality and malnutrition in children by widespread implementation of oral rehydration therapy and improved feeding practices. More than 70 countries have agreed to incorporate the control of diarrhoeal diseases as an integral part of primary health care.

Clinical management of diarrhoea is based on the principle of replacement of lost fluid and electrolytes. The first step in management is the identification of dehydration and the assessment of its severity in the child with diarrhoea. The severely dehydrated child requires parenteral fluid therapy to correct shock by rapid restoration of circulatory volume. Lesser degrees of dehydration can be managed successfully with oral fluids, which if given early in the course of diarrhoea, prevent the development of circulatory failure and the use of expensive equipment and fluids for parenteral therapy. The solution recommended by the World Health Organisation for oral therapy is oral rehydration salts (ORS) solution containing:

Glucose	110 mmol/l
Na^+	90 mmol/l
Cl^-	80 mmol/l
K^+	20 mmol/l
HCO^-_3	30 mmol/l

The solution is made from glucose 20 g, sodium chloride 3.5 g, sodium bicarbonate 2.5 g and potassium chloride 1.5 g dissolved in one litre of clean drinking water. This ORS solution is satisfactory for the management of hypo-osmolar dehydration found in most developing countries, but its content of sodium is too high for use in young infants or children suspected of hyper-osmolar dehydration.

Initial oral rehydration should be complete within 4–6 hours when skin turgor and pulse will return to normal and urine flow will have begun. Mild to moderate cases, passing stool every 2 hours, will require 100–200 ml of ORS solution per kg body weight daily. After 4–6 hours the same amount of oral fluids is given if signs of dehydration persist. As stool frequency decreases, less ORS solution is offered until the patient returns to normal. Infants with diarrhoea are encouraged to breast feed during oral rehydration. Vomiting is not a contra-indication to oral therapy.

Oral rehydration with ORS solution is effective, simple and safe in the management of acute diarrhoea worldwide. When provided early in the disease, it substantially reduces death rates and hospitalisation.

Amoebiasis

This disease caused by the protozoon, *Entamoeba histolytica* causes a severe illness in malnourished young children in the tropics and was the fourth most important cause of death found at autopsy in Mexico City. The parasite invades the large intestine producing mucosal ulcers from the terminal ileum to the perineum. Haematogenous spread to the liver with abscess formation occurs even in mild infections. Most children present with mild diarrhoea which may become chronic or relapsing; the stools are loose, containing excess mucus and some blood. Fever and constitutional disturbance may not be evident, but abdominal discomfort, tenesmus and tenderness over the colon are present. The severest form of amoebiasis may be acute, simulating bacillary dysentery, and be complicated by colonic perforation and peritonitis with a high mortality. Cutaneous ulceration in the perineum is another complication.

Women with untreated amoebic dysentery can infect their newborn infants during parturition.

Diagnosis of amoebiasis is made by examination of a fresh warm stool for haematophagenous trophozoites of *E. histolytica*.

Metronidazole 40 mg/kg body weight given orally in three divided doses daily (maximum 2400 mg) for 7 days is safe and effective treatment; the parasites disappear from the stools within 24 hours.

Giardiasis

Giardia lamblia is a flagellate protozoon which lives in the duodenum and jejunum of the host. Surveys of primary schoolchildren in Rangoon and Mexico City showed prevalence rates of 21 per cent and 13.7 per cent respectively. Symptoms vary from mild to severe diarrhoea which may become prolonged and result in failure to thrive. Giardia infection is associated with malabsorption and the passage of pale, frothy, offensive stools. Diagnosis is made by finding oval cysts or, sometimes trophozoites, in freshly voided stools. When stool examination is negative, duodenal juice aspirates should be examined for trophozoites.

Transmission of the parasite is by the ingestion of contaminated food and water.

Metronidazole 20 mg/kg body weight daily (maximum 1200 mg) in three divided doses for 7–10 days gives a cure rate in excess of 80 per cent.

Shigellosis

Shigellae are Gram-negative bacilli that can invade the mucosa of the colon and cause dysentery, acute severe diarrhoea with mucus, pus and blood in the stools. There are four sub-groups: *Sh. dysenteriae, Sh. flexneri, Sh. boydii* and *S. sonnei*, listed in order of severity of illness produced in man. *Shigella flexneri* tends to be the dominant species in the tropics, although *Sh. dysenteriae* has been responsible for epidemics in Central America; *Sh. sonnei* is the dominant species in the UK. After a short incubation (2–3 days) there is an abrupt onset of fever, abdominal cramps and pain, vomiting and diarrhoea. Initially the stools are loose and yellow-green but later, mucus, pus and blood are passed. Young children may present with febrile convulsions and signs of meningeal irritation.

A very severe form of infection with *Sh. shigae, (subtype of Sh. dysenteriae)* may produce gangrene of the colon and prove rapidly fatal.

When diarrhoea is the main symptom, the illness can be distinguished from salmonellosis, *E. coli* enteritis and staphylococcal food poisoning by culturing the stools.

The most important aspects of treatment is the early recognition and correction of dehydration and shock and restoration of fluid and electrolyte balance. In severe infection with *Sh. dysenteriae* and *Sh. flexneri* subtypes, antimicrobial agents, chloramphenicol, ampicillin or co-trimoxazole should be adminsitered for 5–7 days. Control of cross-infection is necessary.

Salmonellosis

Salmonellae are motile, non-lactose fermenting Gram-negative bacilli; there are more than 1000 species. *Salmonella typhi, S. paratyphi A* and *S. paratyphi B* cause typhoid or enteric fever while the other species are associated with food poisoning. These pathogens are heat sensitive. Food poisoning results when frozen poultry and meat are not completely thawed before cooking.

Typhoid Fever

Typhoid fever reported in the UK is an imported disease, 80 to 85 per cent of cases having acquired the infection in the Indian subcontinent and the Mediterranean. Around one-half of cases occur in children, mainly from immigrant households who have visited the Indian subcontinent.

The infection is usually acquired from food and drink contaminated by a human carrier. *Salmonella typhi* invades the mucous membranes and Peyer's patches of the upper small intestine to enter the reticuloendothelial system and blood, producing bacteraemia. Fever is high and persistent associated with delirium, the temperature seldom returning to normal. The child has anorexia, vomiting and diarrhoea. Headache is a frequent complaint and signs of meningeal irritation are present in some cases. A palpable spleen is almost always found in typhoid fever. Complications are rare if treatment is instituted early, but may include toxic myocarditis, detectable by electrocardiography, and perforation and haemorrhage in the small intestine. Leucopenia is present in 25 per cent and thrombocytopenia in 15 per cent of patients. Although typhoid fever is a major illness, some untreated cases may resolve spontaneously.

Laboratory diagnosis of typhoid fever depends upon culture of *S. typhi. S. paratyphi A or B* from blood and stools. Serology is of limited value because the Widal reaction is useful in patients not normally resident in typhoid endemic areas who have not been given TAB vaccine. A rise in O antigen titre suggests an active infection but a rise in H antigen titre suggests previous infection or immunisation.

Management consists of symptomatic treatment of fever and the use of antimicrobial agents, namely, chloramphenicol (50 mg/kg daily) or amoxycillin (100 mg/kg daily) for 3 weeks. In a large series from Durban, amoxycillin was found to be superior to chloramphenicol because there was no recurrence of fever, no persistent carriers and only 2 per cent failure of response in African children.

It is important to realise the association between schistosomiasis and persistent salmonella infection in children from the tropics. Salmonellae reside in the integumen of schistosomes but will be eradicated with treatment for schistosomiasis. There is also a high frequency of salmonella osteomyelitis in West African children with sickle cell disease, probably due to tissue hypoxia from thrombotic crises.

Viral haemorrhagic fevers

The media have drawn attention to the hazards of Lassa fever, Marburg and Ebola virus diseases being imported from Africa. The high mortality and infectivity of these diseases have prompted the establishment of high security isolation units in England. In fact, these exotic diseases are rarely encountered in the UK when compared with cases of imported malaria, tuberculosis and typhoid. Fever and rash, often haemorrhagic, are features of these diseases and dengue haemorrhagic fever which is a major public health problem affecting children in South East Asia. These diseases should be suspected in children with fever who have recently arrived from endemic areas. However, it is important that malaria and typhoid be excluded by blood examination.

INHERITED DISORDERS

There are three major genetic disorders involving the red cell prevalent in the tropics and subtropics: thalassaemias, haemoglobinopathies and glucose-6-phosphate-dehydrogenase (G6PD) deficiency (Table 25.2). These inherited disorders are found in Africa, South East Asia, the Mediterranean and Middle East, and wherever there are migrants from these areas e.g. the Caribbean, the Americas, Australia and the UK. The world distribution of these genetic conditions is similar to that of endemic malaria, past or present. It is postulated that the prevalence of these genes is related to the advantage endowed to heterozygous carriers to cope successfully with *P. falciparum* malaria. Evidence from epidemiological and clinical research favour this postulate in heterozygous carriers of sickle cell haemoglobin (HbS). However, homozygous subjects appear to have a distinct disadvantage when exposed to infections, drugs and other environmental factors.

Thalassaemia

Thalassaemia is a genetically determined anaemia found in Cypriots, North Indians, Arabs, Vietnamese and Chinese. It is an inherited disorder of haemoglobin synthesis in which there is a reduction in the rate of synthesis of one globin chain and an excess of the partner chain produced at the normal rate. The chain produced in excess precipitates in the bone marrow and erythrocytes causing ineffective erythropoiesis, decreased red-cell survival and chronic anaemia. There are two main types of thalassaemia: α-thalassaemia and β-thalassaemia, both inherited in an autosomal recessive manner.

Homozygous β-thalassaemia

This is a severe anaemia in children who die unless frequent blood transfusions are given. Although affected infants are normal at birth, anaemia of insidious onset is obvious after the third month together with poor feeding, pallor and splenomegaly. There is stunting of growth and hyperplasia of the maxillae resulting in a charac-

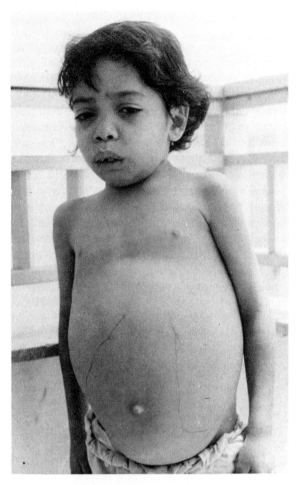

Fig. 25.3 An 8-year-old Arab girl with homozygous β thalassaemia. She has gross hepatosplenomegaly and hypertrophy of the maxillae (producing the thalassaemia facies) as a result of chronic anaemia

teristic appearance, the thalassaemia facies (Fig. 25.3). Regular blood transfusions are needed but these and the increased intestinal iron absorption lead to haemosiderosis and death from cardiac failure in the second and third decades. This dismal outlook has been modified by early diagnosis and the regular use of iron chelating agents. The blood pictures resembles iron deficiency anaemia but with many target cells, tear-drop cells and red cell fragments. Fetal haemoglobin (HbF) concentrations are increased (10–90 per cent). The basis of treatment is the correction of anaemia without inducing iron overload. The haemoglobin concentration should be raised to the normal range and maintained by blood transfusions. Excess iron is removed by desferrioxamine administered by overnight subcutaneous infusion with a syringe pump. Ascorbic acid is given to enhance the action of desferrioxamine. Young children have been maintained in negative iron balance by this method.

Haemoglobin H

This disease is a form of α-thalassaemia prevalent in some Mediterranean countries and South East Asia. Most subjects have moderate anaemia (haemoglobin 8–9 g/dl), splenomegaly and a normal life expectancy. Anaemia may be severe during infection, pregnancy or from haemolysis induced by oxidant drugs e.g. sulphonamides. The red cells are hypochromic and microcytic with fragmentation, basophilic stippling and target cells. The mean cell volume (MCV) and mean cell haemoglobin (MCH) are low. On incubation of the red cells with brilliant cresyl blue for 30 minutes, numerous HbH inclusion bodies are visible.

Haemoglobinopathies

A haemoglobinopathy is a structural haemoglobin variant resulting from substitution of an amino acid in one of the globin chains e.g. HbS (sickle cell haemoglobin) in which glutamic acid is replaced by valine in position 6 of the β chain. Haemoglobinopathies are transmitted by autosomal recessive inheritance; the parents are heterozygous (HbAS) and the affected child is homozygous (HbSS).

Sickle cell disease

Sickle cell disease occurs in the homozygous individual (HbSS) who does not possess any normal adult haemoglobin (HbA). Sickling or polymerisation of HbS molecules into filaments occurs when the erythrocyte is deoxygenated. Anaemia is obvious in the 3-month-old infant in whom fetal haemoglobin concentration is declining and insufficient to protect red cells from sickling. Other clinical features in infancy include dactylitis, pneumococcal infections and anaemic crisis from acute splenic sequestration (sudden splenic enlargement and circulatory collapse). The latter two complications contribute to a mortality rate of 10 per cent in Jamaican infants with sickle cell anaemia. Older children suffer vaso-occlusive crises consisting of sudden onset of bone pain in the limbs, joints, spine and chest, or abdominal pain accompanied by nausea and vomiting. The child will resent examination of the affected part because of pain. Symptoms are due to ischaemia and may last from hours to days. Infection (particularly malaria) is often a precipitating factor, with accompanying fever, dehydration and tachycardia. Aplastic crises are serious, occurring when marrow erythropoiesis suddenly ceases, and are related to viral infections or folate deficiency. Severe anaemia develops rapidly to precipitate life-threatening cardiac failure.

Diagnosis of sickle cell disease depends on identifying sickle cells on blood film and electrophoresis of haemoglobin which shows the presence of HbS and absence of HbA.

Prompt treatment of any infection or fever is most important in the prevention of vaso-occlusive crises. The child with pain should be given bed rest, hydration, analgesics and antimicrobial agents. Blood transfusion is required in the presence of severe anaemia. Folic acid supplements and prophylactic penicillin should be provided.

Prognosis is good in the UK. Symptoms tend to decrease as the child grows older. The disease is mild in Saudi Arabs and those who have high concentrations of fetal haemoglobin in adulthood.

Haemoglobin E

Haemoglobin E found mainly in South East Asians is the next most frequent abnormal haemoglobin. The homozygous individual has mild anaemia (haemoglobin 9–10 g/dl), decreased red-cell lifespan and microcytosis. Anaemia may be marked in the presence of infection, pregnancy and nutritional deficiency .

Glucose-6-phosphate-dehydrogenase (G6PD) deficiency

More than 100 million people with glucose-6-phosphate-dehydrogenase deficiency are to be found in South East Asia, Mediterranean and Middle Eastern countries, Africa, the Caribbean, and wherever these peoples have emigrated. Deficiency of this red-cell enzyme is associated with neonatal hyperbilirubinaemia, acute haemolytic anaemia and chronic haemolytic disease.

The enzyme G6PD catalyses the conversion of glucose-6-phosphate to 6-phosphogluconate and the reduction of nicotinamide adenine dinucleotide (NADP) to NADPH. The latter participates in the production of reduced glutathione which protects the red-cell membrane from damage by oxidative products (e.g. hydrogen peroxide) of metabolism.

Neonatal hyperbilirubinaemia

Neonatal hyperbilirubinaemia due to G6PD deficiency has been observed in Chinese, Greek and African infants. Jaundice appears on the second day, usually in male infants (G6PD deficiency is an X-linked inherited condition), and hyperbilirubinaemia is frequent on the third to fifth days but sometimes occurs in the second week in Chinese infants. Kernicterus develops rapidly particularly in preterm infants and those with severe infections. Anaemia is variable and splenomegaly uncommon. Serum bilirubin concentration is usually high (350 μmol/l) and unconjugated. In the tropics serum bilirubin concentrations of 700 μmol/l have been recorded in infants on admission to hospital. There is a simple test for detecting G6PD enzyme using a few drops of blood and based on a colour change when NADP is converted to NADPH. Management of these severely jaundiced babies is with blood exchange transfusions and phototherapy. It is important to identify the agent which induced the haemolysis. In South East Asia and West Africa, naphthalene in mothballs is usually responsible as it can be absorbed through the skin and lungs. Infants in contact with linen stored in naphthalene develop hyperbilirubinaemia rapidly leading to kernicterus and permanent neurological sequelae.

Acute haemolytic anaemia

This condition is precipitated when G6PD deficient children are prescribed drugs or exposed to certain chemicals, listed in Table 25.5. Other agents like vitamin K and aspirin have not been proven to induce haemolysis. Symptoms are

Table 25.5 Drugs and chemicals causing clinically significant haemolysis in G6PD deficiency

Acetanilid	Naphthalene
Nalidixic acid	Trinitrotoluene
Nitrofurantoin	Diaphenylsulphone (Dapsone)
Niridazole	Sulphanilamide
	Sulphacetamide
Phenylhydrazine	Sulphapyridine
	Sulphamethoxazole
Primaquine, Pamaquine	Fava beans, Methylene
Pentaquine	blue, Toluidine blue

similar to those of favism but the outcome is seldom fatal.

Favism is a disorder of young children, usually male, who suffer acute haemolysis following inhalation of the pollen or ingestion of the beans of *Vicia fava*. It has been recognised since antiquity in Greece and China, and is a serious complication of G6PD deficiency. There appears to be a familial predisposition as only some G6PD deficient children develop favism while others are unaffected. Symptoms consist of headache, dizziness, nausea, vomiting, chills, fever, pallor and lumbar pain. Haemoglobinuria appears within a few hours followed by jaundice. A typical attack lasts for 2–6 days and deaths occur within the first 48 hours.

Anaemia is usually severe in acute haemolysis and renal failure is a potential complication.

Prevention of haemolysis

There is a case for screening newborn infants of susceptible genetic origin for G6PD enzyme and to give advice about the avoidance of potentially harmful drugs, chemicals and food to those who have G6PD deficiency.

MEDICAL ADVICE AND IMMUNISATIONS FOR TRAVEL TO THE TROPICS

Protection should be given against the major diseases of childhood prevalent in the tropics and sub-tropics such as malaria, tuberculosis, poliomyelitis, tetanus, diphtheria, pertussis, measles and yellow fever.

Immunisations should be given as follows:

Vaccine	Age
BCG	Neonatal period onwards
Diphtheria/pertussis tetanus (DPT)	The first dose can be given at 2 months. Two further doses given at monthly intervals in the tropics. Booster dose at 12–18 months
Poliomyelitis	Both killed and live vaccines can be given simultaneously with DPT
Measles	9–2 months
Yellow fever	After 9 months

Smallpox vaccination is no longer mandatory for travel abroad now that the disease has been eradicated worldwide. The vaccine causes complications in children with eczema and skin eruptions. Cholera and typhoid vaccinations are not recommended for infants.

Malaria chemoprophylaxis is essential when travelling to endemic areas (see p 00).

Personal hygiene and health can be maintained by giving infants extra fluids in the tropics, boiling suspect water for drinking, avoiding bathing in infected rivers and pools and wearing shoes outside the house.

FURTHER READING

Hendrickse R G (ed) 1981 Paediatrics in the tropics: current review. Oxford University Press. Oxford
Lobo E de H 1978 Children of immigrants to Britain: their health and social problems. Hodder and Stoughton. London

26

Emergency procedures

Acute medical emergencies are common in young children and may be caused by illness or accident. In 1976 accidents and injuries caused 13 per cent of deaths in childhood, 14.6 per cent of hospital admissions in children aged 0–4 years and 20.5 per cent of hospital admissions in the 5–14-year-old age group. Ill children should be transfered to hospital but medical assistance in the home, the clinic or at the site of an accident may be life-saving.

CARDIORESPIRATORY ARREST

The child appears blue or very pale; there are no respiratory movements, the carotid and femoral pulses are not palpable and the heart sounds are inaudible. Events preceding the cardiorespiratory arrest should be determined; a history of illness, drug intake, respiratory difficulty, blood loss or accident may be helpful in management.

Management

Prompt resuscitation is vital in order to maintain cerebral circulation (Table 26.1). This is ideally carried out by a team in a hospital setting but may need to be attempted anywhere. Equipment for paediatric resuscitation is listed in Table 26.2; the basic items should be kept in all family doctors' surgeries and childrens' clinics.

Establish ventilation

Lie the child on a hard flat surface. Suck out the mouth and pharynx and insert airway. Pull the chin forwards by lifting the angle of the mandible

Table 26.1

Management of cardiorespiratory arrest

Cardiorespiratory arrest	— Lie flat — Clear airway	
Ventilation	—	Mouth-to-mouth Bag + Mask + O_2 Endotracheal intubation + IPPV + O_2
Circulation	—	External cardiac massage (4 compressions:1 breath)
I.v. infusion	—	sodium bicarbonate (8.4% 2–3 ml/kg)
ECG monitor	—	Drugs i.v. or intracardiac

Table 26.2 Equipment for management of cardiac arrest

Suction apparatus or mucus extractor
Airway
Bag and mask e.g. Ambubag, Penlon bag
Paediatric laryngoscope
Endotracheal tube with connections (sizes 3.0–7.5 mm)
Oxygen
ECG machine
Defibrillator
Intravenous cannulae sizes 18, 20, 22, FG
Paediatric infusion set
Cutdown pack
Infusion pump

and begin mouth-to-mouth ventilation; for young children use only a mouthful of air. Endotracheal intubation and positive pressure ventilation should be performed; bag and mask ventilation using oxygen or air should however be sufficient. Chest wall movements will be visible if adequate ventilation is taking place. Tracheostomy is rarely needed, but may be necessary, for example, after foreign body inhalation or severe upper airways obstruction.

Restore circulation

External cardiac massage (ECM) should begin at once with rhythmic compression of the sternum at a rate of 60–100 per minute; the faster rate is used in infants. The pressure of two fingers on the lower sternum is sufficient in young infants. A palpable femoral pulse is a sign of adequate cardiac output. The rate of ECM to artificial ventilation is 4 to 1. An intravenous infusion of dextrose/saline or plasma should be started immediately. The antecubital fossa is often the easiest site for insertion of a cannula; the jugular and scalp vein sites may interfere with the giving of artificial respiration; if a cut-down is needed the long saphenous vein at the ankle, anterior to the medial malleolus is the best site. Sodium bicarbonate (2–3 mmol/kg) is given to correct any metabolic acidaemia caused by inadequate peripheral circulation (Table 26.3); further alkali administration should be determined by blood gas status. In young children care must be taken not to give excessive volumes of fluid as this may cause circulatory overload.

If there is evidence of serious blood loss or severe dehydration then plasma (10–20 ml/kg) or blood should be given to restore blood volume.

Drugs

Drugs (Table 26.3) should be given intravenously or if necessary intracardiac, there is no place for intramuscular administration. An ECG machine should have been attached so that any arrhythmia may be identified and treatment monitored. Adrenaline and calcium gluconate are useful for asystole; if there is ventricular fibrillation a DC

Table 26.3 Drugs which may be used during resuscitation at cardiac arrest

Sodium bicarbonate 8.4%	—	2–3 ml/kg (2–3 mmol/kg)
Adrenaline 1:*10 000*	—	0.1–0.2 ml/kg (1 ml/year up to 10 ml)
Calcium gluconate 10%	—	0.1–0.2 ml/kg (1ml/year up to 10 ml)
Lignocaine	—	0.5–4 mg/kg dose (then continuous infusion at 0.5–3 mg.kgh^{-1}
Dopamine	—	5–20 µg.kgmin^{-1}

shock starting at 10 J/sec (or 2 joules/sec/kg) is given; with ventricular tachycardia lignocaine can be tried, while dopamine or isoprenaline infusions are used to maintain circulation and restore blood pressure.

PROLONGED CONVULSIONS

Convulsions, particularly those precipitated by fever, are common in childhood.

The child should be laid semi-prome to maintain a clear airway. It is not necessary to place anything between the teeth. Remember the risk of aspiration if there is vomiting.

Prolonged fits may lead to cerebral oedema and thus be self-perpetuating. Anticonvulsant treatment is therefore urgent, while tepid sponging should be given if there is a high fever.

Drug management outside hospital

Rectal diazepam or intramuscular paraldehyde are the safest and most appropriate anticonvulsant drugs. Rectal diazepam is well absorbed and can be given by a syringe without a needle in a dosage of 0.6–0.8 mg/kg. A repeat dose may be necessary. Paraldehyde (0.2 ml/kg) is given by deep intramuscular injection; although a glass syringe is often used; a plastic syringe can be used if the solution is in the syringe for only a very short while. If the convulsion does not stop the child should immediately be transferred to hospital.

Drug management in hospital

Bolus intravenous diazepam (0.3 mg/kg) can be tried; there is a danger of respiratory depression if large doses are used. Intramuscular diazepam is ineffective. If the convulsion persists a diazepam infusion (0.04 mg.kg.h^{-}) may be given. Intravenous phenytoin, phenobarbitone, chlormethiazole or induction of anaesthesia are alternatives in persistent epilepticus.

Advice for parents of children who have recurrent febrile convulsions

If the child develops a high fever but has not yet had a convulsion a tepid sponge with lukewarm water and an appropriate dose of a medicine to reduce the fever (paracetamol elixir or aspirin suppository) are used. Administration of rectal diazepam can be taught to parents and should be used if they feel there is an impending convulsion or during a convulsion. Should a fit occur the child should be laid on his side in the semi-prone position and the airway cleared, and medical attention should be sought urgently if the convulsion does not stop within 5 minutes. The general practitioner should be told about 'the fit whether or not it stops quickly.

UPPER AIRWAYS OBSTRUCTION

The common causes in childhood include laryngotracheobronchitis, croup, epiglottitis, foreign body inhalation, pharyngeal oedema due to allergy, burns or trauma and retropharyngeal abscess. The clinical features are inspiratory stridor, signs of respiratory distress, drooling and sitting forward, cyanosis, drowsiness and respiratory arrest.

In severe cases transfer to hospital is urgent; the doctor should accompany the child and give oxygen if necessary. *The throat must not be examined*, unless there is an anaesthetist and resuscitation equipment available as respiratory obstruction may be precipitated.

When obstruction is severe it must be bypassed. This should be carried out by an experienced anaesthetist or surgeon; appropriate endotracheal intubation under general anaesthesia is used but tracheostomy may be necessary. In extreme cases of emergency and when experienced staff are not available a large bore canula (size 14 Medicut) can be inserted safely into the trachea in the midline just below the thyroid cartilage.

SHOCK

This is a clinical syndrome resulting from poor tissue perfusion. Shock may become irreversible and prove fatal even though the underlying cause is corrected. Clinical features include pale, cold skin, poor capillary return, hypotension, tachycardia and tachypnoea. There is initial agitation followed by progressive confusion and coma. Causes of shock include hypovolaemia due to haemorrhage or burns, dehydration from gastroenteritis or diabetic ketoacidosis, septicaemia (from meningococcus, staphylococcus or Gram-negative organisms), meningitis, peritonitis, cardiogenic conditions (e.g. myocarditis, paroxysmal arrhythmia, cardiac tamponade), anaphylaxis, neurogenic agents (e.g. overdose of hypnotics, tranquillisers or anaesthetic agents, or spinal cord injuries), adrenocortical insufficiency (e.g. congenital adrenal hyperplasia), poisoning particularly with salicylates or iron, or respiratory disease causing profound hypoxia (e.g. epiglottitis, staphylococcal pneumonia).

Immediate treatment

1. Lie the child flat
2. Establish an airway
3. Endotracheal intubation where appropriate with intermittent positive pressure ventilation
4. Oxygen
5. Elevate the legs except when the cause is respiratory in origin
6. Start an intravenous infusion; a cut-down may be necessary, administer normal saline or plasma up to 20 ml/kg
7. Monitor the central venous pressure
8. Catheterise the bladder
9. Nurse in intensive care area
10. Treat underlying cause
11. Monitor therapy

Anaphylactic shock

This is an extreme form of allergy causing respiratory distress and circulatory collapse. The offending antigen leads to the release of histamine and related substances resulting in increased capillary permeability and bronchial constriction. Common causes include drugs (e.g. penicillin or anaesthetics), injections (e.g. desensitisation material, radiological contrast media), immunisations, incompatible blood transfusions and insect stings.

Clinical features include erythema, urticaria, itching, angioneurotic oedema, sweating, vomiting, diarrhoea, colicky abdominal pain and cough.

Bronchospasm, laryngeal oedema and cardiac arrest may follow.

Management

Remove the suspected agent. Apply a tourniquet above the local site. Adrenaline (0.01 ml/kg of 1:1000 strength to a maximum of 0.5 ml) can be given subcutaneously, together with intravenous or intramuscular antihistamine (0.25 mg/kg of chlorpheniramine or 0.5 mg/kg of promethazine).

In life-threatening situations with circulatory collapse ensure an adequate airway, give oxygen, give adrenaline intravenously (0.01 ml/kg of 1:1000, maximum 0.5 ml or 0.1 ml/kg of 1:10 000 maximum 5 ml) and give plasma expander (20 ml/kg) or saline intravenously. Aminophylline (4 mg/kg) by slow intravenous injection is used for bronchospasm, while intravenous hydrocortisone (50–100 mg) is given if there is a poor response or laryngeal oedema.

HYPOGLYCAEMIA

Hypoglycaemia is most frequently a problem in diabetic children on insulin, but may occur in salicylate, alcohol or oral hypoglycaemic poisoning. Spontaneous hypoglycaemia occurs in glycogen storage disease, ketotic hypoglycaemia, adrenocortical insufficiency, hypopituitarism, pre-diabetes or if there is excess insulin production such as by an islet cell tumour.

Hypoglycaemia is defined as a blood glucose concentration less than 2.2 mmol/l. Early symptoms include headaches, dizziness, pallor, sweating and associated irritability and mood changes; nightmares may occur. Profound hypoglycaemia causes drowsiness, coma and convulsions.

Mild attacks respond to oral glucose in the form of glucose tablet, sweets, sugar lumps or a sugary drink. All diabetics should have some form of glucose available at all times. If there is impairment of consciousness then the ideal treatment is an intravenous infusion of 10 per cent dextrose (5 ml/kg, 0.5 g/kg) as a bolus, followed by a slow infusion. Stronger glucose solutions are available, but should never exceed 20 per cent. Outside hospital, an intramuscular injection of glucagon (1 mg) should reverse hypoglycaemia.

BURNS

Burns are common in toddlers, usually as a result of of domestic accidents. The classification, clinical features and common causes of burns are shown in Tables 26.4 and 26.5. If more than 10 per cent of the body surface area is involved with second or third degree burns then shock may ensue from fluid loss.

Burns are sometimes due to non-accidental injury, but more often are related to overcrowded, disorganised or careless management of the child. Appropriate investigation of the circumstances is necessary and help given to the family.

Table 26.4 Classification of burns

Type	Skin layers involved	Features	Common causes
First degree	Superficial epidermis	Erythema Pain	Scalds Sunburn
Second degree	Entire epidermis	Erythema Pain Blistered and moist areas	Scalds Contact with hot objects
Third degree	Entire dermis including nerve endings ± underlying tissue	Dry lesion White or charred painless	Open flames Chemicals Electricity Steam

Table 26.5 Percentage surface area of different parts of the body

	surface area (per cent)		
	1 year	3 years	10 years
Head	17	15	9
Trunk	36	36	36
Both arms	16	16	18
Both legs	30	32	36
Genitalia	1	1	1

First aid measures

If there is only involvement of small areas of skin, the affected area may be immersed in cold water. It should then be covered with a sterile, but non-adhesive, dressing and bandaged. The dressing should be changed after 48 hours.

Chemical burns, particularly those involving the eye, must be thoroughly irrigated with water; clothes and all traces of the offending agent should be removed.

For all other types and more extensive burns the affected area may be immediately cooled by immersion in cold water, blisters should be left intact and clothes should not be removed. The burns should then be covered with a clean sheet and the child transferred to hospital for assessment.

Burns involving the eye or mouth, genitalia, hands and feet should receive specialist attention even when only a small area is involved.

Emergency hospital management

Maintain the airway; any burn involving the mouth or neck may produce oedema and respiratory obstruction. Emergency intubation or tracheostomy may be needed. If more than 10 per cent of the body surface is involved intravenous fluids will be required to prevent shock from fluid loss. Plasma should be given (10 ml/kg), half in the first 8 hours and the other half during the following 12 hours. Maintenance fluids should also be given. Packed cell volume, blood urea, electrolytes, blood group and urine specific gravity should be monitored serially. A urinary catheter may be needed to monitor urinary output. Some form of analgesia is usually required for the first 48 hours; intravenous pethidine (0.5 mg/kg) may be needed.

The child is barrier nursed in a warm cubicle lying on sterile towels with the burn exposed until it has dried. Antibiotics are not usually necessary unless there is evidence of secondary infection.

The parents will need help and support because of the anxiety and long-term management often required; plastic surgeons must be consulted early.

DEHYDRATION

In the UK and worldwide the commonest cause of dehydration in childhood is gastroenteritis. Dehydration may be classified as hypotonic, isotonic or hypertonic depending on the proportion of water and electrolyte lost and the blood sodium measurement. The physical signs become increasingly obvious as the severity increases (see Tables 26.6 and 26.7).

Management outside hospital

Mild gastroenteritis can be treated with oral, clear electrolyte-containing about 50 mmol sodium/l, (e.g. Dioralyte), solutions of flat Coca-Cola or lemonade. Older children who show evidence of 5 per cent dehydration may be treated at home as long as they are able to take fluid by mouth and are carefully monitored; dehydration, however, may appear rapidly in infancy, and babies with diarrhoea and vomiting may require admission to hospital even if there is no overt evidence of dehydration. Even a single diarrhoea stool can cause dehydration; it must be remembered also that liquid stool in a baby can be mistaken for urine. Hypernatraemia is a problem of the first year of life; many of the signs of dehydration appear late in the illness because of the relative preservation of the intravascular compartment. Fortunately, it is now uncommon, because of the low solute milks which are used for babies and the popularity of breast feeding.

Management in hospital

Clinical assessment; check weight against recent known weights; monitor blood electrolytes,

Table 26.6 Features of different types of dehydration

	Hypernatraemic dehydration	Isotonic dehydration	Hypotonic dehydration
Plasma Na (mmol/l)	>150	130–150	<130
Losses	Na < H_2O	Na = H_2O	Na > H_2O
Skin texture	Rubbery + thick	Reduced elasticity	Reduced elasticity
Skin colour	Grey	Grey	Grey
Anterior fontanelle	Depressed	Depressed	Very depressed
Pulse	Rapid	Rapid	Rapid
Blood pressure	Normal until late in illness	Low	Very low
Sunken eyes	Not obvious	Present	Present
Convulsions	Yes	No	$\pm$
Replace fluid deficit	slowly + steadily over 48 hours	$\frac{1}{3}$ in 4 hours, $\frac{2}{3}$ in next 16 hours	$\frac{1}{3}$ in 4–6 hours, $\frac{2}{3}$ in next 16 hours
Type of fluid	0.45% saline with 2.5% glucose not 5% dextrose	0.45% saline or 4% dextrose/ physiological saline	0.9% (normal) saline with 5% dextrose

Table 26.7

	Mild	Moderate	Severe
Degree of dehydration	5%	10%	15%
Loss (m/kg body weight)	50	100	150
Rehydration	Oral	Intravenous	Intravenous
Replacement volume	Maintenance + 50 ml/kg	Maintenance + 100 ml/kg	Plasma 20 ml/kg then maintenance + 150 ml/kg

haematocrit and urine specific gravity. Send appropriate bacteriology including blood culture.

With 10 per cent dehydration or persistent vomiting intravenous rehydration is required;

Table 26.8 Maintenance fluid requirements at different ages

Age	Volume (ml.kg24h^{-1})
1 week–6 months	150
6 months–1 year	120
1–2 years	100
2–4 years	90
4–8 years	80
8–12 years	70
Over 12 years	60

plasma (20 ml/kg) or saline should be given initially if there is evidence of shock. Rehydration is based on the extent of dehydration, type of dehydration (as indicated by blood electrolytes), age and weight, maintenance requirements (Table 26.8), and whether fluid losses continue.

POISONING

In England and Wales in 1976 there were 32 child deaths caused by the ingestion of drugs and other poisonous substances (excluding carbon monoxide); 20 per cent of hospital admissions of children under 15 years of age were due to poisoning or suspected poisoning. Accidental poisoning is common in young children (less than 4 years old) but is rare among older children of normal intelligence. Intentional drug overdose becomes more common at puberty.

Loss of consciousness or odd behaviour may be presenting symptoms and poison must always be considered in the differential diagnosis of such problems. Young children, fortunately, spill more poison than they swallow. Most deaths, however, occur in the young age group. Poisoning often occurs during periods of domestic upheaval (e.g. moving house, family illness, pregnancy), or in disorganised families where poisons are unwisely left within the reach of toddlers. All parents should be counselled about the risk of poisons when discussing childhood safety and hazards.

Management

Maintain the airway; if there is any sign of respiratory difficulty endotracheal intubation and assisted ventilation may be necessary.

The general condition of the child should be assessed with special attention to the level of consciousness, adequacy of respiration, blood pressure and other vital signs. If blood pressure is low or consciousness is impaired an intravenous infusion should be started. Local effects of corrosive poisons may be evident from burns on the mouth or skin or there may be signs of systemic effects of an ingested agent. Examples include pinpoint pupils due to barbiturates, cardiac dysrhythmias due to tricyclic antidepressants, hyperventilation due to salicylate overdosage, and dilated pupils, flushed skin and tachycardia due to atropine-like substances. The nature and time of ingestion are important clinical details. Careful enquiry into circumstances surrounding the poisoning should also be made.

Identification of the poison is important. A MIMS colour identification chart, which should be kept in all casualty departments, may give a clue. The regional poison centre should be consulted regarding contents of mixtures, toxicity of substances and also for information about treatment.

Removal of poison should be induced if the child is fully conscious and the substance is not corrosive or oily. Ipecachuana syrup (15 ml) is given with a drink and usually produces vomiting within 20 minutes. The dose may be repeated if this fails. Gastric lavage is usually reserved for children who have ingested iron-containing medicines, but may also be used when there is a large overdose of drugs. The contra-indications to gastric lavage are as with ipecachuana emesis; lavage may be carried out in an intubated child who has a cuffed endotracheal tube in situ. Haemoperfusion and dialysis may be required with certain toxic drugs (Table 26.9). Forced alkaline diuresis may be of use if phenobarbitone, barbitone or salicylates have been ingested; this should, however, be used with caution in young children because of the risk of metabolic upset. Specific antidotes (Table 26.10) may be available.

Table 26.9 Drugs which may be removed by haemodialysis and haemoperfusion

Barbiturates
Ethchlorvynol
Glutethimide
Meprobamate
Methaqualone
Salicylates
Chloral hydrate (trichlaethanol derivative)
Theophylline

Table 26.10 Specific antidotes for certain poisons

Poison	Antidote
Carbon monoxide	Oxygen
Opiate (morphine, pethidine)	Naloxone
Cyanide	Cobalt
Paracetamol	Methionine
Thallium	Prussian Blue

Hospital observation is advisable even if there are no apparent ill effects; 6-hours observation is adequate in most cases. Blood levels of drugs such as paracetamol, salicylate and barbiturates together with blood biochemistry should be estimated. If poisoning is suspected, but is not proven, urine should be sent to the local poisons centre for chromatography testing in order to confirm the diagnosis.

Poisoning with specific agents

Paracetamol

Paracetamol may cause hepatic necrosis; more than 150 mg/kg may cause severe but often reversible liver damage, over 300 mg/kg may cause irreversible liver necrosis and has a high mortality.

Clinical features include on day one, vomiting, on day one to two, abdominal pain, increased serum bilirubin, aspartate transaminase and prothrombin time, progressing to hepatic failure with jaundice, encephalopathy and acute renal failure on days two to seven.

Management. Induce emesis, give methionine, or N-acetyl cystine, give vitamin K if the prothrombin time is prolonged, treat any hepatic failure and provide supportive care. Methionine or N-acetyl cystine will prevent irreversible hepatic damage by paracetamol if given within 12 hours of ingestion. The likelihood of damage can be predicted from plasma paracetamol levels; if the plasma paracetamol level is above the line joining 200 mg/l at 4 hours and 70 mg/l at 12 hours after ingestion, then the following agents should be given over a 4 -hour period. Methionine 2.5 g orally every 4 hours to a total of 10 g, or N-acetyl cystine 150 mg/kg i.v. over 15 minutes, then 50 mg/kg in the next 4 hours, and 100 mg/kg over the following 16 hours. Intravenous glucose should be given (as 5% dextrose initially) in order to prevent hypoglycaemia. Paracetamol overdosage should not be regarded lightly.

Dextropropoxyphine

This substance is usually in a combination with paracetamol (e.g. Distalgesic). The signs are similar to those of opium poisoning, pinpoint pupils, depressed respiration and loss of consciousness. Respiratory failure may occur rapidly, naloxone (0.005–0.01 mg/kg intravenously or intramuscularly) will specifically reverse the effects. The response should be immediate.

Salicylates

Salicylate poisoning in children has become a little less common presumable due to the introduction of child-resistant tablet containers and other restrictions on packaging. Methyl salicylate or oil of wintergreen is highly dangerous; about 4 ml may be fatal for infants. The therapeutic administration of salicylate to sick children may cause poisoning because of cumulative effects. Infants are as a rule more susceptible, with the same blood level, to toxic effects than older children. A blood level greater than 30 mg/100 ml (2.2 μmol/l) suggests moderate or severe poisoning.

The clinical features include epigastric pains, nausea and vomiting, pyrexia, sweating, tremor, hyperventilation, oedema and dehydration. The laboratory data includes hyperkalaemia, hypernatraemia or hyponatraemia, respiratory alkalosis, metabolic acidosis (though not in young children), hyperglycaemia, hypoglycaemia and hypoprothrombinaemia.

Management. Up to 12 hours after ingestion induce emesis; an intravenous infusion should be started if the blood salicylate level is greater than 30 mg/dl or there are signs or symptoms as above. Blood salicylate level, electrolytes, glucose, prothrombin time and blood gases should be monitored and any electrolyte, acid-base or blood glucose imbalance treated. Vitamin K should be given. Alkaline diuresis may be used in adolescents while haemoperfusion and dialysis may be required in severe cases (salicylate level greater than 90 mg/dl, 6.6 μmol/l).

Barbiturates

These drugs cause respiratory depression, coma and hypotension. Induce emesis if the child is fully conscious; if drowsy observe in an intensive-care area, artificial ventilation may be necessary. The barbiturate blood level confirms the diagnosis. Blood biochemistry should be monitored. Forced alkaline diuresis is useful in barbitone or phenobarbitone poisoning; haemodialysis may be required in severe cases.

Phenothiazines

This group includes chlorpromazine, perphenazine, (Fentazin) and prochlorperazine (Stemetil); metoclopramide (Maxolon) is a related compound.

Clinical features include drowsiness, facial grimacing, oculogyric crisis, rigidity, tremor and hypotension.

Management is by symptomatic support; induce emesis, while dyskinesia can be treated with benztropine (Cogentin) 0.03 mg/kg i.v.

Belladonna akaloids

Atropine, deadly nightshade and lomotil are in this group. A dry mouth and skin, flushing, fever, tachycardia and dilated pupils are seen. Lomotil causes small pupils.

Management is by inducing emesis, symptomatic care and giving naloxone (0.02 mg/kg).

Tricyclic antidepressants

These drugs are now the commonest cause of death by accidental poisoning in young children; ingestion of more than 10 mg/kg will cause severe symptoms, while more than 20 mg/kg may be fatal.

The major toxic effects are on the cardiovascular (CVS) and central nervous systems (CNS). The drugs are believed to act by blocking re-uptake of noradrenaline and 5-hydroxytryptamine in neurones and by blocking the parasympathetic nervous system (PNS) and peripheral uptake of noradrenaline, plus a quinidine-like action on the heart.

The clinical features include: 1. CVS — all forms of arrhythmia plus hypotension; 2. CNS — hallucinations, convulsions, pyramidal and extra-pyramidal signs, coma; 3. PNS — dry mouth, blurred vision, dilated pupils, retention of urine, pyrexia; and 4. respiratory system — respiratory depression, apnoea.

Management. Up to 12 hours after ingestion emesis is induced if the child is fully conscious. The cardiac rhythm, blood gas status and biochemistry should be monitored. Hypoxia and acidosis (these potenteiate arrhythmias) and hypovolaemia should be treated. Dopamine is used if hypotension persists without arrhythmia; arrhythmias should be treated after correction of acidosis. Physostigmine (0.5 mg) may be given by slow intravenous infusion in prolonged coma but may cause convulsions or bradycardia.

Iron

Iron tablets are commonly eaten by toddlers when their mothers are pregnant; as few as three ferrous sulphate tablets may be fatal. Serum iron levels greater than 90 µmol/l indicate severe poisoning.

Clinical features include vomiting, gastrointestinal haemorrhage (gastric mucosal necrosis), hypotension if bleeding is severe and grey stools or melaena; after 24 hours encephalopathy (convulsions, coma), metabolic acidosis, renal failure and pulmonary oedema occur, while hepatic necrosis may develop later.

Management. Intramuscular desferrioxamine (1 g) as a chelating agent, gastric lavage with 1 per cent sodium bicarbonate solution and 5 g of oral desferrioxamine. The serum iron level should be monitored. If there are symptoms or a serum iron level greater than 90 µmol/l then intravenous infusion of desferrioxamine (15 mg/kg every 4 hours, up to 80 mg/kg total) is given. Desferrioxamine may cause hypotension if given too fast.

Lead

Lead is a common environmental contaminant; poisoning is usually an insidious processes resulting from repeated and often unsuspected exposure. In addition to clinically evident poisoning, it is now suggested that increased blood and tissue lead concentrations may be associated with behaviour disorder, lowered intelligence and minor neurological dysfunction.

Lead may be absorbed from the gut, lungs, and skin; it is bound to erythrocytes, redistributed to liver and kidney and finally excreted or is deposited in bones and teeth. Iron deficiency, common in toddlers, potentiates lead absorption from the gut.

Clinical features of lead excess include lassitude, colicky abdominal pain, constipation, pallor from anaemia and later impaired consciousness, convulsions and raised intracranial pressure. Blue lines in the gums and peripheral nerve palsies are rare. Blood lead levels are, in part, correlated with symptoms:

0–40 µg/dl   0–2 µmol/l — 'normal'
40–60 µg/dl   2–3 µmol/l — asymptomatic

60–100 µg/dl   3–5 µmol/l — symptomatic
> 100 µg/dl   >5 µmol/l — encephalopathy

Investigations may show hypochromic anaemia with normal serum iron, haemolytic anemia, aminoaciduria and glycosuria, radio-dense metaphyseal bands at growing ends of long bones and opaque material may be evident on abdominal X-ray. There may be evidence of raised intracranial pressure on skull X-ray and CT scan.

Management. The management of lead poisoning depends on symptoms: the source of lead intoxication should be identified (pica, old paint), supportive care should be given for convulsions and raised intracranial pressure, and chelating agents to lower the blood lead concentrations. The chelating agents are calcium versenate (calcium — EDTA, 1500 mg/m^2 daily i.v. or i.m.), dimercaprol (BAL, 500 mg/m^2 daily i.m.) and penicillamine (600 mg/m^2 daily orally or i.m.) As a rough guide penicillamine is adequate if the blood lead is 3–4 µmol/l, (60–80 mg/dl), calcium versenate is used if there is a higher concentration. Remember the child may be returning home to re-exposure unless the cause is identified and removed.

Poisoning with household products

These substances are generally accidentally ingested by toddlers: most are surprisingly harmless but should nevertheless be kept locked safely out of reach. The National Poisons Information Service will provide details of toxicity and management.

Bleach

Bleach is 3–6 per cent hypochlorite and causes burning sensation, vomiting and abdominal pain; it may produce pharyngeal and laryngeal oedema. Chlorine gas is produced in the stomach and may produce pulmonary oedema. Oral fluids should be encouraged if small amounts are ingested. Gastric lavage should be considered for large quantities.

Abrasive agents

These include oven cleaners (30 per cent caustic soda), kettle descaler (formic acid), dishwashing machine powders (silicates and metasilicates), drain cleaners (caustic soda or sulphuric acid), car battery acid (concentrated sulphuric acid).

All cause ulceration and necrosis of the tissues they contact. Laryngeal oedema and gastric perforation may occur. Formic acid may cause acute renal failure. *Gastric lavage and emesis are contraindicated.* Contrast radiography then endoscopy should be performed if there is evidence of serious damage and laparotomy considered. Antibiotics and steroids should be given for severe cases.

Cleaning products containing surfactants

These include carpet shampoo, dishwashing liquid, fabric conditioner, washing powder, general purpose household cleaners, scouring liquids, creams and powders.

Effects include skin irritation, vomiting and diarrhoea. Liberal fluids are given by mouth with demulcent (milk or antacid preparation).

Lavatory cleaners

These contain paradichlorobenzene which causes vomiting and diarrhoea. Purgation is necessary if more than 1 g is ingested.

Disinfectants

Disinfectants may consist of up to 40 per cent isopropyl alcohol (double the potency of ethyl alcohol). They cause local irritation, depression of respiration, drowsiness, stupor and coma; 100 ml of isopropyl alcohol can be fatal in adults. Haemodialysis can be used in severe cases.

Ethyl alcohol poisoning

Ethyl alcohol is contained in many cosmetics as well as beverages. It is rapidly absorbed through the gastric mucosa. It is a nervous system depressant and causes hypoglycaemia by inhibiting gluconeogenesis.

Blood alcohol level and glucose should be measured and emesis induced if the child is fully conscious; if drowsy, an intravenous infusion of 10 per cent dextrose should be started. The blood glucose should be monitored and corrected if required; naloxone may improve the level of consciousness, while haemodialysis and haemoperfusion may be needed in severe cases.

Paraffin poisoning

The danger here is from pulmonary aspiration and severe chemical pneumonitis. Do not induce emesis or perform gastric lavage but rather treat symptomatically.

Solvent abuse

Glue and petrol sniffing are becoming major sociological problems; it usually occurs among male teenagers but even younger children are now involved. It causes drunken behaviour and may be suspected from typical smell on clothes and unexplained mood changes. Glue sniffing has relatively few complications but can cause neurological damage and occasional deaths, while petrol sniffing causes more chronic than acute problems but may cause coma and cardiac arrhythmias.

FURTHER READING

Alpert J J, Reece R (eds) 1979 Paediatric emergencies. Paediatric Clinics of North America 26: 4

Black J A 1979 Paediatric emergencies. Butterworths, London

Grosfield J L (ed) 1975 Childhood trauma. Pediatric Clinics of North America 22: 2

Gutgesell H P, Tacher W A, Geddes L A, Davis J S, Lie J T, McNamara D G 1976 Pediatrics 58: 898

Knusden F U 1979 Rectal administration of diazepam in solution in the acute treatment of convulsions in infants and children — anticonvulsants effect and side effects. Archives of Disease in Childhood 54: 855–857

Lissauer T 1980–81 Paediatric emergencies. Hospital Update 6 and 7

McLean W 1980 Child poisoning in England and Wales. Some statistics on admissions to hospital 1964–76. Health Trends 12: 9–12

Vale J A S Meredith T J (eds) 1981 Poisoning. Update Books Ld, London

Valman H B 1979 Accident and emergency paediatrics, 2nd edn. Blackwell Scientific Publications, Oxford

27

Pharmacology and prescribing of drugs

The number of children who reach adolescence without having received any drugs must be few; over 60 per cent of children in hospital and nearly 5 per cent of all newborn babies receive drugs. There are no adequate data on the extent of paediatric prescribing by general practitioners although it is known to be considerable.

There are marked differences in the way children and adults handle drugs, but more particularly, there are also differences between children of different ages. Children are in a continuous state of development; more marked changes occur in the first few weeks and months of life. Children are not scaled down adults. Information on the way that children handle individual drugs is still limited and it is necessary to supplement what is known with adult data. This approach is less than satisfactory but without it, the basis of the present approach to prescribing in children would be too narrow. There is even less available information about the beneficial or adverse effects of drugs on children. It is clear, however, that some differences exist between children and adults.

This chapter describes the pharmacological basis for a rational approach to paediatric prescribing and therapeutics.

DRUG HANDLING PROCESSES

Absorption, distribution and elimination of the drug determine the time dependent changes in serum concentration of the drug and its metabolites. The mathematical expression of these changes is called pharmacokinetics. The study of pharmacokinetics forms the basis for rational use of dosages and frequency schedules.

Absorption

Entry into the circulation is essential for the action of most drugs and the rate and extent of absorption depends on the route of administration, the physiochemical properties of the drug, such as pKa, molecular weight and lipid solubility, and the site and area of the absorbing surfaces. If the drug is in a solid form, the rate of its disintegration and dissolution will also be important. Age-related differences in these factors are probably minimal. As far as is known, there are no functional differences between older infants, children and adults that may affect absorption from the gastrointestinal tract. Liquid preparations, however, have been traditionally used for children, often without good cause, and these tend to be absorbed at greater rates, but not to greater extents, than tablet or capsule formulations.

In the newborn, the stomach is less acid and the gastric emptying time and intestinal transit time considerably slower than at other ages. Drugs which are partially inactivated in acidic conditions, e.g. the penicillins, will tend to have greater absorption and those drugs absorbed in the stomach will have increased absorption. Most drugs are absorbed from the small intestine, and their rate of entry will be reduced by the slower gastric emptying time. The prolonged contact with the small bowel absorbing surfaces because of the long transit time, may enhance the absorption of many drugs.

Absorption from intramuscular and subcutaneous sites depends mainly on tissue perfusion; if this is adequate, there should be no differences between children of different ages. It might be expected that the apparent vasomotor instability of the newborn baby could delay absorption of drugs, but in practice this does not seem to be so.

Absorption of drugs through the skin is generally poor, although it may be slightly greater in children than adults, and is certainly increased when the skin is inflamed or broken.

The term, systemic bioavailability, describes the rate and relative amount of drug that reaches the systemic circulation from a particular dosage form. Different preparations of the same drug may vary considerably in their bioavailability and this may be an argument for proprietary drug name prescribing but the case seems to have been overstated.

Distribution

Distribution is the process which regulates the amount of drug reaching specific body compartments or tissues and therefore the concentration of drug at the receptor site. Tissue mass, fat content, membrane permeability, blood flow, and the degree of protein binding influence the extent and pattern of the process.

Most drugs are bound intracellularly, but distributed freely through body water compartments. The relative proportions of these compartments vary with age through childhood. The largest volume relative to body weight is in the first few months of life while the greatest change with age is in the extracellular compartment (Fig. 27.1).

Water-soluble drugs whose distribution is mainly confined to extracellular water, for example the penicillins, sulphonamides, cephalosporins and aminoglycosides, are affected by these changes. Water-soluble drugs require to be given in larger weight-related doses in early infancy, especially in preterm babies, to reach concentrations similar to those in older children.

The relative body fat content is lowest in the newborn especially in preterm and small-for-dates babies. The subcutaneous fat mass increases to a maximum at 9 months, subsequently decreasing towards 6 years, and later increasing again towards adolescence; there are, however, marked differences within similar age ranges. Very lipid-soluble drugs such as thiopentone and other inhalational anaesthetic agents, accumulate preferentially in fat tissue, including the brain. Changes in relative body fat affect the concentration, and therefore the activity, of these agents.

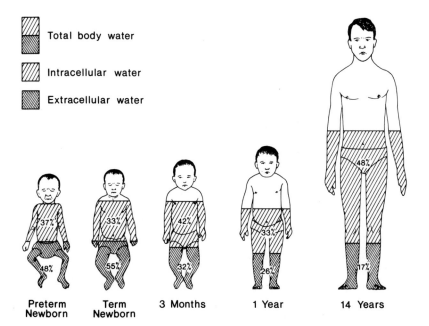

Total body water

Intracellular water

Extracellular water

Preterm Newborn — Term Newborn — 3 Months — 1 Year — 14 Years

Fig. 27.1 Body fluid compartment proportions

The passage of drugs across biological membranes is an important part of the distribution process. The blood-brain barrier is more permeable in the newborn period when an increased passage of drugs into the cerebrospinal fluid is likely. Some drugs reach particularly high concentrations in specific tissues, for example, digoxin in cardiac muscle.

The degree of extracellular binding of drugs to plasma proteins, especially albumin, determines the amount of the pharmacologically active fraction (unbound) of each drug. The reduction in protein binding in the newborn, compared with older children and adults, results mainly from their low and qualitatively different plasma albumin, and is further modified by the displacement of drugs because of the higher free fatty acid and bilirubin concentrations. Drug protein binding is lower in the newborn and perhaps infancy, but after one year of age is similar to adults. Lower protein binding has been shown in the newborn for a number of drugs including phenobarbitone, phenytoin, salicylates, sulphonamides, diazoxide, phenylbutazone and ampicillin. It is not easy to predict the net effect of this increase in the pharmacologically-active free fraction. There is more free drug available to receptor sites and therefore more activity, but there is also more available for metabolite breakdown and excretion.

Drug distribution is expressed in kinetic terms as an apparent volume of distribution (Vd). This describes, theoretically the volume of fluid into which the drug appears to be distributed in a concentration equal to that in plasma and therefore indicates the extent to which the drug passes from the vascular space into peripheral tissues. Its usefulness lies in that the dosage requirement (D) to produce a desired plasma concentration (C) can be calculated using the expression: $D = Vd \times C$ provided that the drug is totally absorbed or given intravenously.

Apparent volumes of drug distribution in children are greatest in the newborn period and reduce progressively throughout childhood, most rapidly in the first year of life, but remain relatively greater than adult values. This presumably reflects the age-dependent variation in the extracellular fluid compartment (Fig. 27.1) which forms part or whole of the distribution volume.

Elimination

Elimination is the process by which the drug is removed from the body. It is effected by either metabolism or excretion of the parent drug. The rates of drug elimination vary greatly with age throughout childhood.

Metabolism

The rate of drug metabolism probably depends on liver size and the metabolising ability of the appropriate microsomal enzyme system. Liver volume per unit body weight is twice as great in the newborn period than in the early teenage years and the relative volume seems to decrease steadily throughout childhood. Little is known about the effects of age on the microsomal enzyme system but, in the newborn period and early infant, it is certainly immature. The deficiency in glucuronidation causing physiological jaundice in the newborn is perhaps the best example of this immaturity. It is also responsible for the cardiorespiratory collapse (grey baby syndrome) seen in preterm newborn babies given similar weight-related doses of chloramphenicol to those used in older children. Pharmacokinetic differences between immature, more mature babies and infants explain this toxic effect. A decreased rate of glucuronidation has also been shown for salicylates and nalidixic acid in newborns. There is a similar decrease in the rate of oxidation of paracetamol, phenylbutazone, phenobarbitone, phenytoin and diazepam in the first few weeks of life. These two processes increase in efficiency during the first year of life, reaching and sometimes overtaking adult levels (Fig. 27.2). Some processes, e.g. demethylation and sulphation, proceed at adult rates from birth.

Liver size and the degree of enzyme system immaturity probably determine drug metabolising rates in early infancy and thus the result and effect are not predictable. Some drug metabolic processes in later infancy and childhood proceed at greater rates than those in adults and faster clearance rates in children have been reported for many drugs including carbamazepine, diazepam, phenobarbitone, sodium valproate, theophylline, and diazoxide. As the enzyme system ability

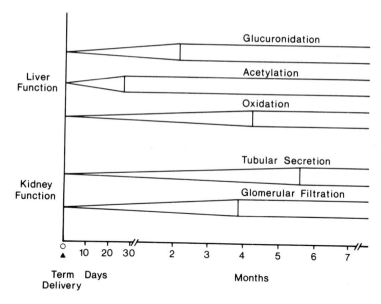

Fig. 27.2 Age-dependent maturity of drug elimination mechanisms

in children is similar to that in adults, it seems likely that the faster rates of metabolism of these drugs is due to the relatively greater liver volumes in children.

Some drugs are extracted and metabolised by the liver and intestinal wall during the first circulation of the drug through these organs. This effect reduces the systemic bioavailability of drugs such as terbutaline, propranolol, methyldopa, pentazocine and imipramine.

Excretion

Most drugs are ultimately eliminated via the kidney, and age-dependent developmental changes in glomerular filtration and tubular secretion are therefore important. Glomerular filtration rates reach adult values, corrected for surface area, between 3 and 5 months of age. Digoxin, gentamicin and tobramycin are excreted by this process and their elimination is therefore slower in the newborn and early infancy periods compared with later infancy and childhood. Tubular secretion reaches adult values (per unit surface area) between 5 and 7 months. The penicillins are excreted in this way and their elimination is therefore slower in the first few months of life.

The rate of drug elimination is best described by the concept of total body clearance which is a measure of the apparent volume from which drug is removed in a given time; this determines dosage requirements. A more convenient expression of the rate of elimination is the drug half-life which is the time over which the concentration of a drug in plasma is reduced by half. It is dependent on both the clearance and the volume of distribution and has important implications for dose-frequency. Compared with adults, the half-lives of most drugs are considerably longer, while their clearance rates are markedly slower in the newborn period and early infancy. In later infancy and throughtout childhood, the situation for most drugs is reversed with faster clearance rates and shorter half-lives than in adolescence and adulthood.

PHARMACODYNAMICS

Pharmacodynamics is the measurement of what the drug does to the body. It includes the mechanism of drug action and the relationship between drug effect and the dosage or plasma concentration. Pharmacodynamics of most drugs may be similar in adults and children, but this cannot be always assumed and well known paradoxical effects do occur, for example phenobarbitone tends to excite in children and sedate in adults, whereas amphetamines tend to produce almost the reverse effect.

ADVERSE REACTIONS

These are the undesirable effects of drugs or their metabolites and often represent extensions of the usual pharmacological effects, for example the anticholinergic effect of atropine which increases the heart rate, may also cause dryness of the mouth and blurred vision. Adverse effects may also arise because of dose-related toxicity, idiosyncratic reactions, or allergic effects. Deafness due to toxic concentrations of gentamicin is an example of dose-related toxicity. Malignant hyperpyrexia with suxamethonium is a genetically-determined

abnormal reaction and is therefore idiosyncratic. Penicillin anaphylaxis and the many skin rashes which directly follow the use of drugs are examples of allergic effects which arise from disturbances of the normal immunological response.

The incidence of all adverse effects is considerable and occurs in approximately 10–15 per cent of all drug-exposed children. The incidence in newborn babies is significantly greater (25 per cent) and may reflect dose-related toxicity problems arising from slower drug elimination rates. As there is likely to be under reporting of adverse reactions in the newborn because they tend to exhibit similar responses to a variety of insults and, therefore, may not be thought to be related to drug therapy, this figure may be higher. Adverse reactions in older children may also be under reported but for different reasons. Few

Table 27.1 The most frequently observed drug reactions and the likely causes in infants and children outside the newborn period

System	Effect	Drug
Gastrointestinal	Nausea and vomiting	Most drugs
	Diarrhoea	Ampicillin
	Monilial infection	Ampicillin
	Stained teeth	Tetracycline
	Hypersalivation	Clonazepam
Haematological	Bone marrow depression	Chloramphenicol
		Cytotoxics
	Megaloblastic anaemia	Co-trimoxazole
		Phenytoin
Cutaneous	Maculo-papular	Ampicillin
	rash	Phenytoin
	Urticaria	Penicillin
	Alopecia	Sodium valproate
		Cytotoxics
Neurological	Nystagmus	Carbamazepine
		Phenytoin
	Drowsiness	Phenobarbitone
		Clonazepam
		Carbamazepine
	Ataxia	Phenytoin
		Carbamazepine
	Dyskinesia	Metoclopramide
		Prochlorperazine
	Hyperkinesis	Phenobarbitone
Metabolic	Hyperkalaemia	Frusemide
	Hyperglycaemia	Prednisolone
		Thiazides
	Cushingoid syndrome	Corticosteroids
	Short stature	Corticosteroids
Cardiovascular	Bradycardia	Digoxin
	Hypertension	Prednisolone

parents are made aware of the likelihood or possible nature of reactions and they may not then recognise them as related to drug therapy, but rather attribute them to problems of the underlying disease. The most frequently observed adverse drug reactions in children, the systems involved and the drugs are shown in Table 27.1.

DRUG INTERACTIONS

Drug interactions can occur with food and with other drugs. The presence of food generally delays gastric emptying; this tends not to affect the total amount of drug absorbed but may reduce the rate of absorption. However, for a small number of drugs, for example, erythromycin, rifampicin, isoniazid and penicillins, food reduces to a small extent, the total amount absorbed. The absorption of nitrofurantoin is increased by food, and this with the tendency to produce gastric upset, provides ample reason for only administering the drug with or after meals. Drug interactions unrelated to food occur less commonly but are generally more important.

Pharmacodynamic interactions occur between drugs which compete for the same receptor site or which act on the same system. They may also occur when one drug induces disease or a change in fluid and electrolyte balance, which then alters the response to another drug, for example thiazide-induced hypokalaemia increases the possibility of digoxin toxicity.

Pharmacokinetic interactions occur by three main mechanisms:
1. Induction of the hepatic microsomal enzyme system by one drug may increase the rate of elimination of another. This is the basis of most anticonvulsant drug interactions. Carbamazepine, phenobarbitone and rifampicin are examples of potent enzyme-inducing agents. The net effect of induced enzyme activity is to reduce the blood levels of concurrently used drugs. Changes in the doses of the initial drug may be required if these enzyme-inducing drugs are added to existing drug regimens and conversely when they are withdrawn.
2. Inhibition of liver enzyme activity usually causes an increase in the drug level of a simultaneously administered drug and therefore an increase in its effect, for example chloramphenicol increases the anticonvulsant effect of phenytoin
3. Displacement of one drug from its protein-binding sites by another drug may cause a greater activity of the displaced drug by an increase in its free fraction, for example an increase in the effect of phenytoin when aspirin is used concurrently.

Of the more common interacting drugs, warfarin and the oral hypoglycaemics are infrequently used in children, and the majority of known interactions will involve the use of anticonvulsant drugs.

DRUG LEVEL MONITORING

Drug concentrations are usually interpreted in relation to a known therapeutic range which, for most drugs, is the concentration range where there is an optimal therapeutic effect with no undue adverse effects. The monitoring of drug levels is important in childhood for several reasons: individual variation in drug response is greater than at other ages; the titration of dose to a therapeutic response is an unsuitable means for most of the commonly prescribed drugs (antimicrobials, anticonvulsants, anti-inflammatory agents); and the difference between a toxic and sub-therapeutic dose (therapeutic index) appears to be narrower in the young. At the present time, however, few reported therapeutic ranges exist for children. Further work is needed; where appropriate, the dose may be monitored with plasma levels and with a small number of drugs using salivary levels. A good case can be made for routine plasma monitoring of the drugs listed in Table 27.2, especially chloramphenicol, gentamicin and tobramycin.

THERAPEUTIC CONSIDERATIONS IN CHILDREN

Is a drug required?

This can be a difficult question, only the patient's doctor can make this decision and it is easy for

Table 27.2 Plasma therapeutic ranges in children

Drug	Therapeutic range (μmol/l unless stated)
Carbamazepine	16–50
Chloramphenicol	15–25 mg/l
Ethosuximide	280–700
Gentamicin	
peak (15 minutes post i.v. dose)	4–12 mg/l
peak (60 minutes post i.m. dose)	
trough (pre-dose)	<2 mg/l
Phenobarbitone	40–105
Phenytoin	20–100
Salicylate	1000–2000
Theophylline	
asthma	55–110
preterm apnea	30–70
Tobramycin	4–12 mg/l

non-involved personnel or those commenting in retrospect, to doubt the wisdom of the use of a particular drug. It is likely however, that drug use in paediatrics could be considerably reduced by a more rational approach than exists, for example, the routine use of antibacterial therapy in upper respiratory tract infection is unnecessary and it is difficult to justify the widespread use of oral and nasal decongestants in this condition. The efficacy of oral anti-emetic drugs in children is doubtful, although intramuscular and rectal preparations may be useful. Drug therapy for diarrhoea in the young child is not to be recommended; the appropriate approach is to withdraw food while substituting a suitable fluid and electolyte solution. Widespread use of aspirin and paracetamol for fevers is not necessarily beneficial to the child, and the use of tricyclic antidepressants for nocturnal enuresis, which is self-limiting, is arguable because of the problems of accidental overdose, or of accidental ingestion by siblings. Children who sleep little and are frequently, but falsely, labelled hyperactive are inappropriately and mostly unsuccessfully given sedatives. The benefits of withholding drug therapy should be carefully considered and, however strong the parental pressure for treatment, it should be resisted if there is no likely advantage.

Prophylaxis

Drugs may be used to prevent disease and below are listed the major indications and most useful drugs as prophylaxis for:

1. Recurrent urinary tract infections — co-trimoxazole, trimethoprim nitrofurantoin
2. Contacts of meningococcal disease — rifampicin
3. Further rheumatic fever — phenoxymethyl penicillin
4. In post-splenctomy children and those with sickle cell disease — phenoxymethyl penicillin to prevent infection with pneumococci
5. For the unvaccinated child after contact with pertussis — erythromycin
6. Bacterial endocarditis in children with a known valve lesion during dental procedures, bladder catheterisation and other procedures likely to result in bacteraemia — phenoxy-methyl, penicillin, cloxacilin, gentamicin
7. The newborn baby exposed to tuberculosis — isoniazid-resistant BCG and isoniazid therapy

Choice of drug

As in adult practice one should prescribe the minimum number of drugs to limit adverse effects and interactions, and aid patient compliance. The chosen drug should be one of low cost, low toxicity, high therapeutic ratio, with available kinetic information in children, and one which can be given easily. If no stronger choices exist, drugs with established therapeutic ranges, such as theophylline and phenytoin, should be used preferentially. The use of antibacterial therapy is governed by considerations such as the likely or known casual organism. For example, in acute otitis media, the most likely organism varies with the age of the child, if under 5 years, it is *Haemophilus influenzae*, whereas over 5 years it is *Streptococcus pneumoniae*, and the antibiotic can then be chosen accordingly. The risks to young siblings if drugs such as tricyclics and opiates are accidentally ingested should also be considered. Some drugs should, if possible, never be used in children for example, tetracycline, which causes tooth staining and inhibition of bone growth.

Choice of route and formulation

The objective of any therapeutic approach is to achieve an effective drug concentration at the expected site of action as quickly and conveniently as possible. This can usually be achieved by the oral route, although the parenteral route is more appropriate for children who are vomiting or gravely ill, for those in whom compliance is uncertain, or where drugs are poorly absorbed from the gastrointestinal tract.

In the younger child, liquid oral preparations are generally preferred, although even young children can usually manage to swallow tablets or capsules, which have advantages, provided they have appropriate parental encouragement. The longer shelf-life of tablets and capsules lengthens the time necessary between prescription renewal which may mean better compliance and less danger of sudden withdrawal problems which occur with anticonvulsants, should prescriptions not be replenished on time. Most liquid preparations are absorbed more rapidly than capsules or tablets, although in practice, this is not important otherwise the parenteral route should be chosen. The more rapid absorption of liquids may, however, increase the fluctuation in plasma drug concentrations which normally occurs between doses, and may lead to a greater tendency for adverse reactions or subtherapeutic levels.

It is now accepted that with chronic administration, sucrose-based liquid medicines cause dental caries and ginigivitis and their use should be discouraged. Information on the base of each liquid drug should be available from regional drug information centres or pharmacies. Phenytoin suspension is a good example of a preparation requiring vigorous shaking prior to administration as the drug tends to settle towards the bottom of the bottle.

Rectal administration is frequently unpleasant for the child and parents, and it cannot be relied upon to produce adequate blood levels of some drugs, for example theophylline, without risk of dangerous toxicity. This route, however, can be useful in children who are convulsing or those about to receive cytotoxic therapy. Anyone who has tried to give diazepam intravenously to a convulsing child will realise the difficulties, and appreciate the place of rectal administration; diazepam solution can be introduced into the child's rectum using a syringe with a plastic tube attached to a nozzle, or by a proprietary rectal tube. Parents can be taught this way to arrest what might have otherwise been a long-lasting convulsion. Prochlorperazine suppositories given before cytotoxic therapy can prevent subsequent vomiting.

The topical application of drugs has only limited therapeutic possibilities other than in the treatment of skin conditions. The enhanced absorption of topical steroids in young infants with the inflamed or broken skin of relatively mild napkin rashes may lead to Cushingoid facies and, more worrying, adrenal insufficiency and retarded growth.

Parenteral therapy is indicated in the ill or vomiting child and the intravenous route is generally the most convenient and least painful, particularly if repeated administration is necessary. Poor peripheral circulation and small muscle mass in the newborn baby makes the intramuscular route unreliable and, in ill babies, intravenous therapy is essential.

Inhalation of some drugs can be useful. Administering salbutamol by this route produces a considerably greater effect than when the drug is given orally. This may be because of a significant first pass metabolism in the gut wall or liver reducing the amount of drug reaching the systemic circulation.

Dosage problems

Dose size

There are many formulae which have been devised to aid calculations of dosage for children. Most involve fractioning the adult doses but those based on age or weight are not always appropriate for all children. After a single dose, the drug concentration in blood or other body tissue depends on the dosage size, route of administration and the apparent volume of distribution. Similar weight-related doses will produce lower blood concentrations in the newborn compared with older children because of their relatively large apparent volumes of distribution. When the dose, however, is related to surface area, then similar dosage is required to produce similar drug levels. Since, for most drugs, volumes of distribution relate to water compartments which are more related to body surface area than weight, surface area related dosage ought to be more useful in children,

although this considers only the kinetics after a single dose and does not take into account potential dynamic differences between children and adults such as tissue responsiveness. It is not practical because of the need to assess two parameters, height and weight, in order to determine surface area and because of the need to state and remember doses to more than one decimal place.

In most circumstances, children require multiple doses and then the steady-state plasma concentration of the drug depends on the systemic clearance (reflecting the sum of all eliminating processes) and the rate of replenishment. The plasma half-life is not important in determining the eventual steady-state concentration of the drug, but is critical to the time taken to reach the mean steady-state level which approximates five half-lives of the drug (Fig. 27.3). The half-lives of most drugs in the newborn period tend to be longer than at any other time in childhood, frequently longer than in adults, and perhaps similar to those in the elderly. This reflects the greater apparent volume of distribution and the slower clearance rate as a result of immature microsomal enzymes and reduced renal elimin-

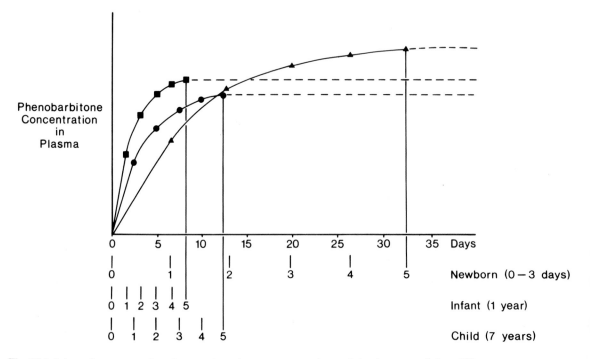

Fig. 27.3 Schematic representation of eventual steady-state concentration and the time to reach it at different ages

ation mechanisms. The clearance rates of drugs later in infancy and in childhood tend to be greater than in adults and as apparent volumes of distribution are only slightly larger at this age, half-lives of drugs tend to be considerably shorter than in adults or the newborn. The time taken to reach a mean steady-state concentration therefore differs in these ages. Figure 27.3 illustrates a schematic representation of the accumulation of phenobarbitone in different ages after administering the same weight-related dose at intervals approximating the half-life; the mean concentration is shown and the variation in mean steady-state concentration reflects to some extent the difference in apparent volumes of distribution. The difference in times to reach this concentration, has obvious implications for the time of assessment of drug therapy either clinically or by measuring drug plasma level.

Dose frequency

Drugs are usually administered at intervals which approximate to their elimination half-lives, limiting fluctuation between doses unless the absorption phase is short. Half-lives of most drugs in babies and children are such that longer intervals are required between doses in the newborn,

and considerably shorter intervals between doses in later infancy and early childhood compared with those required for adults. If these drugs are given at the same frequency to older infants and children as to adults, large fluctuations in drug concentration between doses occur with the increased risk of adverse effects or decrease in efficacy.

Many commonly used drugs in children have relatively short half-lives for example theophylline, which is less than 6 hours. If three or more equal dose and time intervals are planned, it is not possible to administer these drugs according to the principles outlines. A relatively long sleep period and the rigidity of the school system mean that children have a shorter day during which drugs may be given, and dose intervals of 4, 8 and 12 (or 8, 4 and 12 hours) punctuating school and sleep are required if drugs are to be given three times a day (Fig. 27.4). It is usual to compromise by using a less frequent dose regimen or unequal dose interval pattern; this leads to increased variability of plasma drug concentration. Sustained release preparations may help in reducing the concentration fluctuation but relatively few are available.

The effects on dose and dose-frequency of the differences in apparent volumes of distribution and clearance rates of drugs between individuals of different age means that the average weight-

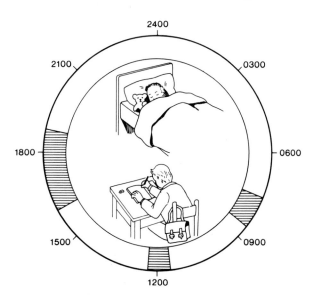

Fig. 27.4 Practical dosing times

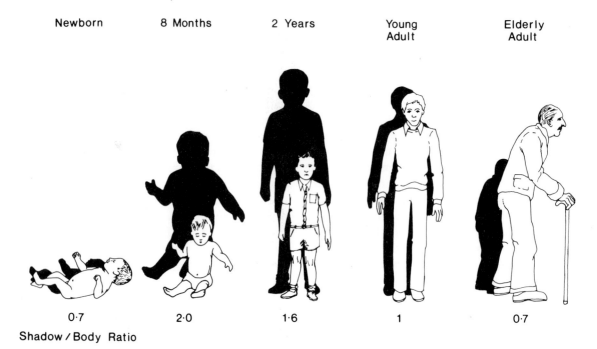

Newborn	8 Months	2 Years	Young Adult	Elderly Adult
0·7	2·0	1·6	1	0·7

Shadow / Body Ratio

Fig. 27.5 Differences in appropriate weight-related doses of most drugs (shadow indicates relative dose)

related daily drug dose for the newborn is lower than that for the normal young adult and perhaps similar to that required for the elderly adult. The dose needed by the infant is considerably greater, but this progressively decreases towards adolescence when similar adult weight-related doses are appropriate (Fig. 27.5).

MODIFICATION OF DOSE REGIMENS ACCORDING TO PHYSIOLOGICAL AND PATHOLOGICAL STATES

There are little data on the effects of normal physiology and disease states on drug handling and response by children. It should not be assumed that similar concepts of such data apply to children and adults. What are the likely and known considerations for paediatric therapeutics?

Renal insufficiency

In this situation, the dose of a drug which is partially or totally eliminated by the kidney should be reduced to some extent either by decreasing the amount given at each dose interval, by lengthening the dose interval, or by changing both. Relative to older infants, children and adults, the newborn baby exhibits a 'physiological' renal insufficiency with respect to drug clearance. Appropriate consideration is especially necessary for gentamicin and digoxin. Renal toxicity due to gentamicin therapy has been reported when trough levels exceed 2 µg/ml. In the newborn, it may be difficult to avoid exceeding this level while at the same time achieving adequate peak levels without extending the recognised 12-hour dose interval. The times during which the minimum inhibitory concentration (MIC) of the organism is exceeded during the therapy course will therefore be less than in older children and adults. In children with renal failure similar considerations as with adults apply.

Liver disease

The effects of liver disease on drug elimination in children are not easily quantified. There may be reduced hepatic blood flow, impaired hepatocellular function and reduced protein binding. The clearance of drugs with a high hepatic extraction ratio and which tend to be removed on 'first pass' through the liver should be reduced in situations such as congestive heart failure and cirrhosis. The clearance of drugs which have a low hepatic extraction ratio and a low affinity for plasma protein depends on the degree of heptocellular function. These drugs will be cleared less rapidly in hepatitis, but also in the newborn, especially preterm babies, when there is immaturity of the microsomal enzymes. Lower or less frequent doses of theophylline and chloramphenicol are necessary at this age. Impaired glucuronidation of paracetamol is compensated for by a relative increase in sulphation in early infancy.

In drugs which are highly protein bound, such as phenytoin, decrease in protein binding as a result of a quantitative reduction of proteins in nephrotic syndrome, or a relative decrease as in a term or preterm neonate, may cause a small absolute change in free drug which represents a large percentage change in drug activity. The increase in free unbound drug, however, leads to an increase in clearance, and the overall effect is unpredictable. The inability of the newborn to clear this increased fraction has implications for dosage at this age.

More importantly, hyperbilirubinaemia resulting from the immaturity of the glucuronyl transferase system in the newborn, and its relationship to drugs and protein-binding requires consideration. The problems of using sulphonomides or salicylates at this vulnerable period with possible displacement of albumin-bound bilirubin with subsequent brain damage are well recognised, but other drugs may displace bilirubin from its complex with albumin in vitro, for example frusemide, ethacrynic acid and indomethacin, and some preparations of gentamicin. Of equal importance is the fact that hyperbilirubinaemia may influence drug protein-binding by displacement and subsequently increase the free and pharmacologically active fraction of the drug.

Gastrointestinal disease

The absorption of drugs in children with alimentary tract disease is variable and unpredictable. For most drugs studied, absorption seems to be unimpaired in acute enteritis, coeliac disease and cystic fibrosis.

Fever

This is a common symptom in childhood, but although the rate of hepatic metabolism seems to decrease in fever, little information is available for children.

Duration of therapy

Therapy is usually given for similar periods in both children and adults for most acute conditions. Developmental changes in the young, however, influence the duration of therapy for some chronic conditions. The most notable example of this difference is the developmental change in the brain which allows cessation of anticonvulsant drug therapy about 2 years after the last of a series of epileptic convulsions in the child.

Compliance

This is the ability of individuals to take drugs as prescribed, to take the right drug in the right dose at the right time and for the right length of time. The degree of compliance in the young largely reflects parental attitudes. Most children are dependent on their parents for drug administration, or they adopt their behaviour and attitude towards therapy. Poor compliance should always be considered if the response to drugs is inadequate or if adverse reactions occur. It can be improved by using the minimum number of drugs, simplifying drug regimens and using appropriate dosage times, carefully monitoring progress to reduce adverse effects, and by giving a full and adequate explanation of the realistic aims and possible drawbacks of the therapy.

PRESCRIBING IN CHILDHOOD

Drug doses are expressed, for convenience, on a body weight basis while recognising the disadvantage of this approach. The dose suggested (Appendix 2) refers to the total daily dose which should then be divided according to the suggested number of doses per day. The dosage guidelines are based upon data from kinetic and clinical studies and empirical use, and cannot be assumed to be totally appropriate for all children.

Prescriptions should be clearly written using approved abbreviations. In general, single drugs should be prescribed and the approved name should be used wherever possible. If a particular brand is required, it should be stated thus: Diazepam — 'Valium brand' only.

The drug name should be printed in block letters. Metric doses must be used and, wherever possible, decimal points should be avoided. The approved abbreviation of gramme is g, of milligramme is mg and of microgram µg, even so it is advisable for micrograms to be written in full. Except for compound formulations, substitutes for dose weights, for example Caps, Tabs, Vials, should be avoided.

Abbreviations such as 'prn' and 'sos' should not be used. The symptom or sign to be relieved must be written in prescribing instructions of this nature and the maximum frequence of administration should be clearly stated, e.g. 'As required for headache — maximum 4 hourly'. Only the following routes of administration should be abbreviated:

Intravenous	— IV	Intradermal	— ID
Intramuscular	— IM	Per rectum	— PR
Topical	— TOP	Subcutaneous	— SC
Inhalation	— INHAL	Intrathecal	— IT

Oral and other routes of administration should be written in full. All prescriptions should bear the full signature of the prescriber and, in hospital practice, this should be repeated when drugs are discontinued.

A choice of route, for example oral i.m./i.v. should never be offered and no amendment to dose or dose frequency should be made to any existing prescription. In both cases, a change means that the prescription must be rewritten.

Although it has been recommended that liquid drug doses should be supplied in 5 ml volumes, it may be necessary because of stability and palatability, to prescribe the required dose and for the pharmacist to decide on the appropriate volume.

Prescriptions for controlled drugs must state the name and address of the patient, dosage and total number of doses written in both figures and letters, and the frequency of administration.

FURTHER READING

Bochner F, Carruthers G, Kampmann J & Steiner J (eds) 1978 Handbook of clinical pharmacology. Little, Brown and Company (Inc), Boston

Mirkin B L (ed) 1978 Clinical pharmacology and therapeutics. A pediatric perspective. Year Book Medical Publishers Inc, Chicago.

Rylance G W & Moreland T A 1980 Drug level monitoring in paediatric practice. Archives of Disease in Childhood 55: 89–98

Shirkey H C 1980 Paediatric clinical pharmacology and therapeutics. In: Avery G S (ed) Drug Treatment, 2nd edn. Adis Press, Sydney ch 4, p 97

28

The dying child

A dying child has two main needs: to be relieved of distress and to be understood. In response, members of the caring team must know when to substitute palliative for active treatment and learn the likely level of the child's understanding. Inclusion of the parents is vital.

PALLIATIVE TREATMENT: SYMPTOM CONTROL

If the threat of death comes suddenly, active intervention is likely to continue almost to the end. Even so, parents must be allowed access and involvement. If the child is dying of an illness known to be fatal, much suffering to both child and family will result from a doctor's inability to give up striving for cure instead of concentrating on comfort. When the course of the illness is clearly downhill, the prescription chart should be reviewed with a check-list of symptoms. Treatment designed for cure, such as cytotoxic therapy, may stop, and drugs for symptomatic relief take over.

Common symptoms in terminal illness are pain or dyspnoea, nausea and vomiting. All these can be kept away if the principle of *round-the-clock* medication is followed together with the recognition that severe symptoms warrant potent drugs, including opiates. Drug cocktails are to be avoided, as each symptom must be titrated against its own appropriate treatment to achieve control. The commonest error in terminal care is to prescribe *as required*. This produces a pattern of acute distress followed by oblivion. The aim is rather to keep the child enjoying what remains of life with as clear a mind as possible. Sensitive vigilance is required.

Anxiety will be reduced as distressing symptoms are controlled. Diverting play helps to pre-occupy both patient and parents, yet may give an opportunity for hidden anxieies to surface. Daily blood tests or the nuisance of a drip are unnecessary worries for a terminally-ill child. Thirst is usually satisfied by drinks or ice chips and parents are freer to hold a child who has no intravenous line.

THE CHILD'S LEVEL OF UNDERSTANDING

Proper medical care involves undestanding personal needs as well as prescribing drugs. Parents may need anticipatory guidance as to how to inform or answer their dying child and his siblings. Those working with them should be able to explain how a child's mind works. Just as there are normal sequences for locomotor development or physical growth, so there are recognisable stages in conceptual development before adult thinking is achieved. Young children may quietly accept facts whose implications greatly upset older minds, but which are beyond their present ability to comprehend. They are also likely to misinterpret statements with a double meaning.

A child of less than 2 years is egocentric, regarding medical procedures entirely as personal attacks during which close parental support is needed. A normal child of under 6–7 years old still takes things at face value. Thus, a 4-year-old child took fright at the offer to 'show him his bones after the X-ray' and adamantly refused to be X-rayed at all. Fears are of pain and isolation rather than to do with dying. Under-fives frequently regard death as a reversible process, although experience will hasten conceptual understanding regardless of age. The illness and death of another patient may thus heighten a child's insight into his own relapsing illness, so that even a 4-year-old may recognise that he is dying. Parents should be warned that trust depends on truth. Because in a child's terms time has little meaning, awkward questions may be satisfied by giving an immediate rather than a longterm answer. 'It's not going to happen today and we won't leave you', may well be sufficiently reassuring. Children who confidently expect a personal welcome to Heaven comfort their care-givers as well as themselves.

By early teens the ability to reason in abstract terms has developed and there is a much greater awareness of the implications of death. Reactions of denial, rage or depression may be evident and the dying teenager may deliberately thwart attempts at communication. There may be fears now about the mode of dying which remain unexpressed, sometimes for fear of adding to the parents' grief. To help bring openness between such family members is a painful process, requiring tact and time, but when it can be achieved the tranquillity of having come to terms with what is happening brings real consolation.

FAMILY AND TEAM SUPPORT

When adequate support is available, thought should be given as to whether the child should be allowed to die at home. This may bring advantages to other children in the family whose sorrows are often overlooked in the hospital setting. Their needs should be included in bereavement counselling offered to the parents afterwards.

Staff as well as parents find the care of a dying child emotionally taxing and all have their own special needs. Strength may be gained from contact with the hospital chaplain, a psychiatrist or simply others who have passed this way before.

Suffering shared and accepted can be a growing point towards maturity, and many parents and professionals have discovered the paradox that to be with a child facing death has been an experience of enrichment as well as of loss.

FURTHER READING

Bluebond-Langner M 1978 The private worlds of dying children. Princeton University Press, Princeton

Chapman J A & Goodall J 1980 Helping a child to live whilst dying. Lancet 1: 753–756

Chapman J A & Goodall, J 1980 Symptom control in ill and dying children. Journal of Maternal and Child Health 5: 144–154

Cotton G et al 1981 A brother dies at home. Journal of Maternal and Child Health 6: 288–292

Donaldson M 1978 Children's minds. Fontana/Collins, Glasgow

Easson W M 1968 Care of the young patient who is dying. Journal of the American Medical Association 205: 203–207

Friedman S B 1967 Care of the family of a child with cancer. Paediatrics 40: 498–504

Green M 1967 Care of the dying child. Paediatrics 40: 492–503

Kubler-Ross E 1969 On death and dying. Macmillan, New York

Piaget J 1926 The language and thought of the child. Routledge and Keegan Paul, London

Rothenburg M B 1967 Reactions of those who treat children with cancer. Paediatrics 40: 507–510

Saunders C M 1978 Management of terminal diseases. Edward Arnold, London

Zorza R & Zorza V 1980 A way to die: living to the end. Andre Deutsch, London

29

Examination technique

TAKING THE EXAMINATION

The hints in this section would apply to most examinations but are based on personal knowledge of the DCH both as a candidate and as an examiner.

There is no substitute for careful preparation, in both theory and practice. A candidate must read as much as possible about all aspects of the subject, but it is very important not to become obsessed with the minutiae of rare illnesses. For the DCH, one should know about the care of well children and the problems of those with chronic handicap in addition to acute illnesses.

An examination like the DCH cannot be taken with book knowledge alone. An examining board may not require a candidate to have had a clinical post in paediatrics or there may not be a clinical part to the examination. This does not mean that a candidate should take the exam without having spent some time in the clinical practice of childhood. It would be unwise to sit for the examination without at least 6 months' preparation — a year would be better. It is particularly important to read fairly extensively about the problems of the children you have seen in clinical practice. This is usually the best way of learning, since the information gained from books and colleagues will allow one to manage that child's problems, help to manage the next one with a similar illness, and stand one in good stead for the examination. One should never forget that prevention is the best form of cure and therefore should think how the disease might have been prevented in the patient or how it might have been discovered earlier. With thorough attention to clinical practice, and constant discussion and arguement with colleagues,

it is possible both to become a good clinician and to prepare for the examination.

Written questions

Before sitting for a written examination, all candidates should look carefully at their handwriting; it would be even better to ask a colleague to criticise it. Is it legible? If it is not, there is not much hope of impressing the examiner. There is nothing more maddening for an examiner than struggling to understand what a candidate has written. Many candidates seem to make the mistake of writing too fast so that their writing deteriorates. It is better to write less, but clearly, rather than a lot which is illegible. If the view of a candidate's friends is that his writing is awful, it would be wise for him to take some professional advice about improving it.

At the top of the examination paper there will be instructions on how to answer it. These must be read very carefully, in order to answer the right number of questions and to know if any of them is compulsory. One should read each question more than once. A plan can then be made for the time available for answering them.

A candidate who does not have English as a first language must make certain of having sufficient command of it to answer the questions easily. If not, it could be sensible to take some instruction in improving it. There are now a number of correspondence courses which are aimed at helping doctors to sit examinations, and some are particularly useful for the DCH. It is not necessary to worry too much about spelling; it is, of course, useful to spell correctly, but it is more important to write down information clearly and precisely.

Multiple choice questions (MCQ)

Many candidates seem confused by these questions, but they have been shown to test knowledge more satisfactorily than other methods.

Before answering the question, one should be certain of what is being asked. It is usually wise to read the question more than once, perhaps three times would be best. Almost all MCQs have a basic statement which is called the stem, and there are several questions based on it. The stem may be only one word, but is more likely to be a short sentence.

There are several different types of MCQ. One variety asks several, usually five, questions about the stem and only one is correct. The MCQ most commonly used in the United Kingdom is known as the "true, false or don't know" type. There are usually five questions about the stem, but any of the statements can be correct; sometimes all of them are correct, sometimes none, or any other combination. It is important to understand this type of MCQ, which is used in this book, as they are the commonest in the DCH. A mark is given for each of the five questions about the stem. If the statement is false and it is answered as false, a mark will be given; similarly if a true statement is answered as true. But a mark will be lost if the answer is wrong. A mark is not lost when a statement is marked as don't know. It is therefore very important *not* to guess. Questions should only be answered as true or false by a candidate who is almost certain of being correct.

MCQs are fairly difficult to set accurately. They are always discussed carefully by the examiners and are evaluated after they have been used to discard any which are ambiguous or do not seem to discriminate well between good and poor candidates. There is no point in having questions which are so difficult that none can answer them or so easy that every candidate gets them right.

It is a good idea to practise MCQs, which is why some have been included in this book. They should be answered against the clock, in order to mimic the time restraints of a real exam.

Short note questions

It is common to find some questions which start with "Write short notes on. . . ." or "Write a brief account of. . . ." One should not be tempted to write too much; it is especially easy to do this when one of the questions is on a subject about which one knows a great deal. It is easy to write too much and to spend so much time that the other questions are skimped; because they are more difficult, they need more thought.

It sometimes helps to make lists or underline some words to draw attention to them. The aim should be to get information over to the examiner in the shortest and clearest fashion.

Essay questions

These seem to be going out of fashion in favour of MCQs and short questions. However, some examinations still expect candidates to write a long account of a subject and to spend about 45 minutes on the answer. It is always possible to find out the type of questions which are asked by writing to the Examining Board which is organising the exam. They will usually be prepared to send old examination papers, so that candidates can practise.

Whereas a short question can be answered with only short phrases, an essay should be written in normal English prose, with proper sentences. It will be necessary to spend a little time planning what needs to be written. The answer should have a short introduction, then cover the subject in a logical fashion and end with some sort of conclusion. It is quite permissable to include lists or even to draw diagrams to illustrate something which cannot be described easily in words. A judicious amount of underlining may help the examiner.

Clinical examination

This is usually the most difficult part of the examination. The candidate will be given a time to take the history and examine the child; then the examiner will listen to a presentation of the findings. A statement of the child's problems and a plan for their management will be expected. There is usually not enough time for the history and examination, rarely as much as in an out-patient clinic, so it is important to move fast. This is why a candidate should prepare for the exam by developing a plan of history taking and examination by the constant practice of seeing children. One must not forget important parts of the history, such as the birth, the family's illnesses and living conditions, development and immunisation. If these items are always included in one's daily work, they will not be forgotten in the fluster of the exam. That, after all, is the point of the clinical — to see if the candidate's technique of clinical practice is satisfactory.

Every moment free should be used to do a complete examination of the child, not forgetting important things like taking the blood pressure of older children. If it is impossible to do certain things, this should be explained to the examiner; examples are that one would like to measure a child accurately and to test the hearing.

Ward rounds are good practice. It is not necessary to present every small point in the history, but to mention the salient points and to demonstrate that a full history and examination have been done. It is permissable, for example to say "There were no important features in the family history" or "The rest of the examination was normal". The examiner can always ask for more details.

If it does not seem possible to make one diagnosis, the examiner should be told so. It is usually more useful to list the child's problems, if any, and to make a plan for management. One should not expect every child to be abnormal; many children in ordinary clinical practice are normal and they appear in an exam. If a candidate thinks that a child is normal, he should say so. After the long case, another examiner will show the candidate some short cases. The children will usually have some obvious clinical signs, which allow a straightforward diagnosis to be made. Sometimes the examiner may want a demonstration of clinical ability, so the question may be "Please examine the cardiovascular system". One must watch out for other related physical signs; thus if a large liver is found, a search should be made for jaundice.

The short cases allow a candidate to demonstrate the ability to approach children properly. It is wise to get down to their level and to remember the dictum that "Never take your child to a paediatrician with a good pair of trousers, because it means that he doesn't kneel on the floor".

It is difficult to make a recommendation about what to wear for the exam. There are no rules, except to look clean and tidy. Some examiners do not like dress which is too informal, but one should not wear anything too formal and uncomfortable as it might hinder a relaxed attitude to the children. A middle way would seem best.

The viva voce

The oral examination is also less popular with examiners than it was. Certainly some candidates perform less well than they should, because they are so nervous.

The examiners will ask questions or may show X-rays or pictures of patients. They are keen to have practical replies and will pay less attention to esoteric information gleaned from a textbook than knowledge drawn from common clinical work.

As in most parts of the exam, one can only perform well with practice and rehearsal. A good way of preparing oneself is to show X-rays to colleagues who are also taking the exam and to demand quick answers to questions. The questioning can then be reversed. Only by getting used to aggressive questioning can one become used to the nerve-racking pressure of the oral.

Changes in the examinations

New techniques are constantly being introduced. For example, it is possible to show videotapes of children and these can be used to replace parts of the clinical examination. When parts of the exam are shown to be unsatisfactory, they are dropped and replaced by a new type of assessment. One should always check with the Examining Board to be certain that they have not made any changes.

30

Multiple choice questions

1 *Cot deaths*:
   A are more likely to occur in babies of low birth-weight
   B are more likely to occur in those whose sibling was previously a cot death
   C could have been avoided in 50% of cases
   D are usually caused by parental failure
   E are associated with negative postmortem findings in over 90% of cases

2 **Vaccines in common use against the following infectious disease contain live organisms:**
   A measles
   B diphtheria
   C rubella
   D tuberculosis
   E typhoid (monovalent)

3 **Cystic fibrosis is a disease characterised by:**
   A changes in exocrine glands
   B small bowel mucosal villous atrophy
   C fat globules in the stool on microscopy
   D a low sweat sodium and chloride concentration
   E recessive inheritance

4 **The following statements are true:**
   A a steady state concentration will be reached earlier when regular large doses are administered
   B drugs eliminated by the kidney should not be given to patients in renal failure
   C the grey baby syndrome should not occur if chloramphenicol levels are maintained within the therapeutic range
   D the timing of samples for monitoring drugs is unimportant if the drug is in a steady state
   E most children require larger weight related doses of most drugs than adults

5 Pertussis (whooping cough):

A is only mildly contagious

B is characterised by a spasmodic cough and is often accompanied by vomiting

C is always due to an infection with *Bordatella pertussis*

D may produce subconjunctival haemorrhages

E is hardly ever seen in the first 3 months of life due to passive immunity provided by the mother

6 In measles:

A the rash starts peripherally and spreads towards the face

B the rash may desquamate

C Koplik spots appear at the same time as the rash

D blindness is a recognised complication

E viral pneumonitis with tachypnoea may occur before the appearance of the rash

7 Long-term immunity follows naturally acquired infection with:

A measles

B rubella

C tetanus

D pertussis

E mumps

8 The duration of the incubation period of:

A rubella is 7–10 days

B measles is 8–11 days

C chickenpox is 3–5 days

D mumps is 7–10 days

E malaria is 9–30 days

9 Viruses involved in respiratory tract infection of infants include:

A adenovirus

B parainfluenza

C herpesvirus hominis

D respiratory syncytial virus

E cytomegalovirus

10 Pubertal development is abnormal when:

A testicular enlargement occurs in a boy of 8 years

B there are no signs of testicular enlargement in a boy of 12 years

C menarche does not occur until 16 years

D there are no signs of breast enlargement in a 14-year-old girl

E pubic hair appears in a 9-year-old girl

11 **The following conditions are more common in patients of immigrant origin compared with those of indigenous origin:**
A unsatisfactory housing
B unemployment
C threadworms
D non-pulmonary tuberculosis
E iron deficiency anaemia

12 **Which of the following could cause an infant not to bend the right elbow and shoulder?**
A lumbar meningomyelocele
B hydrocephalus
C right Erb's palsy
D fracture of right humerus
E right cephalohaematoma

13 **Frank blood in the stools of a 6-month-old child may be due to:**
A anal fissure
B intussusception
C Meckel's diverticulum
D appendicitis
E shigella gastroenteritis

14 **Abdominal pain in childhood may be associated with:**
A lobar pneumonia
B Henoch-Schönlein purpura
C school phobia
D diabetes insipidus
E lead poisoning

15 **Congenital dislocation of the hip:**
A is commoner in girls than boys
B is commoner in infants with spina bifida
C cannot be detected at birth
D may run in families
E always requires an operation

16 **Deafness occurs following:**
A meningococcal meningitis
B measles
C mumps
D 'glue' ear
E congenital syphilis

17 **In the following 3 questions indicate whether each statement is true or false.**
A conductive nerve deafness is a sign of kernicterus
B hypothyroidism may cause prolonged neonatal jaundice

C plasma unconjugated bilirubin levels below 340 μmol/l are not associated with kernicterus in preterm infants

D bruising may cause hyperbilirubinaemia

E hypoglycaemic convulsions have a better prognosis than hypocalcaemic convulsions

18 A cyanosis of hands and feet occurs in many healthy babies

B subconjunctival haemorrhage is associated with intracranial haemorrhage

C infants of poorly-controlled diabetics are prone to respiratory distress syndrome

D anaemia may cause respiratory distress

E meconium aspiration indicates intrapartum asphyxia

19 A small-for-gestational-age term infants are liable to intraventricular haemorrhage

B cow's milk has a higher protein content than human milk

C cow's milk has a higher vitamin D content than human milk

D *Staphylococcus aureus* is the commonest cause of neonatal septicaemia

E modern artificial baby milks are not allergenic

20 Which of the following could cause bile-stained vomiting?

A overfeeding

B malrotation of the gut

C oesophageal atresia

D pyloric stenosis

E Hirschsprung's disease

21 Hydrocolpos:

A usually presents during the neonatal period

B is best managed by abdominal exploration

C may be due to excessive oestrogen secretion in the child

D regresses spontaneously in many instances

E causes retention of urine

22 Evaluation of every child who has enuresis should include the following:

A family history

B urine culture

C intravenous urography

D a test of renal function

E physical examination

23 Immunisation against whooping cough is contra-indicated in:

A a child with acute otitis media

B a child whose birth weight was less than 2500 g

C the child who is allergic to eggs

D a child with a history of neonatal convulsions

E a child with eczema

24 In rubella:

A the rash usually appears on the third day
B the rash spares the face
C arthropathy may occur
D the rash is never vesicular
E the occipital adenopathy is an important diagnostic feature

25 In chickenpox:

A the lesions should heal without scarring
B the rash is centrifugal in distribution
C routine immunisation is offered to all children at one year
D hyperimmune gammaglobulin may be a common adjunct to therapy if the patient is taking steroids
E acquired in the first 5 days of life has approximately a 20% mortality

26 Strawberry naevi:

A are usually present at birth
B are hamartomas
C commonly undergo malignant change
D may be associated with an intracranial haemangioma on the same side
E should be excised

27 In iron poisoning:

A no symptoms occur until 8 hours after ingestion
B may cause an encephalopathy
C penicillamine is the treatment of choice
D if symptom free after 24 hours the patient may be discharged
E scarring of the pylorus may occur as a late complication

28 The risk of developing malignant disease in childhood is:

A 1:100
B 1:200
C 1:600
D 1:2000
E 1:10 000

29 The health visitor:

A can be a state enrolled nurse (SEN)
B is an employee of the general practitioners with whom she works
C must have some experience in obstetric nursing
D works solely with antenatal mothers and children up to the age of 15
E can prescribe treatment for simple medical conditions

30 An infant's size at birth:

A relates equally to maternal and parental size
B may be greater than expected if mother is diabetic

C correlates well with his adult height
D is not affected by sex
E is likely to be reduced if there is a congenital malformation

31 Vaginal bleeding in childhood is:

A commonest between 4 and 6 years of age
B often due to a blood dyscrasia
C caused by a foreign body in the vagina
D often associated with precocious puberty
E sometimes due to a malignant tumour of the vagina

32 Would you be worried about a child's development if:

A there was head lag on pull to sit at 5 months
B he was not sitting alone by 7 months
C he was not speaking in sentences by 18 months
D he was not walking alone by 18 months
E there was no tuneful babble with consonants by 10 months

33 The commonest malignant solid tumour of childhood is:

A nephroblastoma
B brain tumour
C Hodgkin's disease
D rhabdomyosarcoma
E osteogenic sarcoma

34 Vulvovaginitis in a child is:

A common in the neonatal period
B usually due to vaginal foreign bodies
C the results of poor vaginal acidity
D responsive to local oestrogen cream
E an allergic phenomenon

35 A 3-year-old cannot sleep at night and goes into his parents' bed. You should:

A admit him to hospital
B use a night sedative as first line of treatment
C discuss with the parents what has been happening in the family
D help the parents to be firm in putting the child back to bed
E explain that this is normal

36 Cystic fibrosis:

A occurs in one in 4000 Caucasian infants
B is commoner in African than Chinese peoples
C is commoner in males than females
D is inherited as an autosomal recessive
E has a gene carrier rate of one in 100

37 The common sites of presentation of soft tissue sarcomas in childhood are:

A head and neck
B retroperitoneum
C genito-urinary tract
D CNS
E lung

38 In the neonatal period:

A breast swelling in little girls is a serious problem calling for early treatment
B a vaginal discharge is often evident
C vaginal bleeding is never encountered
D cystic vulval swellings call for early excision
E vulval congestion and oedema are common

39 Most children of 3 years should:

A speak using short sentences
B give name and address
C play appropriately with miniature toys
D build a bridge of three cubes from memory
E remain clean and dry, day and night

40 Acute leukaemia in childhood may mimic:

A rheumatoid arthritis
B streptococcal tonsillitis
C irritable hip syndrome
D iron deficiency anemia
E infectious mononucleosis

41 The following features suggest handicap:

A Moro reflex present at 6 months
B easily elicited asymmetrical tonic neck reflex
C hand preference present by 2 years
D Mouthing toys at 18 months
E hand regard at 3 months

42 Significant bacteriuria:

A is indicated by $>10^3$ bacteria/ml urine
B is always accompanied by pyuria
C may be asymptomatic
D in most cases involves the upper urinary tract as well as the bladder
E is an indication for a micturating cysto-urethrogram

43 In normal pubertal development:

A the pubertal growth spurt occurs earlier in boys than in girls
B testicular enlargement is the first sign of puberty in the male

C at the time of onset of menstruation in girls the height spurt is almost
    complete
D gynaecomastia may occur in boys
E aprocrine sweat activity, oiliness of the hair and acne are androgenic
    changes

44 In immunological reactions:
A T lymphocytes manufacture antibodies
B IgG may mediate type 1 hypersensitivity
C histamine is released from eosinophils
D IgA reduces antigen absorption through epithelial surfaces
E activation of the complement system produces cell lysis

45 The prescriber should:
A generally use liquid preparations for children under 8 years
B limit tetracyclines to topical use only in children under 12 years
C only use inhalational drug forms if oral forms are unavailable
D always check the weight and age of the child before prescribing
E use parenteral preparations in only those occasions when the child
    is vomiting

46 Rickets is more common in the following immigrant groups than in the indigenous population:
A Asian children over the age of two
B Chinese children
C African children
D Asian mothers
E Asian babies around the age of 6 months

47 The following vaccines are normally given by subcutaneous or intramuscular injection:
A measles
B poliomyelitis
C tuberculosis
D smallpox
E tetanus

48 Infantile eczema:
A may improve on a cow's-milk-free diet
B is less common in breast-fed babies
C is made worse by frequent baths
D on the face should never be treated with topical fluorinated steroids
E is made worse by heat

49 Children on cytotoxic chemotherapy are at particular risk from:
A nutritional deficiency
B skin infections

C Chickenpox and measles
D sleep disturbance
E fungal infections

50 A five-year-old-boy has never spoken. You should:
A refer him for hearing tests
B see if there is any abnormal behaviour such as stereotypies
C take a detailed developmental history
D take a detailed family history
E check maternal rubella antibody titres

51 The following are associated with hypertension:
A coarctation of the aorta
B end-stage renal disease
C acute renal failure
D acute post-streptococcal glomerulonephritis
E acute gastroenteritis

52 A 6-year-old girl has been dry at night but is now wetting again. You should:
A restrict her night time fluid intake
B discuss possible family upsets with her parents
C keep her home from school
D set up an award system for dry nights
E culture her urine

53 The following are common precipitants of wheeze in asthmatic children:
A *Dermatophagoides pteronyssinus*
B exercise
C *Aspergillus fumigatus*
D adenovirus
E egg ingestion

54 Three months after entering the UK a 3-year-old girl from a rural community in Pakistan develops a fever 39°C, vomiting and loose stools. She passed five roundworms in her stool:
A her symptoms are due to heavy infestation with *Ascaris lumbricoides*
B she should be suspected of suffering from *P. vivax* malaria and this must be confirmed by examining a blood film
C she should be given a course of chloroquine immediately as cerebral malaria is a likely complication
D stool examination for *Giardia lamblia* and *Entamoeba histolytica* are unlikely to be positive
E she should be investigated for salmonellosis and shigellosis.

55 In acute haemolysis:

A the urine is brown due to methaemoglobin

B loin pain and myalgia occur

C reticulocytes and nucleated red cells are seen in the blood in the acute phase

D ascorbic acid as an antioxidant can limit the haemolysis in G6PD deficient patients

E testing for G6PD deficiency is best done during the acute haemolytic episode

56 Vesico-ureteric reflux:

A is an abnormal finding

B may disappear spontaneously

C is attributed to an abnormally long intramural course of the ureter

D should always be corrected surgically

E implies bladder neck obstruction

57 In a retarded child with bilateral cataracts you might expect to find the following:

A aminoaciduria and glycosuria

B a continuous heart murmur

C polydactyly

D warts

E deafness

58 The children of social class IV parents:

A include the sons of hotel porters

B make more use of immunisation services than do children of social class I parent

C make more use of the diagnostic and therapeutic services that the general practitioner offers, than do children of social class I parents

D have a greater chance of dying in the first year of life than do children of social class I parents

E are more likely to suffer from dental caries than the children of social class I parents

59 The following conditions fufill the criteria necessary for screening:

A undescended testes

B hypothyroidism in the newborn

C plantar warts

D hypertension

E conductive deafness

60 A 14-year-old is missing school, because of abdominal pain. You should:

A see his parents and discuss ways of getting him to school

B admit him to hospital for investigations

C see if his mother is depressed or anxious

D test his urine

E contact educational welfare officer

61 In an infant with a ventricular septal defect:

A the shunt of bood through the VSD is from left to right

B there maybe a diastolic murmur in the left mid-parasternal area

C the murmur is soft in quality and occupies only the first half of diastole

D the pulmonary circulation is congested on chest X-ray

E failure to thrive is common

62 In rheumatic fever:

A there may be a rash consisting of rings of normal skin surrounded by a raised erythematous margin

B an apical diastolic murmur might be heard

C there may be a prolonged PR interval on ECG

D the knees are often swollen for some weeks

E steroids are the treatment of choice

63 In infancy, heart failure:

A never occurs in the first day of life

B commonly presents with peripheral oedema

C causes enlargement of the liver

D may be caused by paroxysmal tachycardia

E should never be treated with digoxin

64 The following may occur in childhood lead poisoning:

A purpura

B reticulocytosis

C anaemia

D abdominal colic

E blue lines on the gums

65 The following diseases are correctly placed against their causes:

A neonatal tetanus: hypocalcaemia

B acute infantile bronchiolitis: respiratory syncytial virus

C *Haemophilus influenzae* meningitis: influenza virus

D oral thrush: *Oxyuris vermicularis*

E infective hepatitis: Epstein-Barr virus

66 Which of the following may be features of hypothyroidism in an 8-week-old infant?

A umbilical hernia

B dry skin

C prolonged physiological jaundice

D poor peripheral circulation

E hypotonia

67 Atopy:

A may be reduced by breast feeding
B may be influenced by month of birth
C is common in cystic fibrosis
D is associated with high IgD levels
E is always symptomatic

68 In haemolytic disease of the newborn which of the following are true?

A blood film showing 4 per cent nucleated red cells is diagnostic
B death *in utero* may be due to cardiac failure associated with haemolytic anemia
C Rhesus haemolytic disease is completely preventable by antenatal screening
D ABO disease occurs when maternal IgM antibodies are involved causing complete red cell lysis
E exchange transfusion may have to be repeated several times in severe cases of Rhesus disease

69 Defects of immune systems:

A frequently lead to development of atopy
B may be associated with absent tonsils and adenoids
C commonly occur in cystic fibrosis
D may occur following measles infection
E can be detected by a positive tuberculin test

70 Feeding:

A Breast-fed infants are seldom grossly obese
B cereals should be introduced in the second month of life
C gastroenteritis is less common in bottle-fed babies
D infants with phenylketonuria should not be fed with goat's milk
E phenindione anticoagulant therapy in the mother is a contra-indication to breast feeding

71 The steroid-responsive nephrotic syndrome is associated with:

A microscopic haematuria
B reduced albumin synthesis
C highly selective proteinuria
D hypovolaemia if the PCV falls
E girls more commonly than boys

72 The following statements are true of imported childhood disease in the UK:

A visceral leishmaniasis can mimic acute leukaemia
B folate deficiency anaemia is associated with heavy hookworm infestation
C iron deficiency anaemis, tenesmus and rectal prolapse are features of heavy infestation with *Trichuris trichiuria*

D the majority of childhood malaria cases are due to *P. falciparum*

E anaemia and splenomegaly are features of haematological inherited disease

73 In β-thalassaemia:

A dietary iron deficiency frequently exacerbates the anaemis of β-thalassaemia trait

B when both parents have β-thalassaemia trait no normal offspring will be produced

C blood transfusions should be avoided in β-thalassaemia major to prevent iron overload

D in β-thalassaemia major death commonly occurs in the second or third decade from heart failure

E a serum ferritin of 13 μg/l is diagnostic of β-thalassaemia major

74 After a cot death, parents:

A usually receive much support from a variety of social and medical agencies

B will blame themselves for their child's death

C will continue to hear their child crying, especially at night

D Soon recover from their grief, especially if another pregnancy quickly follows

E usually talk openly about their loss

75 Which of the following are associated with constipation:

A sugar intolerance

B anal fissure

C pyloric stenosis

D hypothyroidism

E Crohn's disease

76 Antihistamines are useful treatment for:

A contact dermatitis

B angio-oedema

C asthma

D coeliac disease

E chronic granulomatous disease

77 An 8-month-old male Chinese infant born in Vietnam is failing to thrive because he is not taking his feeds. He is listless, pale and underweight and his spleen is palpable 1 cm below the costal margin:

A he should be investigated for primary disseminated tuberculosis

B a blood film should be examined and a specimen sent for haemoglobin electrophoresis

C thalassaemia is not likely, if both parents are not anaemic

D his parents should be asked about exposure of their baby to naphthalene because of the danger of haemolysis in G6PD deficient infants

E If this baby was not jaundiced during the neonatal period, he is unlikely to be G6PD deficient

78 **In an 8-year-old child complaining of recurrent episodes of mid-abdominal pain without obvious cause, it would generally be accepted as wise to:**

A examine the urine for infection

B review the child's emotional and psychological status

C remove the appendix

D reassure the parents

E X-ray the spine

79 **In unilateral talipes equinovarus:**

A the forefoot is adducted

B the heel is everted

C there is overactivity of tibialis anterior muscle

D there may be an associated myelodysplasia

E a posteromedial release operation may be required

80 **A 16-year-old girl has secondary amenorrhoea: You should:**

A weigh her

B put her on the 'pill'

C arrange an immediate psychiatric opinion

D reassure her and her parents

E do a pregnancy test

81 **Undiluted fresh cow's milk when compared with human breast milk contains more of the following:**

A protein

B lactose

C fat

D phosphorus

E sodium

82 **A 5-year-old English boy develops headache, vomiting cough and fever 40°C, 5 weeks after a holiday in Kenya. He had taken chloroquine 150 mg weekly whilst on holiday and for 3 weeks on return to the UK:**

A he is unlikely to be suffering from malaria because he has been taking chloroquine

B malaria should be suspected as the most likely diagnosis

C Lassa fever is a likely diagnosis

D the presence of anaemia and splenomegaly on examination support the diagnosis of *P. falciparum* malaria

E if he has continuous fever and jaundice he probably has hepatitis

83 Rickets:

A always responds to oral vitamin D
B is less common in Asian immigrant children
C is excluded if the serum calcium level is normal
D may be associated with retarded motor development
E causes an angular stomatitis

84 Congenital adrenal hyperplasia of the 21-hydroxylase type:

A is inherited as an autosomal dominant
B can be diagnosed pre-natally
C may present as primary amenorrhoea
D if inadequately treated the excess androgens cause rapid linear growth and tall stature as adults
E may cause neonatal death due to severe hyponatraemic dehydration

85 Headache:

A the longer the history of headache the more serious is the cause likely to be
B erogotamine derivatives do not make a major contribution to the treatment of headache in childhood
C headaches due to raised intracranial pressure are acute but often brief
D the pain associated with tension headache in childhood has no organic basis
E the treatment of choice for headache in children under the age of 10 is soluble aspirin

86 Clumsy children:

A do not usually have an abnormal birth history
B are usually of normal birth weight
C are best identified by the performance scale of the WISC
D are difficult to identify reliably at the age of school entry
E respond well to stimulant drugs

87 The 3-week-old baby should:

A gain 20–30 g daily
B require 50 ml of milk/kg daily
C require 10 μg (400 iu) vitamin D daily
D take 5 minutes for a feed
E be given iron supplements routinely

88 Nasal polyps:

A occur commonly in cystic fibrosis
B are always bilateral
C are associated in some cases with an increased sensitivity to aspirin
D are associated with intestinal polyps
E may be mistaken for a meningocele

89 In juvenile rheumatoid arthritis (IgM Rh factor positive):

A boys are more affected than girls
B chronic arthritis is common
C the commonest age of onset is less than 2 years
D erosions may occur on X-ray
E HLA B27 tissue type antigen is present in 75 per cent

90 Iron deficiency in children:

A is less common than megaloblastic anaemia
B is sometimes a presenting feature of coeliac disease
C is common in preterm infants
D causes a macrocytic hypochromic anaemia
E may be associated with hookworm infestation

91 Feeding difficulties in the neonatal period may be due to:

A prematurity
B hiatus hernia
C cerebral birth trauma
D intrauterine growth retardation
E congenital heart disease

92 Stridor in the first 2 weeks may be caused by:

A subglottic stenosis
B haemangioma of trachea
C laryngomalacia
D milk allergy
E cystic hygroma

93 Reduced height velocity in the pre-pubertal child may be a feature of:

A hypothyrodidism
B congenital adrenal hyperplasia
C long-term steroid therapy
D simple obesity
E coelic disease

94 Nephroblastoma occurs with increased frequency in association with the following anomalies:

A imperforate anus
B hemihypertrophy
C aniridia
D hypoplastic lung
E phocomelia

95 Which of the following agents are B_2 stimulants and useful in asthma:

A disodium cromoglycate
B beclomethasone propionate

C terbutaline
D aminophylline
E salbutamol

96 In bleeding disorders:

A prolonged prothrombin time, kaolin cephalin coagulation time and low platelet count suggest disseminated intravascular coagulation
B fresh frozen plasma is the treatment of choice in an acute joint bleed in a patient with haemophilia
C in a child with spontaneous bruising a platelet count of $202 \times 10^9/l$ suggests that non-accidental injury is a more likely cause than thrombocytopenia
D heparin treatment has dramatically reduced the mortality of the haemolytic-uraemic syndrome
E a history of recent viral infections should be sought in children presenting with thrombocytopenia

97 Childhood asthma:

A is always associated with atopy
B may be confused with an inhaled foreign body
C invariably remits in adolescence
D may respond to atropine
E is associated with eczema in less than 20% of cases

98 Immediate priorities in the management of severe gastroenteritis are:

A give a broad spectrum antibiotic
B stop oral feeding
C use an anti-emetic drug
D begin to restore fluid and electrolyte balance
E administer intravenous potassium

99 The following activities represent secondary prevention:

A Immunisation against poliomyelitis
B amniocentesis for spina bifida
C the Guthrie test for phenylketonuria
D screening for hypertension
E the administration of anti D gammaglobulin postnatally in the Rhesus-negative mother who has given birth to a Rhesus-positive baby

100 Which of the following statements are true:

A most drugs are metabolised at faster rates in children than adults
B for most drugs, mothers on therapy should be discouraged from breast feeding
C oxytetracycline is one of the drugs of choice for children with *Haemophilus influenzae* infections

D tricyclic antidepressant drugs are the first line in the general management of nocturnal enuesis

E An appropriate fluid and electrolyte mixture, rather than using mixture. Kaolin paediatric mixture, is the better approach to viral gastroenteritis management in the infant

101 The majority of tumours of the central nervous system in childhood:

A occur in structures above the tentorium

B are glioblastomas

C present with severe headaches

D cause a block in the CSF pathway

E respond well to cytotoxic chemotherapy

102 Under the National Health Service in the UK, a general practitioner:

A is employed by the local health authority

B is responsible for the care his patients receive from his deputy, even when he himself is not on call

C is more likely to be working single-handed than in partnership

D is responsible for providing the premises from which he works

E can obtain from the local district hospital the simple diagnostic equipment that he needs to do his work

103 The following statements are true:

A antibacterial prophylaxis should be limited to children with recurrent urinary tract infections or previous rheumatic fever

B most commonly used drugs are best given after meals

C intramuscular therapy will always prove more effective than that given by the oral route

D children generally require less frequent drug dosing than adults

E compliance should be better with single rather than multiple therapy

104 Which of the following are associated with Turner's syndrome:

A dysplastic nails

B short stature

C pulmonary stenosis

D cubitus valgus

E primary amenorrhoea

105 In the treatment of imported diseases:

A chloroquine is the drug of choice for all types of acute malaria

B piperazine citrate is the drug of choice for ascaris infestation

C piperazine citrate is a safe drug and can be given in multiple doses

D thiabendazole is effective against hookworm and trichuris

E metronidazole is effective against *Entamoeba histolytica* and *Giardia lamblia* but a higher dose is required for the former

106 The following may cause malabsorption:

A threadworm infestation
B tuberculosis of the gut
C *Giardia lamblia* infection
D gluten sensitivity
E Hirschsprung's disease

107 The following convey a greater than 10 per cent risk of epileptic seizures in later childhood and adolescence:

A reflex anoxic seizures in the first year
B two febrile convulsions in the first 3 years
C one parent affected by idiopathic epilepsy
D idiopathic infantile spasms
E head injury aged 5 with post-traumatic amnesia of 6 hours

108 The following are recognised adverse effects of sodium valproate:

A permanent alopecia
B thrombocytopenia
C induction of barbiturate metabolism
D liver failure
E depression and irritability

109 Febrile convulsions:

A can be prevented by intermittent treatment with phenobarbitone
B are the commonest seizure type under the age of 6 months
C are commoner in children with history of perinatal problems
D affect the sexes equally
E a positive family history favours a better outcome

110 A 25-year-old woman develops rubella during the third month of her pregnancy:

A the chances of a major fetal abnormality are greater than 50 per cent
B cardiac abnormalities in the fetus are unlikely
C the affected baby may excrete the virus for more than one year
D deafness is the commonest congenital abnormality at this stage
E giving immunoglobulin prevents any complication

111 In primary tuberculosis in children:

A the infection may be silent
B miliary TB cannot result
C erythema nodosum is never a feature
D the treatment of choice is isoniazid on its own for at least one year
E Mantoux conversion takes 3 weeks

112 The following are classical features of congenital rubella infection:

A jaundice
B hypoglycaemia
C purpura
D microphthalmia
E patent ductus arteriosus

113 Infantile gastroenteritis:

A is due to bacterial infection in over 70 per cent of cases
B may be caused by coliform organisms
C is rare in wholly breast-fed infants
D is usually associated with metabolic alkalosis
E may present with meningism

114 Croup:

A is never a serious condition
B is characterised by expiratory stridor
C is often associated with an upper respiratory tract infection
D principally affects children over the age of 3 years
E may be caused by an acute epiglottitis

115 Cerebral palsy:

A in school age the incidence is about 2.5 per 1000
B spasticity is present from birth
C sensory loss is always present
D in bilateral hemiplegia the upper limbs are more severely affected than the lower
E hearing impairment occurs more frequently in dyskinesia than other forms of cerebral palsy

116 Transposition of the great vessels:

A is a form of non-cyanotic heart disease
B produces pulmonary oligaemia
C is incompatible with life unless there is also a VSD or a patent ductus arteriosus
D is associated with an increased heart size
E requires urgent treatment in the first few days of life

117 The following are associated with non-accidental injury to children:

A the degree of injury is out of keeping with the history
B bruises that appear to have a similar time aetiology
C retinal haemorrhages
D no delay between the injury and the seeking of medical advice
E spiral fractures of the long bones

MCQ ANSWER KEY

Q	1	2	3	4	5	6	7	8	9	10	11	12	13	14	15
A	T	T	T	F	F	F	T	F	T	T	T	T	F	T	T
B	T	F	F	F	T	T	T	T	T	F	T	F	T	T	T
C	F	T	T	T	F	F	F	F	F	F	T	T	T	T	F
D	F	T	F	F	T	T	F	F	T	T	T	T	F	F	T
E	F	F	T	T	F	T	T	T	T	F	T	F	T	T	F

Q	16	17	18	19	20	21	22	23	24	25	26	27	28	29	30
A	T	F	T	F	F	T	T	T	T	T	F	F	F	F	F
B	T	T	F	T	T	F	T	F	F	F	T	T	F	F	T
C	T	F	T	T	F	F	F	F	T	F	F	F	T	T	F
D	T	T	T	F	F	F	F	T	T	T	F	F	F	F	F
E	T	F	T	F	T	T	T	F	T	T	F	T	F	F	T

Q	31	32	33	34	35	36	37	38	39	40	41	42	43	44	45
A	F	T	F	F	F	F	T	F	T	T	T	T	F	F	F
B	F	F	T	F	F	T	F	T	F	F	T	F	T	T	T
C	T	F	F	T	T	F	T	F	T	F	T	T	F	F	F
D	T	T	F	T	T	T	F	F	F	F	T	F	T	T	T
E	T	T	F	F	T	F	F	T	F	T	F	F	T	T	F

Q	46	47	48	49	50	51	52	53	54	55	56	57	58	59	60
A	T	T	T	T	T	T	T	T	F	T	T	T	T	T	T
B	F	F	T	F	T	T	T	T	F	T	T	T	F	T	F
C	F	F	F	T	T	T	F	F	F	T	F	F	T	F	T
D	F	F	T	F	T	T	T	F	F	F	F	F	T	T	T
E	T	T	T	T	F	F	T	F	T	F	F	T	T	T	T

Q	61	62	63	64	65	66	67	68	69	70	71	72	73	74	75
A	T	T	F	F	F	T	T	F	T	T	F	T	T	F	F
B	T	T	F	F	T	T	T	T	T	F	F	F	F	T	T
C	F	T	T	T	F	T	T	F	F	F	T	F	F	T	T
D	T	F	T	T	F	T	F	F	T	T	F	F	T	F	T
E	T	F	F	F	F	F	F	T	F	T	F	T	F	F	F

Q	76	77	78	79	80	81	82	83	84	85	86	87	88	89	90
A	F	T	T	T	T	T	T	F	F	F	T	T	T	F	F
B	T	T	T	F	F	F	T	F	T	T	T	F	F	T	T
C	F	F	F	F	F	F	F	F	T	T	F	T	T	F	T
D	F	T	T	T	F	T	T	T	F	F	T	F	F	T	F
E	F	F	F	T	T	T	F	F	T	F	F	F	T	F	T

Q	91	92	93	94	95	96	97	98	99	100	101	102	103	104	105
A	T	T	T	F	F	T	F	F	F	T	F	F	F	T	F
B	T	F	F	T	F	F	T	T	T	F	F	T	F	T	T
C	T	T	T	T	T	F	F	F	T	F	F	F	F	F	T
D	F	F	F	F	F	T	T	T	F	F	T	T	F	T	T
E	T	T	T	F	T	T	F	F	F	T	F	F	T	T	T

Q	106	107	108	109	110	111	112	113	114	115	116	117
A	F	F	F	F	T	T	T	F	F	T	F	T
B	T	F	T	F	F	F	T	T	F	F	T	F
C	T	F	F	T	T	T	T	T	T	F	F	T
D	T	T	T	F	T	T	T	F	F	T	T	F
E	F	F	T	T	F	T	T	T	T	T	T	T

Appendix 1

Normal paediatric values

BIOCHEMICAL AND PHYSIOLOGICAL DATA

The Système International d'Unités (or SI unit system) is now commonly used in the UK. Reference values are given in SI units followed by traditional units. A multiplication factor is included; traditional units are multiplied by this factor to convert to SI units (thus, if the values in SI Units are divided by this factor, the result will be given in traditional units). The unit of volume commonly used is the litre.

The SI unit of quantity is the mole.

Normal blood, serum and plasma values

	Traditional units normal ranges	Multiplication factor	SI units normal ranges
Bicarbonate or total CO_2 (plasma)			
Newborns	18–23 mEq/l	1.0	18–23 mmol/l
Thereafter	18–25 mEq/l		18–25 mmol/l
Bilirubin (serum)			
Cord blood	Up to 2.9 mg/100 ml	17.1	Up to 50 μmol/l
Cord blood (preterm infants)	Up to 3.4 mg/100 ml		Up to 58 μmol/l
First 24 hours (higher in preterm infants)	Up to 6.0 mg/100 ml		Up to 103 μmol/l
2–5 days	Up to 12 mg/100 ml		Up to 205 μmol/l
(In the newborn period virtually all the bilirubin is present as free (unconjugated) bilirubin)			
After 1 month (mainly conjugated)	0.1–0.8 mg/100 ml		1.7–14 μmol/l
Calcium (serum)			
Cord blood	9.3–12.2 mg/100 ml	0.25	2.33–3.05 mmol/l
1st week — breast fed	8.2–12.2 mg/100 ml		2.05–3.05 mmol/l
— bottle fed	7.4–11.0 mg/100 ml		1.85–2.75 mmol/l
Thereafter	8.8–11.0 mg/100 ml		2.20–2.75 mmol/l
Carbon dioxide PCO_2 (arterial)	35.–45	0.133	4.7–6.0 kPa
Chloride (serum)	98–106 mEq/l	1.0	98–106 mmol/l
Cholesterol (serum)			
Cord blood	23–135 mg/100 ml	0.0259	0.6–3.5 mmol/l
1–6 weeks	93–217 mg/100 ml		2.4–5.6 mmil/l
Increasing gradually until 1 year and older	119–263 mg/100 ml		3.1–6.8 mmol/l
Cortisol (plasma)			
Children 0800 h	8–26 μg/100 ml	27.6	200–720 mmol/l
2200 h (usually less than 50 per cent of 0800 h value)	below 10 μg/100 ml		below 275 mmol/l

Normal blood, serum and plasma values

	Traditional units normal ranges	Multiplication factor	SI units normal ranges
Creatinine (serum)	0.4–1.3 mg/100 ml	88.4	35–106 μmol/l
Glucose (blood)			
Fasting	60–100 mg/100 ml	0.0556	3.3–5.5 mmol/l
Newborn	40–80 mg/100 ml		2.2–4.4 mmol/l
Transiently low values below 2.2 mmol/l are commonly seen on the first day of life. Persistently low values should be investigated			
Iron (serum)			
3 years of age	60–175 μg/100 ml	0.179	10.7–31.3 μmol/l
Iron binding capacity (serum) — (TIBC)			
after 6 months	250–500 μg/100 ml	0.179	44.8–89.5 μmol/l
Lead (blood)	Up to 40 μg/100 ml	0.0483	Up to 1.9 μmol/l
Magnesium (serum)			
Newborns	1.40–2.45 mg/100 ml	0.41	0.58–1.00 μmol/l
Older children	1.45–2.32 mg/100 ml		0.60–0.95 mmol/l
Osmolality (serum)	275–295 mosmol/kg	1.0	275–295 mmol/kg
pH (arterial blood)	7.35–7.42		
PO_2 — oxygen tension (arterial blood)			
Umbilical vein	12.8–32.0 mmHg	0.133	1.7–4.3 kPa
Newborns after first 24 hours	77–100 mmHg		9.3–13.3 kPa
Older children	85–100 mmHg		11.3–13.3 kPa
Phenylalanine (plasma)			
Newborns	0.7–2.8 mg/100 ml	60.5	42–170 μmol/l
Transient values above 2.8 mg/100 ml may be found in the newborn period. Plasma concentrations are usually maintained at between 84 and 300 μmol/l in the treatment of phenylkentonuria			
Phosphorus, inorganic (serum)			
Newborns, 1st week	5.8–9.0 mg/100 ml		1.87–2.91 mmol/l
Newborns, 2nd week	4.9–8.9 mg/100		1.58–2.87 mmol/l
Up to 1 year	4.8–6.2 mg/100 ml		1.55–2.00 mmol/l
Thereafter	3.6–5.9 mg/100 ml		1.16–1.91 mmol/l
Phosphorus values in the newborn period vary greatly depending very much on the type of milk feed; lower values are found in breast-fed infants			
Potassium (plasma)			
Newborns	4.3–7.6 mEq/l		4.3–7.6 mmol/l
Older children	3.5–5.6 mEq/l		3.5–5.6 mmol/l
Proteins (serum)			

(values in g/100 ml)	Total	Albumin	Globulins x^1	x^2	β	γ
1 year	5.6–7.3	3.5–5.0	0.2–0.4	0.4–1.0	0.5–1.0	0.5–13
4 years and over	6.4–7.5	3.7–5.0	0.2–0.4	0.4–1.0	0.6–1.1	0.5–1.8
1 year (values in g/l (using multiplication factor of 10))	56–73	35–50	2–4	4–10	5–9	4–12
4 years and over	64–75	37–50		4–10	6–10	5–12

Immunoglobins (serum)	IgG mg/100 ml	IgG g/l	IgA mg/100 ml	IgA g/l	IgM mg/100 ml	IgM g/l
Newborns	650–1450	6.5–14.5	0–10	0–0.1	0–20	0–0.2
1–3 months	200–650	2.0–6.5	5–40	0.05–0.4	10–50	0.1–0.5
4–6 months	150–800	1.5–8.0	10–60	0.1–0.6	10–80	0.1–0.8
1 year	300–1200	3.0–12.0	20–80	0.2–0.8	20–100	0.2–1.0
3 years and older	500–1500	5.0–15.0	30–300	0.3–3.0	40–200	0.4–2.0

Immunoglobin values vary widely in children particularly in the first 6 months of life. Care should be taken in interpreting marginal differences from the normal

	Traditional units normal ranges	Multiplication factor	SI units normal ranges
Sodium (plasma)	136–145 mEq/l	1.0	136–145 mmol/l
Standard bicarbonate (blood)			
Newborns	18–25	1.0	18–25
Thereafter	21–25		21–25

Normal blood, serum and plasma values (continued)

	Traditional units normal ranges	Multiplication factor	SI units normal ranges
Thyrotrophin or thyroid stimulating hormone (TSH) (serum) (1 represents the lower level of sensitivity of most present assay methods. Many euthyroid children may have TSH values which are less than 1 μU/l)	<1–5.8 μU/l	1.0	<1–5.8 μU/l
Thyroxine — T4 (serum)			
Cord blood and newborns	5.5–18.2 μg/100 ml	12.9	71–235 nmol/l
Thereafter	5.8–11.6 μg/100 ml		75–150 nmol/l
Urea (blood)	14–40 mg/100 ml	0.166	2.5–6.6 mmol/l
Higher values are commonly seen during the first 6 months of life in infants on unmodified milks i.e., those whose protein concentration is substantially above that of breast milk			

Normal haematological values (all values shown are means with the ranges in parentheses)

Age	Red blood cells per litre	Red blood cells per mm^3	Haemoglobin %	Haematocrit %	White blood cells per litre	White blood cells per mm^3	Neutrophils %
Birth	5.0–6.0 × 10^{12}	5.0–6.0 × 10^6	17 (14–20)	55 (45–65)	18 × 10^9 (9–30 × 10^9)	18 000 (9–30 000)	60 (40–80)
1 week	Values fall within 3 months to	Values fall within 3 months to	17 (13–21)	54 (43–66)	12 × 10^9 (6–22 × 10^9)	12 000 6–22 000)	39 (30–50)
2 weeks			16.5 (13–20)	50 (42–66)	12 × 10^9 (5–21 × 10^9)	12 000 (5–21 000)	40 (30–50)
6 months–6 years	3.5–5.6 × 10^{12}	3.5–5.6 × 10^6	12 (10.5–14)	38 (33–42)	10 × 10^9 (6–15 × 10^9)	10 000 (6–15 000)	42 (35–52)
Adult F	3.9–5.6 × 10^{12}	3.9–5.6 × 10^6	14 (12–16)	42 (37–47)	7.5 × 10^9 (5–10 × 10^9)	7500 (5–10 000)	60 (40–75)
M	4.5–6.5 × 10^{12}	4.5–6.5 × 10^6	16 (14–18)	46 (42–52)			

Lymphocytes %	Eosinophils %	Monocytes %	Reticulocytes %	Platelets per litre	Platelets per mm^3	MCV fl	MCH pg	MCHC g/dl
32	2	7–14	5 (3–7)	100 × 10^9 300 × 10^9	100 000 300 000	94–118	32–40	34–36
46	3	7–14	2 (0–4)			88–108	32–40	34–36
48	3	6–12	1 (0–2)	150 × 10^9 to	150 000 to	86–106	32–40	34–36
51	2–3	4–8	1 (0–2)	450 × 10^9	450 000	76–88	24–30	30–36
						76–98	27–32	30–35
30 (20–45)	1–6	2–10	0–2			76–96	27–32	30–35

(See also Matoth, Zaizov and Varsano, 1971)
Up to 34 to 36 weeks of fetal life 90 to 95 per cent of haemoglobin is fetal haemoglobin. Thereafter the proportion of fetal haemoglobin decreases at rate of 3 to 4 per cent per week, until 40 weeks when mean is 75 per cent and range 50 per cent to 85 per cent.
Thereafter slow fall to < 60 per cent at 2 months after birth (range 40 to 60 per cent)
Then more rapid fall to < 30 per cent at 3 months after birth
    < 15 per cent at 4 months after birth
    < 5 per cent at 6 months after birth
    < 2 per cent at 3 years after birth

Appendix 2

Common drugs

Drug	Route	0–4 weeks	Total daily dose 4 weeks– 1 year	1–14 years	Doses per day	Comments
Adrenaline injection 1:1000	s.c. (slow)	← 0.01 ml/kg →			Single dose	Inject over 5–10 minutes
Aluminium hydroxide	Oral (mixture)	—	—	15–20 ml	Single dose	Most effective 60–90 minutes after feeds
Aminophylline						See theophylline
Amitriptyline						
depression	Oral	—	—	1.5–2 mg/kg	2	
nocturnal enuresis	Oral	—	—	1–2 mg/kg	1 (at night)	Not indicated before 5 years Caution: dangerous accidental ingestion
Amoxycillin	Oral	30 mg/kg	25 mg/kg	25 mg/kg	3	Preferred to ampicillin because of reduced dose frequency
Amphotericin	Oral (buccal cavity)	← 200–400 mg →			4	Lower dose should be left in mouth after each feed in 0–1 year of age
Ampicillin	Oral i.v., i.m.	← 50–100 mg/kg →			4	400 mg/kg for meningitis
Aspirin						
analgesic/antipyretic	Oral	—	—	15 mg/kg	3 or 4	0–1 years use paracetamol
rheumatic fever or rheumatoid arthritis	Oral	—	—	50–75 mg/kg	4–6	Monitor blood levels Adjust to 1–2 µmol/l
Atropine sulphate	Oral or s.c.	← 15 µug/kg →			Single dose	Pre-operative dose
Beclomethasone dipropionate						
asthma	Oral inhalation	—	—	200–400 µg	2–4	Metered dose, 50 µg
hay fever	Nasal inhalation	—	—	200–400 µg	2–4	Metered dose, 50 µg
Bisacodyl	Oral	—	—	5–10 mg	1	Suppository
	p.r.	—	—	5–10 mg	1	
Calciferol (Vitamin D2)						
— rickets	Oral	← 1500–3000 units →			1	Vitamin D sensitive dose
1α-hydroxycholecalciferol	Oral	← 15 ng/kg →			1	Monitor phosphate level to maintain below 1.9 mmol/1
Carbamazepine	Oral	—	—	10–25 mg/kg	2 or 3	Give more frequent dose (3 per day) for 7 years
Cefuroxime	i.m.	← 30290 mg/kg →			3	Two doses/day in newborn
Cephalexin		—	75 mg/kg	75 mg/kg	4	
Chloral hydrate						
sedative	Oral	← 90 mg/kg →			3	
hypnotic	Oral	← 50 mg/kg →			1	

Drug	Route	Total daily dose 0–4 weeks	Total daily dose 4 weeks– 1 year	Total daily dose 1–14 years	Doses per day	Comments
Chloramphenicol	Oral	—	75–100 mg/kg	75–100 mg/kg	3 or 4	Therapeutic range 10–25 μg/ml (peak level)
	i.v.	Preterm 15–25 mg/kg Term 25–50 mg/kg	75–100 mg/kg	75–100 mg/kg	3 or 4	Monitor levels. Toxicity = grey baby syndrome
Chlorpheniramine maleate	Oral	—	0.4 mg/kg	0.4 mg/kg	3	Dose may be safely doubled
	i.v.	—	0.2 mg/kg	0.2 mg/kg	Single dose	
Clonazepam	Oral	—	0.1–0.2 mg/kg	0.1–0.2 mg/kg	2	Extreme stupor when given with sodium valproate
	i.v.	0.05 mg/kg	0.05 mg/kg	0.35 mg/kg	Single dose	Respiratory depression. May need short term ventilation
Corticotrophin	i.m.	←——————— 1 unit/kg ———————→			Twice weekly or alternate days	
Co-trimoxazole	Oral	←——————— 8 mg/kg ———————→ (dose of trimethoprim)			2	Caution in newborn, displaces bilirubin from binding sites
	i.v.	←——————— 6 mg/kg ———————→			2	
Dexamethasone	Oral	←——————— 0.5 mg/kg ———————→			3	For cerebral oedema
	i.m., i.v.	←——————— 0.5 mg/kg ———————→			3	
Diazepam	i.v.	←——————— 0.2–0.3 mg/kg ———————→			Single dose	Respiratory depression as with clonazepam
	Rectal (i.v. solution)	—	2.5 mg	5 mg	Single dose	Use syringe inserting attached plastic nozzle extension into rectum
Dicyclomine	Oral	←——————— 2 mg/kg ———————→				
Digoxin	Oral	←——————— 10 μg/kg ———————→			1	No need for digitalisation
	i.m., i.v.	←——————— 10 μg/kg ———————→			1	
Disodium cromoglycate	Oral inhalation	—	—	60–80 mg	3 or 4	
	Nebuliser	—	—	½–1 ampoule	4	1 ampoule = 20 mg in 2 ml
	Nasal inhalation	—	—	60–80 mg	3 or 4	
	Nasal spray	—	—	12 squeezes	6	Squeezes to each nostril
'Dorbanex'	Oral	—	—	2.5–10 ml	1	
Erythromycin	Oral	←——————— 50–100 mg/kg ———————→			4	
	i.v.	←——————— 50–100 mg/kg ———————→			4	
Ethosuximide	Oral	—	—	15–30 mg/kg	1	Therapeutic range 280–700 μmol/l
Ferrous sulphate	Oral	←——————— 20 mg/kg ———————→			2	1 mg ≃ 0.3 mg elemental Fe
Flucloxacillin	Oral	←——————— 50 mg/kg ———————→			4	Treble dose in severe staphylococcal infection
	i.v.	←——————— 50 mg/kg ———————→			4	
Folic acid	Oral	←——————— 0.25 mg/kg ———————→			1	
Frusemide	Oral	←——————— 0.5–2 mg/kg ———————→			1	Give potassium supplements if on digoxin or for liver failure.
	i.m., i.v.	←——————— 1 mg/kg ———————→			1	Do not give supplement within 6 h of frusemide dose
Fusidic acid (sodium salt)	Oral	←——————— 50 mg/kg ———————→			3	
	i.v.	←——————— 50 mg/kg ———————→			3	
Gentamicin	i.m.	6 mg/kg	7.5 mg/kg	7.5 mg/kg	3 2	Monitor levels. Ototoxicity if peak levels > 12 μg/ml
	i.v.	6 mg/kg	7.5 mg/kg	7.5 mg/kg	3 2	Renal toxicity if trough levels > 2.0 μg/ml
Hydrocortisone	i.m., i.v.	25 mg	50–100 mg	50–100 mg	3	

Drug	Route	0–4 weeks	Total daily dose 4 weeks– 1 year	1–14 years	Doses per day	Comments
Imipramine						
depression	Oral	—	—	1.5–2 mg/kg	2	
nocturnal enuresis	Oral	—	—	1–2 mg/kg	Single nightly	Not indicated before 5 years. Caution: accidental ingestion dangerous
Ketovite	Oral	←————— 3 tablets —————→			3	
		and 5 ml			1	
Lactulose 50%	Oral	—	—	5–20 ml	1	
Metoclopramide	Oral	←————— 0.3 mg/kg —————→			3	Extrapyramidal signs of toxicity increased with phenothiazines
	i.m., i.v.	←————— 0.3 mg/kg —————→			3	
Metronidazole						
amoebiasis	Oral	—	—	30–50 mg/kg	3	For 5 days
giardiasis	Oral	—	—	40 mg/kg	1	For 3 days
anaerobic infections	Oral	—	25 mg/kg	25 mg/kg	3	For 7 days. With or after meals
	p.r.	—	—	500 mg	3	Suppository: until oral therapy possible
Nalidixic acid	Oral	—	50 mg/kg	50 mg/kg	4	
Naloxone	i.m.	←————— 60 μg/kg —————→			Single dose	i.v. dose of 10 μg/kg is rarely necessary as i.m. injection is effective rapidly, and ventilation should be used meantime
Neomycin	Oral	—	50 mg/kg	50 mg/kg		
Nitrazepam	Oral	—	0.5–1 mg/kg	0.5–1 mg/kg	2	Sedation, hypersecretion
Nitrofurantoin	Oral	—	5–10 mg/kg	5–10 mg/kg	4	Give with or after food. Prophylactic dose is one-third total dose daily
Nystatin	Oral (buccal cavity)	←——— 200 000–400 000 units ———→			4	Give after each feed in babies
Paracetamol	Oral	—	60 mg/kg	60 mg/kg	4	
Paraldehyde	i.m.	←——— 1 ml/year of age to 5 years then add 0.5 ml/year for each additional year ———→			Single dose can repeated after 30 minutes	Give deep i.m. injection. Safe to use modern plastic syringes if given within 10 minutes
Penicillin						
procaine	i.m.	50 mg/kg	25 mg/kg	25 mg/kg	1	
prolonged action	i.m.	¼ vial	¼ vial	½–1 vial	Once every 3 days	'Triplopen'
G	i.m.	25–50 mg/kg	25 mg/kg	25 mg/kg	4	Treble dose in meningitis
V	Oral	←————— 50 mg/kg —————→			4	
Pethidine	i.m., i.v.	←————— 1 mg/kg —————→			Single dose	Controlled drug
Phenobarbitone	Oral, i.m.	5 mg/kg	4–8 mg/kg	4–8 mg/kg	1	Drowsiness, hyperkinesis, poor school performance, rashes
	i.v.	10 mg/kg	10 mg/kg	8 mg/kg	Single dose	Give slowly possible temporary respiratory depression
Phenytoin	Oral	8 mg/kg	10 mg/kg	4–10 mg/kg	2	Therapeutic range 20–100 μmol/l. Small increase in dose may result in larger increase in blood level

Drug	Route	0–4 weeks	Total daily dose 4 weeks– 1 year	1–14 years	Doses per day	Comments
	i.v.	←————— 10 mg/kg —————→			Single dose	Give slowly, under ECG control, arrhythmias
Piperazine	Oral	—	½–1 sachet	½–1 sachet	Single dose	Repeat after 14 days
Prednisolone	Oral	←————— 1–2 mg/kg —————→			3	'Steroid precautions'
Prochlorperazine	Oral, i.m.	—	0.4 mg/kg	0.4 mg/kg	3	
	Rectal	—	0.8 mg/kg	0.8 mg/kg	3	
Promethazine	Oral	—	1 mg/kg	1 mg/kg	3	
Salbutamol	Oral	—	—	0.3 mg/kg	3	
	Oral inhalation	—	—	400–800 μg	4	100 μg per metered dose
	Oral inhalation	—	—	600–800 μg	3 or 4	'Rota caps'
	Nebuliser	—	—	2.5–5 mg	Single dose: repeat up to 8/day	Solution 5 mg/ml Dilute dose with 2–5 ml saline
Sodium valproate	Oral	—	—	20–50 mg/kg	1 or 2	Give with or after meals. Monitor liver function
Sulphadimidine	Oral	—	150 mg/kg	150 mg/kg	4	Prophylactic dose is
	i.m., i.v.	—	150 mg/kg	150 mg/kg	4	50 mg/kg
Terbutaline	Oral	—	—	0.4 mg/kg	3	Tablets or syrup
	Oral inhalation	—	—	1 or 2 doses	As required: not more than 8/day	Inhaler Metered dose = 0.25 mg
	Oral inhalation	—	—	As above	As above	Spacer
	Nebuliser	—	—	2–5 mg	Single dose: repeat up to 8/day	Solution 10 mg/ml Dilute dose with 5 ml saline
Tetracosactrin zinc injection	i.m.	—	0.5–1 mg	0.5–1 mg	Alternate days or twice weekly	
Theophylline aminophylline	i.v.	—	—	4 mg/kg	Single then	Therapeutic range 55–110 μmol/l
				0.7 mg/kg hourly	continuous	(for theophylline)
aminophylline SR	Oral	—	—	28 mg/kg	2	'Phyllocontin'
theophylline	Oral	—	—	25 mg/kg	4–6	'Nuelin'
theophylline SR	Oral	—	—	24 mg/kg	2	'Rona-Slo-phylline'
choline theophyllinate	Oral	—	—	30 mg/kg	4–6	
Trimeprazine	Oral	—	1 mg/kg	1 mg/kg	3	Pre-medication dose is 3 mg/kg
Triprolidine/ pseudoephidrine	Oral	—	1 mg/kg	1 mg/kg	3	
Vitamin drops compound	Oral	0.3 ml (6 drops)	0.6 ml (12 drops)	0.6 ml (12 drops)	1	

Index